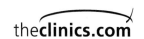

CRITICAL CARE CLINICS

Cardiac Critical Care

GUEST EDITOR
Arthur L. Riba, MD, FACC

CONSULTING EDITORS
Richard W. Carlson, MD, PhD
Michael A. Geheb, MD

October 2007 • Volume 23 • Number 4

SAUNDERS

An Imprint of Elsevier, Inc.
PHILADELPHIA LONDON TORONTO MONTREAL SYDNEY TOKYO

W.B. SAUNDERS COMPANY
A Division of Elsevier Inc.

Elsevier Inc. • 1600 John F. Kennedy Blvd., • Suite 1800 • Philadelphia, Pennsylvania 19103-2899

http://www.theclinics.com

CRITICAL CARE CLINICS
October 2007
Editor: Lisa Richman

Volume 23, Number 4
ISSN 0749-0704
ISBN-13: 978-1-4160-4299-0
ISBN-10: 1-4160-4299-7

The ideas and opinions expressed in *Critical Care Clinics* do not necessarily reflect those of the Publisher. The Publisher does not assume any responsibility for any injury and/or damage to persons or property arising out of or related to any use of the material contained in this periodical. The reader is advised to check the appropriate medical literature and the product information currently provided by the manufacturer of each drug to be administered to verify the dosage, the method and duration of administration, or contraindications. It is the responsibility of the treating physician or other health care professional, relying on independent experience and knowledge of the patient, to determine drug dosages and the best treatment for the patient. Mention of any product in this issue should not be construed as endorsement by the contributors, editors, or the Publisher of the product or manufacturers' claims.

Critical Care Clinics (ISSN: 0749-0704) is published quarterly by Elsevier Inc., 360 Park Avenue South, New York, NY 10010-1710. Months of issue are January, April, July, and October. Business and Editorial Offices: 1600 John F. Kennedy Blvd., Suite 1800, Philadelphia, PA 19103-2899. Customer Service Office: 6277 Sea Harbor Drive, Orlando, FL 32887-4800. Periodicals postage paid at New York, NY and additional mailing offices. Subscription prices are $206.00 per year for US individuals, $339.00 per year for US institution, $103.00 per year for US students and residents, $254.00 per year for Canadian individuals, $411.00 per year for Canadian institutions, $278.00 per year for international individuals, $411.00 per year for international institutions and $140.00 per year for Canadian and foreign students/residents. To receive student/resident rate, orders must be accompanied by name of affiliated institution, date of term, and the *signature* of program/residency coordinator on institution letterhead. Orders will be billed at individual rate until proof of status is received. Foreign air speed delivery is included in all *Clinics* subscription prices. All prices are subject to change without notice. POSTMASTER: Send address changes to *Critical Care Clinics*, Elsevier Periodicals Customer Service, 6277 Sea Harbor Drive, Orlando, FL 32887-4800. **Customer Service: 1-800-654-2452 (US). From outside of the US, call 1-407-345-1000. E-mail: hhspcs@harcourt.com**

Critical Care Clinics is also published in Spanish by Editorial Inter-Medica, Junin 917, 1er A, 1113, Buenos Aires, Argentina.

Critical Care Clinics is covered in *Index Medicus, EMBASE/Excerpta Medica, Current Concepts/Clinical Medicine, ISI/ BIOMED, and Chemical Abstracts.*

Printed in the United States of America.

CONSULTING EDITORS

RICHARD W. CARLSON, MD, PhD, Chairman, Department of Internal Medicine, Marcopia Medical Center; and Professor, Department of Medicine, Mayo Graduate School of Medicine, Phoenix, Arizona

MICHAEL A. GEHEB, MD, Professor, Department of Medicine, and Vice President, Clinical Programs, Oregon Health & Sciences University, Portland, Oregon

GUEST EDITOR

ARTHUR L. RIBA, MD, FACC, Medical Director of the Cardiac Care Units, Cardiovascular Quality Management, Oakwood Hospital and Medical Center, Dearborn, Michigan

CONTRIBUTORS

RAGAVENDRA R. BALIGA, MD, MBA, FRCP, FACC, Director & Chief of Cardiovascular Medicine, University Hospitals East; and Clinical Professor of Medicine, The Ohio State University, Columbus, Ohio

ERIC R. BATES, MD, Professor of Internal Medicine, Division of Cardiovascular Medicine, Department of Internal Medicine, University of Michigan, Cardiovascular Center, Ann Arbor, Michigan

MELIKE BAYRAM, MD, Resident in Internal Medicine, Division of Cardiovascular Medicine, Department of Internal Medicine, University of Michigan, Ann Arbor, Michigan

ROHIT BHATHEJA, MD, Gill Heart Institute; Division of Cardiovascular Medicine, University of Kentucky, Lexington, Kentucky

EDUARDO BOSSONE, MD, PhD, FESC, FACC, Director, Cardiology Division, Cava de' Tirreni; Amalfi Coast Hospital, Salerno; and Via Pr. Amedeo, Lauro (AV), Italy

OLIVER G. CAMERON, MD, PhD, Emeritus Professor of Psychiatry, Department of Psychiatry, University of Michigan Medical Center, Ann Arbor, Michigan

AAMER CHUGHTAI, FRCR, Assistant Professor, Department of Radiology, University of Michigan Health System, Ann Arbor, Michigan

THOMAS C. CRAWFORD, MD, Cardiac Electrophysiology, Division of Cardiovascular Medicine, University of Michigan, Ann Arbor, Michigan

LARRY M. DIAMOND, RPh, PharmD, Clinical Pharmacy Specialist – Cardiology, Oakwood Hospital and Medical Center, Dearborn, Michigan

KIM A. EAGLE, MD, FACC, Albion Walter Hewlett Professor of Internal Medicine, University of Michigan; Clinical Director, University of Michigan Cardiovascular Center, Ann Arbor, Michigan

HITINDER S. GURM, MD, Assistant Professor of Internal Medicine, Division of Cardiovascular Medicine, Department of Internal Medicine, University of Michigan, Cardiovascular Center, Ann Arbor, Michigan

ZACHARY HECTOR-WORD, MD, Resident in Internal Medicine, Division of Cardiovascular Medicine, Department of Internal Medicine, University of Michigan, Ann Arbor, Michigan

DESIKAN KAMALAKANNAN, MBBS, MRCP, Fellow - Cardiology, St. John Hospital and Medical Center, Detroit, Michigan

AMRITA M. KARVE, BS, Research Associate, Duke Clinical Research Institute, Duke University Medical Center, Durham, North Carolina

ELLA A. KAZEROONI, MD, MS, Professor and Director of Cardiothoracic Radiology, Department of Radiology, University of Michigan Health System, Ann Arbor, Michigan

RAJENDRA H. MEHTA, MD, MS, Research Faculty, Duke Clinical Research Institute, Duke University Medical Center, Durham, North Carolina

DEBABRATA MUKHERJEE, MD, MS, Gill Heart Institute; Associate Professor, Division of Cardiovascular Medicine, University of Kentucky, Lexington, Kentucky

JAMES F. NEUENSCHWANDER, II, MD, FACEP, Assistant Professor, Emergency Department, The Ohio State University Medical Center, Columbus, Ohio

HAKAN ORAL, MD, Section Chief, Cardiac Electrophysiology, Division of Cardiovascular Medicine, University of Michigan, Ann Arbor, Michigan

HOWARD S. ROSMAN, MD, FACC, Professor of Medicine/Cardiology, Wayne State University School of Medicine; Program Director – Clinical Cardiovascular Fellowship, St. John Hospital and Medical Center, Detroit, Michigan

MELVYN RUBENFIRE, MD, Professor of Internal Medicine, Division of Cardiovascular Medicine and Department of Internal Medicine, University of Michigan, Ann Arbor, Michigan

CONTENTS

Erratum   xi

Preface   xiii
Arthur L. Riba

Publisher's Note   xv

Acute ST-Segment Elevation Myocardial Infarction: Critical
Care Perspective   685
Amrita M. Karve, Eduardo Bossone, and Rajendra H. Mehta

> More than 1.2 million patients suffer from new or recurrent
> ischemic events occur annually. This includes an estimated 565,000
> cases of first and 300,000 cases of recurrent myocardial infarction
> (MI). Although mortality from acute MI has declined in recent
> years, it still remains high at 25% to 30%. Despite its high mortality,
> prognosis can be improved with timely and effective use of
> evidence-based treatment in the acute setting. This review outlines
> the critical care management strategies for ST-segment MI (STEMI).

Acute Coronary Syndromes: Unstable Angina/Non-ST
Elevation Myocardial Infarction   709
Rohit Bhatheja and Debabrata Mukherjee

> Acute coronary syndrome is a major health problem affecting
> approximately 1.5 million individuals a year. Early diagnosis and
> appropriate evidence-based therapies improve clinical outcomes
> significantly. Current data suggest that an early invasive therapy
> may improve intermediate-term and long-term outcomes, partic-
> ularly in high-risk individuals. The last few years also have seen
> significant advances in antiplatelet and antithrombotic therapies
> for the management of patients who have acute coronary
> syndrome.

Acute Decompensated Heart Failure 737

James F. Neuenschwander, II and Ragavendra R. Baliga

This article defines acute decompensated heart failure. Additionally, it lists common precipitating factors and the clinical presentation. Proper diagnostic technique is highlighted, as are possible treatments.

Cardiogenic Shock Complicating Myocardial Infarction 759

Hitinder S. Gurm and Eric R. Bates

Cardiogenic shock is the primary cause of death among patients hospitalized with acute myocardial infarction. It is defined as tissue hypoperfusion resulting from ventricular pump failure in the presence of adequate intravascular volume. These patients need rapid assessment and appropriate institution of supportive therapies including vasopressor and inotropic agents, ventilatory support, and intra-aortic balloon pump counterpulsation. Emergency coronary artery revascularization is the only therapy that reduces mortality, and this should be provided early to patients to achieve maximal benefit, unless further care is deemed futile. Whereas newer support devices can provide better hemodynamic augmentation, their impact on mortality is limited. Novel therapies are needed to further decrease mortality rates, which remain high despite reperfusion therapy.

Acute Aortic Dissection 779

Desikan Kamalakannan, Howard S. Rosman, and Kim A. Eagle

Acute aortic dissection is an uncommon but potentially catastrophic illness with high mortality. Significant advances in the understanding, diagnosis, and management have been made since the first reported case of aortic dissection 3 centuries ago. This comprehensive review discusses the pathophysiology, classification, clinical manifestations, early diagnosis, and management of this important cardiovascular emergency.

Pulmonary Hypertension in the Critical Care Setting: Classification, Pathophysiology, Diagnosis, and Management 801

Melvyn Rubenfire, Melike Bayram, and Zachary Hector-Word

Pulmonary hypertension (PH) is common in the critical care setting, and may be a target for specific therapy. Moderate degrees of pulmonary hypertension are most often the consequence of acute or chronic heart failure, hypoxemia, or acute pulmonary embolism, and may be relatively rapidly reversible. The consequences of more severe forms of PH, both acute and chronic, can include hypotension; low cardiac output; right heart failure with congestion of the liver, gut, and kidneys; and varying degrees of hypoxemia, each of which can lead to death or severe disability. We review the physiology, definitions, classification, pathogenesis, diagnostic tools, and algorithms for diagnosis and specific treatments for the various causes of PH as seen in the critical care setting.

CT and MRI of Acute Thoracic Cardiovascular Emergencies

835

Aamer Chughtai and Ella A. Kazerooni

A wide spectrum of acute cardiovascular disorders is seen in patients who are hospitalized in a critical care setting. Imaging plays a central role in the diagnosis and management of these conditions. The most frequently used imaging remains chest radiography; however, more advanced modalities, including coronary angiography, echocardiography, and radioisotope scintigraphy, have well established roles in the assessment of patients in the critical care setting. More recently, multidetector row CT (MDCT) and MRI are being used increasingly for evaluation of coronary artery disease, cardiac structure and function, coronary artery anomalies, cardiac masses, pericardial disease, valvular disease, postoperative cardiovascular abnormalities, venous thromboembolism and acute aortic syndromes, often with other ancillary findings that can provide important clinical information. The three most common life-threatening cardiovascular processes in which advanced imaging plays a role, particularly CT, are discussed, including pulmonary embolism, aortic dissection, and coronary artery disease.

Cardiac Arrhythmias: Management of Atrial Fibrillation in the Critically Ill Patient

855

Thomas C. Crawford and Hakan Oral

This article reviews the most relevant information for the hospitalist or intensivist managing patients who have atrial fibrillation (AF) in the acute or critical care setting. Emphasis is placed on clinically useful information, and evidence-based strategies for managing acute and chronic AF.

Cardiopulmonary Resuscitation and Acute Cardiovascular Life Support—A Protocol Review of the Updated Guidelines

873

Larry M. Diamond

For the first time in 5 years, new guidelines for cardiopulmonary resuscitation (CPR) of adults and children were introduced at the end of November 2005. The new CPR guidelines evolved from emerging evidence-based resuscitation studies and the evaluation process included the input of 281 international resuscitation experts who evaluated hypotheses, topics, and research over a 36-month period. The process included evidence evaluation, review of the literature, and focused analysis. This article reviews the four major changes to the guidelines. Changes are currently being made in the training of all new and recertifying ACLS health care providers.

Delirium, Depression, and Other Psychosocial and Neurobehavioral Issues in Cardiovascular Disease 881
Oliver G. Cameron

Understanding relevant psychosocial (neural, behavioral, psychiatric) issues is essential to optimal care of individuals who have cardiovascular disorders. Delirium, a condition of diffuse cerebral dysfunction caused by underlying systemic or central nervous system pathology, and often requiring measures of acute neurobehavioral management with nonpharmacological and pharmacological means, in addition to treatment of the underlying medical disorder, often occurs in association with severe cardiovascular disease. Depression is a psychiatric disorder known to be associated with cardiovascular disease. Substantial improvement in understanding the nature of this association has occurred in the past 10 to 20 years, including very preliminary data suggesting that pharmacological treatment with selective serotonin reuptake inhibitor (SSRI) antidepressants might improve postmyocardial infarction cardiac prognosis. Numerous other factors—anxiety, stress, social support, anger, and other personality factors-also are implicated in the relationship of psychosocial issues to cardiovascular disease.

Index 901

FORTHCOMING ISSUES

January 2008

Neurological Complications in Critical Illness
Robert Stevens, MD, *Guest Editor*

April 2008

Anti Microbial Therapy/Hospital-Acquired Infections
Burke Cunha, MD, *Guest Editor*

RECENT ISSUES

July 2007

Monitoring in the Intensive Care Unit
Mark D. Siegel, MD, *Guest Editor*

April 2007

Mechanical Ventilation
Peter J. Papadakos, MD, FCCM and
Joseph Dooley, MD, *Guest Editors*

January 2007

Early Mobility of the ICU Patient
Peter E. Morris, MD, *Guest Editor*

THE CLINICS ARE NOW AVAILABLE ONLINE!

Access your subscription at:
http://www.theclinics.com

ELSEVIER
SAUNDERS

Crit Care Clin 23 (2007) xi

CRITICAL
CARE
CLINICS

Erratum

In the April 2007 issue of Critical Care Clinics, Volume 23, Number 2, in Dr. Victoria E. Johnson's article, "Special Cases: Mechanical Ventilation of Neurosurgical Patients" starting on page 275, an error was made in the section titled "Hyperventilation as a Therapy". On page 282 the sentence should read, "Hyperventilation results in a decrease in blood CO_2 level."

doi:10.1016/j.ccc.2007.07.008

CRITICAL
CARE
CLINICS

Crit Care Clin 23 (2007) xiii–xiv

Preface

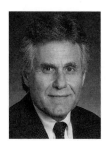

Arthur L. Riba, MD, FACC
Guest Editor

Quality cardiac care results when evidence-based clinical practice guidelines are applied reliably, consistently, and appropriately by competent and dedicated clinicians. Improvement in the care and outcomes for the hospitalized patient with acute cardiac disorders can be achieved by aligning systems, directing care processes, and implementing tools that assure that the clinical practice guidelines are applied in practice, especially those processes that have been shown to be linked to improved clinical outcomes.

It is the intent of this issue of the *Critical Care Clinics* to provide practicing physicians, hospitalists, cardiovascular specialists, and aligned healthcare providers with a state-of-the-art, evidence-based, and clinically relevant overview of acute cardiac disorders encountered in the hospital setting. My distinguished colleagues were asked to review and summarize concepts and practical applications of best cardiovascular care practice, and the evidence-based treatments and diagnostic evaluation and processes of inpatient cardiovascular care, which in turn, would lead to desired outcomes meaningful to patients. In addition, where available, these concepts would provide physicians with the strategies and tools to be successful in translating scientific evidence into effective and rewarding care. Those processes of care that have been linked to improved outcomes, based on evidence and efficacy from randomized controlled trials, are emphasized. Given the accelerating pace in which new treatments, performance indicators, and care processes are evolving from clinical trials, we set a goal to assure that emerging therapies are introduced. It is the expectation that the physician armed with established and updated evidence-based therapies will be most effective

doi:10.1016/j.ccc.2007.09.001   *criticalcare.theclinics.com*

in the day-to-day care of acutely decompensated cardiac patients. The acute
cardiovascular encounter is the best clinical setting to apply evidence-based
therapies, given the link to improved clinical outcomes and sustainable compliance of secondary preventive therapies after discharge.

It has not been possible to be inclusive of all acute cardiovascular disorders in this issue of *Critical Care Clinics*. Chosen for inclusion are topics
supported by the best clinical trial evidence, conditions that are most commonly encountered, and those situations where there is substantial evidence
that when the therapeutic processes are applied, the likelihood of optimal
outcomes will result. I am greatly indebted to the authors of this issue for
the outstanding contributions they have made. Each of the authors is a recognized authority in their respective field. We are also greatly indebted to
Dr. Michael Geheb, Division President of Oakwood Hospital and Medical
Center, and Consulting Editor of *Critical Care Clinics*, who suggested that
we bring together a group of distinguished authors to write a compendium
of state-of-the-art articles on acute cardiovascular care in the inpatient setting. Much gratitude goes to Lisa Richman, Editor of *Critical Care Clinics*,
Elsevier, who has provided outstanding support and guidance for this effort,
and has been most gracious, understanding and patient in keeping us on
track, and focusing us on our goals and missions.

Arthur L. Riba, MD, FACC
*Medical Director of the Cardiac Care Units
and Cardiovascular Quality Management
Oakwood Hospital and Medical Center
18181 Oakwood Boulevard, Suite 402
Dearborn, Michigan 48124, USA*

E-mail address: ribaa@oakwood.org

ELSEVIER
SAUNDERS

Crit Care Clin 23 (2007) xv

CRITICAL
CARE
CLINICS

Publisher's Note

An article entitled "Evidence-Based Performance and Quality Improvement in the Acute Cardiac Care Setting" that was scheduled to publish in this issue of the *Critical Care Clinics* will now be included as an addendum to the January 2008 issue.

0749-0704/07/$
doi:10.1016/j.ccc.2007.09.003

ELSEVIER
SAUNDERS

Crit Care Clin 23 (2007) 685–707

CRITICAL
CARE
CLINICS

Acute ST-Segment Elevation Myocardial Infarction: Critical Care Perspective

Amrita M. Karve, BS[a],
Eduardo Bossone, MD, PhD, FESC, FACC[b,c],
Rajendra H. Mehta, MD, MS[d,*]

[a]Duke Clinical Research Institute, Duke University Medical Center, Suite 7078,
PO Box 17989, Durham, NC 27715, USA
[b]Cardiology Division, Cava de' Tirreni and Amalfi Coast Hospital, Salerno, Italy
[c]Via Pr. Amedeo, 36, 83023 Lauro (AV), Italy
[d]Duke Clinical Research Institute, Duke University Medical Center,
P.O. Box 17969, Durham, NC 27715, USA

Over 1.2 million patients suffer from new or recurrent ischemic events annually [1]. This includes an estimated 565,000 cases of first and 300,000 cases of recurrent myocardial infarction (MI) [1]. Although mortality from acute MI has declined in recent years, it still remains high at 25% to 30% [1]. Despite its high mortality, prognosis can be improved with timely and effective use of evidence-based treatment in the acute setting [2]. This review outlines the critical care management strategies for ST-segment MI (STEMI).

Etiology of STEMI

The most common cause of STEMI is acute plaque rupture and the resultant thrombosis leading to acute closure of coronary arteries. Less commonly, STEMI is caused by abnormalities of coronary vessels, wall, hypercoagulation, and substance abuse as listed in Box 1 [3].

Source of funding: Duke Clinical Research Institute, Durham, NC.
* Corresponding author.
E-mail address: mehta007@dcri.duke.edu (R.H. Mehta).

Box 1. Nonatherosclerotic etiologies of acute myocardial infarction

Arteritis
Takayasu's disease
Polyarteritis nodosa
Kawasaki syndrome
Systemic lupus erythematosus
Rheumatoid arthritis
Ankylosing spondylitis
Trauma to coronary arteries

Metabolic diseases with involvement of coronary arteries
Hurler's syndrome
Homocystinuria
Fabry's disease
Amyloidosis

Other mechanisms of luminal narrowing
Spasm
Aortic dissection involving coronary arteries

Coronary artery emboli
Infective endocarditis
Nonthrombotic endocarditis
Prosthetic valve emboli
Cardiac myxoma
Paradoxical emboli
Papillary fibroelastoma of aortic valve

Congenital anomalies
Anomalous origin of the left coronary from the pulmonary artery
Left coronary artery from anterior sinus of valsalva

Miscellaneous
Carbon monoxide poisoning
Polycythemia vera
Thrombocytosis
Cocaine abuse

Data from Cheitlin MD, McAllister HA, de Castro CM. Myocardial infarction without atherosclerosis. JAMA 1975;231:951–9.

Clinical presentation and evaluation

Symptoms

The classic symptom of a STEMI patient is chest pain. Chest pain unique to a STEMI patient is severe and may manifest as intense pressure in the shoulders or directly under the ribs. Pain may radiate to the jaw, neck, back, shoulders, and arms. Occasionally, there may be no chest pain at all, and patients may report pain localized to any one of the areas described above [2].

Atypical symptoms are often characteristics of the elderly, women, diabetic patients, patients with prior cardiac surgery, and those in the immediate postoperative period of noncardiac surgery. These atypical symptoms include nausea, shortness of breath, diaphoresis and epigastric discomfort, dizziness, syncope, weakness, fatigue, or complaints of indigestion [2].

Physical examination

Physical examination is more important for excluding other causes of chest pain and for risk-stratifying patients with STEMI, but is not helpful by itself for making the diagnosis of STEMI. A thorough baseline and periodic examination allows for identification of patients who present with or who develop congestive heart failure, mechanical complications, and pericarditis. A fourth heart sound is present in most patients, whereas systolic blood pressure, heart rate, rales, and third heart sound provide important prognostic information.

Electrocardiogram

An electrocardiogram should be performed within 10 minutes of arrival to emergency room in patients with chest pain or other ischemic symptoms [2]. Elevation of ST segments greater than 0.1 mV in two consecutive leads is typically indicative of a STEMI, and elevation of greater than 0.2 mV has been shown to be more specific in accurately diagnosing a STEMI. Right-sided leads are desirable in all patients with inferior STEMI to rule out right ventricular infarction (RVI). While new left bundle branch block in presence of ischemic symptoms is considered consistent with the diagnosis of STEMI, the presence of previous left bundle branch block may confound the diagnosis of STEMI. In these patients, a STEMI can be diagnosed by the following criteria: (1) ST elevation greater than or equal to 0.1 mV in leads with a positive QRS; (2) ST depression greater than or equal to 0.1 mV in V1 to V3; and (3) ST elevation greater than or equal to 0.5 mV in leads with a negative QRS [4]. As STEMI evolves, new Q waves develop, ST segment elevation resolves, and new T-wave inversions are evident. Besides helping in diagnosis, ST segment elevations are important for localization of infarct and infarct-related artery. Additionally, they impart important prognostic information, ie, the risk of mortality is proportional to the number of leads showing ST segment elevations and resolution of ST segments with reperfusion therapies suggests establishment of normal myocardial flow and is associated with better prognosis.

Imaging

Transthoracic echocardiography allows bedside confirmation or exclusion of the diagnosis of STEMI, although EKG and availability of cardiac markers have limited its use. Nevertheless, it remains the most valuable tool for evaluation of left and right ventricular function as well as for the diagnosis of mechanical complications. Other imaging modalities such as transesophageal echocardiography, a contrast chest CT scan, or magnetic resonance imaging are predominantly useful for excluding some of the other causes of chest pain, ie, aortic dissection, pulmonary embolism, and so forth.

Cardiac biomarkers

The most commonly used markers in clinical practice to diagnose and assess infarct size include creatine kinase (CK)-MB fraction and cardiac troponins. CK-MB is elevated 3 to 12 hours after onset of ischemia and has a mean peak time of 24 hours. Cardiac troponin I (cTnI) and cardiac troponin T (cTnT) are considered elevated above the 99th percentile of a reference control group. Both troponins are detectable 4 to 12 hours after the onset of ischemia, and peak at 12 to 48 hours. CK-MB may remain elevated for up to 3 days after infarction, while troponins may be elevated for more than a week. CK-MB has proven quite specific for diagnosing a myocardial infarction and only rarely do myocardial infarcts occur without elevated CK-MB levels.

Although an elevated CK-MB has long been considered the "gold standard" for myocardial necrosis, recent studies show that troponin may, in fact, be even more sensitive and specific for detecting necrosis of coronary vessels at the microscopic level [5]. The values of both baseline CK-MB and troponin levels are associated incrementally with risk of mortality in patients with STEMI [6]. However, because of it higher sensitivity and specificity, their measurement has largely replaced CK-MB evaluation for suspected MI and should be measured in all patients with suspected STEMI.

Differential diagnosis

Box 2 shows a list of differential diagnoses that should be considered in patients presenting with ischemic symptoms [2]. Rapid physical examination, laboratory tests, and imaging studies serve to eliminate these diagnoses. An erroneous diagnosis of STEMI among these patients may increase their risk not only related to missed diagnosis, but also because fibrinolytic agents in some of these patients have potential for harm.

Box 2. Differential diagnosis of ST-elevation myocardial infarction

Life-threatening
Aortic dissection
Pulmonary embolus
Perforating ulcer
Tension pneumothorax
Boerhaave syndrome (esophageal rupture with mediastinitis)

Other cardiovascular and nonischemic
Pericarditis
Atypical angina
Early repolarization
Wolff-Parkinson-White syndrome
Deeply inverted T waves suggestive of a central nervous system
Lesion or apical hypertrophic cardiomyopathy
LV hypertrophy with strain
Brugada syndrome
Myocarditis
Hyperkalemia
Bundle-branch blocks
Vasospastic angina
Hypertrophic cardiomyopathy

Other noncardiac
Gastroesophageal reflux (GERD) and spasm
Chest-wall pain
Pleurisy
Peptic ulcer disease
Panic attack
Biliary or pancreatic pain
Cervical disc or neuropathic pain
Somatization and psychogenic pain disorder

Data from Antman EM, Anbe DT, Armstrong PW, et al. ACC/AHA Guidelines for the Management of Patients With ST-Elevation Myocardial Infarction—Executive Summary: A Report of the American College of Cardiology/American Heart Association Task Force on Practice Guidelines (Writing Committee to Revise the 1999 Guidelines for the Management of Patients With Acute Myocardial Infarction) Circulation 2004;110:588–636.

Treatment

Box 3 outlines the initial diagnostic and therapeutic measures. A treatment algorithm is outlined in Figs. 1 and 2 [7]. Important initial goals are

---

Box 3. Diagnostic and treatment measures in patients with STEMI

Initial diagnostic measures
1. Use continuous EKG, automated blood pressure, heart-rate monitoring
2. Take targeted history (for acute myocardial infarction inclusions, thrombolysis exclusions), check vital signs, perform focused examination
3. Start intravenous lines and draw blood for serum cardiac markers, hematology, chemistry, lipid profile
4. Obtain 12-lead EKG
5. Obtain chest x-ray (preferably upright)

General treatment measures
1. Aspirin, 160–325 mg (chew and swallow)
2. Nitroglycerin, sublingual: test for Prinzmetal's angina, reversible spasm; anti-ischemic, antihypertensive effects
3. Oxygen: sparse data; probably indicated, first 2–3 hours in all; continue if low arterial oxygen saturation (<90%)
4. Adequate analgesia: small doses of morphine (2–4 mg) as needed

Specific treatment measures
1. Reperfusion therapy: goal—door-to-needle time <30 min; door-to dilatation time <60 min
2. Conjunctive antithrombotics: aspirin, heparin (especially with fibrin-specific lytic agents)
3. Adjunctive therapies: Beta-adrenoceptor blockade if eligible, intravenous nitroglycerin (for anti-ischemic or antihypertensive effects), angiotensin-converting enzyme inhibitor (especially with large or anterior ST-elevation, heart failure without hypotension [SBP >100 mm Hg], previous myocardial infarction)

Data from Ryan TJ, Antman EM, Brooks RH, et al. ACC/AHA guidelines for management of patients with acute myocardial infarction. A report of the American College of Cardiology/American Heart Association Task Force on Practice Guidelines (Committee on Management of Acute Myocardial Infarction). J Am College Cardiol 1999;34:890–911.

---

to (1) establish indications; (2) rule out any possible contraindications for reperfusion therapy; (3) determine the time to treatment; (4) assess risk versus benefits; (5) quickly decide the mode of reperfusion, ie, fibrinolysis or primary percutaneous coronary interventions (PCIs); and (6) to rapidly

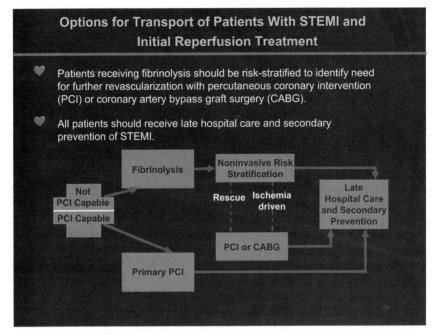

Options for Transport of Patients With STEMI and Initial Reperfusion Treatment

Patients receiving fibrinolysis should be risk-stratified to identify need for further revascularization with percutaneous coronary intervention (PCI) or coronary artery bypass graft surgery (CABG).

All patients should receive late hospital care and secondary prevention of STEMI.

Fibrinolysis

Noninvasive Risk Stratification

Not PCI Capable

Rescue Ischemia driven

Late Hospital Care and Secondary Prevention

PCI Capable

PCI or CABG

Primary PCI

Fig. 1. Treatment and risk stratification algorithm for patients with ST-elevation myocardial infarction. (*Adapted from* Antman EM, Anbe DT, Armstrong PW, et al. ACC/AHA Guidelines for the Management of Patients With ST-Elevation Myocardial Infarction—Executive Summary: A Report of the American College of Cardiology/American Heart Association Task Force on Practice Guidelines (Writing Committee to Revise the 1999 Guidelines for the Management of Patients With Acute Myocardial Infarction). J Am Coll Cardiol 2004;44:671–719; with permission.)

proceed with the chosen mode of reperfusion (Fig. 3). The National Heart Attack Alert Program Coordinating Committee has established a door-to-needle time (for fibrinolysis) to be less than 30 minutes and door-to-balloon time (for PCI) to be less than 90 minutes in which diagnosis is to be completed and reperfusion achieved [8].

Choosing a reperfusion strategy

Patients presenting within 12 hours should undergo reperfusion therapy [2]. An invasive strategy is preferred for high-risk patients (elderly, large MI, cardiogenic shock, or those with comorbid conditions) if the door-to-balloon time can be achieved within 90 minutes, or there is contraindication for fibrinolysis or diagnosis uncertain (see Fig. 3). On the other hand, fibrinolytic therapy remains the principal mode of reperfusion globally because of lack of facilities and accessibility to invasive centers that preclude timely primary PCI [2].

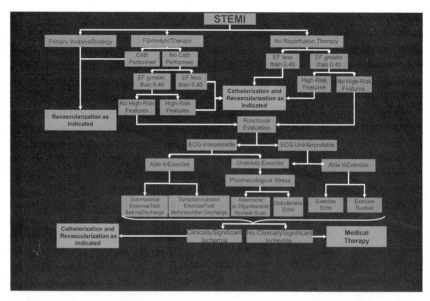

Fig. 2. Evidence-based approach to need for catheterization (cath) and revascularization after ST-elevation myocardial infarction (STEMI). The algorithm shows treatment paths for patients who initially undergo a primary invasive strategy, receive fibrinolytic therapy, or do not undergo reperfusion therapy for STEMI and the use of noninvasive tests to guide further invasive procedures. When clinically significant ischemia is detected, cardiac catheterization and revascularization are indicated; if no clinically significant ischemia is detected, medical therapy is recommended after STEMI. (*Adapted from* Antman EM, Anbe DT, Armstrong PW, et al. ACC/AHA Guidelines for the Management of Patients With ST-Elevation Myocardial Infarction—Executive Summary: A Report of the American College of Cardiology/American Heart Association Task Force on Practice Guidelines (Writing Committee to Revise the 1999 Guidelines for the Management of Patients With Acute Myocardial Infarction). J Am Coll Cardiol 2004;44:671–719; with permission.)

Fibrinolytic therapy

Fibrinolytic therapy represents one of the major advances in the management of STEMI. Fibrinolytic agents dissolve infarct artery thrombus and restore myocardial perfusion, thereby reducing infarct size, preserving left ventricular systolic function, and improving survival. Patients with more than 1 mm ST elevation in two or more contiguous leads or new left bundle branch block within 12 hours of symptom onset should be administered one of the currently available fibrinolytic agents (Table 1) unless contraindicated. The absolute and relative contraindications are outlined in Box 4 [2]. The success of fibrinolytic therapy is largely dependent on timely administration, as early as in the prehospital setting. The most effective fibrinolytic regimens achieve epicardial infarct artery patency rates in 75% of patients within 90 minutes, but requires blood transfusion in 5% and is associated with hemorrhagic stroke in approximately 1% of patients [2,9]. Prehospital fibrinolysis has been shown to have excellent outcomes with no increased

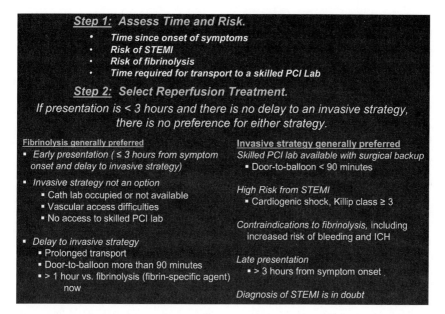

Step 1: Assess Time and Risk.
- *Time since onset of symptoms*
- *Risk of STEMI*
- *Risk of fibrinolysis*
- *Time required for transport to a skilled PCI Lab*

Step 2: Select Reperfusion Treatment.
If presentation is < 3 hours and there is no delay to an invasive strategy, there is no preference for either strategy.

Fibrinolysis generally preferred
- *Early presentation (≤ 3 hours from symptom onset and delay to invasive strategy)*
- *Invasive strategy not an option*
  - Cath lab occupied or not available
  - Vascular access difficulties
  - No access to skilled PCI lab
- *Delay to invasive strategy*
  - Prolonged transport
  - Door-to-balloon more than 90 minutes
  - > 1 hour vs. fibrinolysis (fibrin-specific agent) now

Invasive strategy generally preferred
Skilled PCI lab available with surgical backup
- Door-to-balloon < 90 minutes

High Risk from STEMI
- Cardiogenic shock, Killip class ≥ 3

Contraindications to fibrinolysis, including increased risk of bleeding and ICH

Late presentation
- > 3 hours from symptom onset

Diagnosis of STEMI is in doubt

Fig. 3. Reperfusion options for patients with ST-elevation myocardial infarction. (*Adapted from* Antman EM, Anbe DT, Armstrong PW, et al. ACC/AHA Guidelines for the Management of Patients With ST-Elevation Myocardial Infarction—Executive Summary: A Report of the American College of Cardiology/American Heart Association Task Force on Practice Guidelines (Writing Committee to Revise the 1999 Guidelines for the Management of Patients With Acute Myocardial Infarction). J Am Coll Cardiol 2004;44:671–719; with permission.)

risk compared with in-hospital treatment and in fact outcomes that are similar to primary PCI. The guidelines recommend fibrinolytic therapy within the first hour after symptom onset, since mortality significantly increases every hour thereafter [9]. The benefits of fibrinolytic therapy on STEMI have been well established with overall 18% risk reduction in 30-day mortality relative to control [9]. Furthermore, this reduction in mortality is risk dependent with higher risk subgroups showing the greatest benefit [9].

For no other treatment of STEMI is consideration of risks versus benefits more important than for the use of a fibrinolytic agent. A major concern with the administration of fibrinolytics is the risk of intracranial hemorrhage [2,9]. This is because it is fatal in up to one half to two thirds of patients and associated with permanent disability in a vast majority of patients who survive this event [10,11]. Models for assessment of risk of intracranial hemorrhage have been developed and allowed accurate estimation of risks before administration of fibrinolytic treatment so that risks versus benefits could be appropriately weighed [10,11]. Factors identified with increased risks have included increasing age, African American race, lower body weight, prior transient-ischemic attack or stroke, presenting systolic blood pressure, excessive anticoagulation, and fibrin-specific agents compared with non–fibrin-specific agents. Mental status and neurological signs and symptoms

Table 1
Comparison of approved thrombolytic agents

	Streptokinase	Alteplase[a]	Reteplase	tenecteplase-tPA[b]
Dose	1.5 MU in 30–60 min	100 mg in 90 min	10 U × 2 each over 2 min	30–50 mg based on weight
Bolus administration	No	No	Yes	Yes
Antigenic	Yes	No	No	No
Allergic reactions (hypotension most common)	Yes	No	No	No
Systemic fibrinogen depletion	Marked	Mild	Moderate	Minimal
90-min patency rates, approximate %	≈50	≈75	≈75	≈75
Thrombolysis in Myocardial Infarction grade 3 flow, %	32	54	60	63
Cost per dose (US)	$613	$2974	$2750	$2833

[a] Bolus 15 mg, infusion 0.75 mg/kg for 30 minutes (maximum 50 mg), then 0.5 mg/kg not to exceed 35 mg over the next 60 minutes to an overall maximum of 100 mg.

[b] Thirty milligrams for weight less than 60 kg; 35 mg for 60–69 kg; 40 mg for 70–79 mg; 45 mg for 80–89 kg; 50 mg for 90 kg or more.

Adapted from Antman EM, Anbe DT, Armstrong PW, et al. ACC/AHA Guidelines for the Management of Patients With ST-Elevation Myocardial Infarction—Executive Summary: A Report of the American College of Cardiology/American Heart Association Task Force on Practice Guidelines (Writing Committee to Revise the 1999 Guidelines for the Management of Patients With Acute Myocardial Infarction). Circulation 2004;110:588–636; with permission.

must be monitored closely after administration of fibrinolytic agents. A change in mental status within 24 hours of treatment should be considered to be due to intracranial hemorrhage until proven otherwise, and immediate neurology/neurosurgery consults are recommended so that appropriate management is undertaken to prevent further neurological damage.

Primary PCI

Primary PCI with patency rates greater than 90% and few contraindications is an attractive reperfusion strategy. This mode of reperfusion has been shown to decrease mortality, nonfatal reinfarction, and hemorrhagic stroke when compared with fibrinolytic therapy [12]. Thus, primary PCI is a preferred reperfusion strategy when performed in a timely manner (90-minute "door-to-balloon time" after arrival to the emergency department [ED]) by individuals skilled in this procedure (performed more than 75 PCI procedures/y) and supported experienced personnel in high-volume centers (more than 200 PCI/y). Major limitations of primary PCI include the lack of availability and the delay in time to treatment. It is the reperfusion strategy of choice in patients with cardiogenic shock. The efficacy of PCI decreases as time to perfusion increases. In fact, in patients with STEMI, particularly those at high risk, presenting to ED, longer door-to-balloon times are associated

---

Box 4. Contraindications and cautions for fibrinolysis in ST-elevation myocardial infarction

Absolute contraindications
Prior intracranial hemorrhage
Known structural cerebral vascular lesion (eg, arteriovenous malformation)
Known malignant intracranial neoplasm (primary or metastatic)
Ischemic stroke within 3 months EXCEPT acute ischemic stroke within 3 hours
Suspected aortic dissection
Active bleeding or bleeding diathesis (excluding menses)
Significant closed-head or facial trauma within 3 months

Relative contraindications
History of chronic, severe, poorly controlled hypertension
Severe uncontrolled hypertension on presentation (SBP greater than 180 mm Hg or DBP greater than 110 mm Hg)
History of prior ischemic stroke greater than 3 months, dementia, or known intracranial pathology not covered in contraindications
Traumatic or prolonged (>10 minutes) cardiopulmonary resuscitation or major surgery (less than 3 weeks)
Recent (within 2 to 4 weeks) internal bleeding
Noncompressible vascular punctures
For streptokinase/anistreplase: prior exposure (more than 5 days ago) or prior allergic reaction to these agents
Pregnancy
Active peptic ulcer
Current use of anticoagulants: the higher the prothrombin time, the higher the risk of bleeding

---

Adapted from Antman EM, Anbe DT, Armstrong PW, et al. ACC/AHA Guidelines for the Management of Patients With ST-Elevation Myocardial Infarction—Executive Summary: A Report of the American College of Cardiology/American Heart Association Task Force on Practice Guidelines (Writing Committee to Revise the 1999 Guidelines for the Management of Patients With Acute Myocardial Infarction). J Am Coll Cardiol 2004;44:671–719; with permission.

---

with increased late mortality (more than 3 hours after presentation). Efforts to reduce the door-to-balloon time (prehospital EKG, transmission of the EKG to the ED, administration of antithrombotic agents by the paramedics, notifying the catheterization laboratory staff of an incoming STEMI patient, and preparing the catheterization laboratory by the time the patient arrives) are expected to improve survival significantly in those undergoing primary

PCI. If a longer delay in door-to-balloon time is anticipated, use of full-dose fibrinolytic agents may be more appropriate. Facilitated PCI (use of half- or full-dose lytics, glycoprotein IIbIIIa receptor antagonists or combination of the two followed by immediate PCI) have not proven to be effective strategies and in fact may be associated with increased risks of complications. Potential limitations of primary PCI include arterial access site complications; adverse reactions related to contrast, volume loading, and antithrombotic agents; and reocclusion (5%) and restenosis (20%) [12].

Coronary artery bypass surgery in STEMI

Coronary artery bypass surgery (CABG) as primary reperfusion strategy is rarely needed in the current era of fibrinolytic therapy and PCI and may be considered appropriate in patients with STEMI and suitable anatomy who are not candidates for fibrinolysis or primary PCI and are within 12 hours of symptom onset. Emergency CABG is also indicated for patients with failed PCI and recurrent ischemia or hemodynamic instability; at the time of surgical repair for ventricular septal rupture, mitral valve insufficiency, or cardiac rupture; cardiogenic shock in patients with STEMI within 36 hours of symptom onset (18 hours of shock) having multivessel or left main disease; and in those with severe life threatening ventricular arrhythmias and multivessel or left main disease [2]. Finally, guidelines for elective CABG in patients with STEMI do not differ from those for other patients and include spontaneous or stress-induced ischemia in patients with left main or multivessel disease, particularly those with significant left ventricular (LV) dysfunction [2].

Adjunctive management

Supplemental oxygen is indicated for those patients with O2 saturations less than 90%; those with ongoing ischemia, hemodynamic instability, or pulmonary congestion; and during first 2 to 3 hours in all patients with STEMI. Vasodilators such as morphine and nitroglycerin can decrease oxygen requirement, decrease anginal pain, and prevent further myocardial necrosis. Nitroglycerin can be administered sublingually or as a spray. If pain is still not alleviated, or for patients with uncontrolled hypertension, left ventricular dysfunction, or pulmonary congestion, intravenous nitroglycerin should be administered and continued for 24 to 48 hours. Nitroglycerin is contraindicated in those with hypotension, bradycardia, or those who have received sildenafil in the preceding 24 hours. It should be used with caution in patients with right ventricular infarction. While symptomatic benefit is seen in most patients, no studies have conclusively shown a significant mortality benefit from nitroglycerin.

Antiplatelet therapy

Patients should chew 162 to 325 mg of aspirin unless otherwise contraindicated and continued indefinitely. Use of aspirin alone has been shown to be associated with 23% relative risk reduction, similar to that seen with streptokinase alone and combination of aspirin and streptokinase results in an even greater 42% relative risk reduction among STEMI patients. Clopidogrel or ticlopidine is a reasonable alternative for patients allergic to aspirin [13]. Aspirin should be administered as soon as patients complain of symptoms presumed to be ischemic in origin [2].

Pretreatment with clopidogrel 600 mg or ticlopidine 500 mg (in addition to aspirin) is indicated as soon as a decision regarding primary PCI is made and this treatment continued for minimum of 1 to 6 months depending on the type of stent used during primary PCI [2]. Recent data indicate a benefit of clopidogrel even among patients treated with fibrinolysis. In patients receiving fibrinolytic therapy, aspirin and clopidogrel together may improve reperfusion and coronary flow. In the ClOpidogrel and Metoprolol in Myocardial Infarction Trial (COMMIT), patients received 75 mg clopidogrel in addition to 165 mg aspirin, versus clopidogrel alone. Patients receiving dual therapy with fibrinolytic regimen had significantly reduced risk of in-hospital outcomes, including mortality [14]. Similarly, the CLARITY-TIMI 28 investigators demonstrated that in STEMI patients younger than 75 years who received aspirin and standard fibrinolytic therapy, addition of clopidogrel (300 mg load, 75 mg/d) versus placebo resulted in a significantly lower combined end point of occluded infarct artery on angiography or death or recurrent infarction before angiography in the clopidogrel group by 36% and 30-day end point of cardiovascular death, recurrent infarction, or myocardial ischemia requiring urgent revascularization by 20%. There was no increase in major bleeding in the clopidogrel group [15]. Thus, clopidogrel pretreatment is reasonable in most patients with STEMI in the emergency department along with aspirin, unless contraindicated. Moreover, for patients undergoing PCI, clopidogrel reduces mortality before and after revascularization, without any increase in major or minor bleeding risk [15].

Antithrombotic agents

Unfractionated heparin is indicated for all STEMI patients, except those receiving streptokinase. The recommended heparin regimen with fibrinolysis is a bolus of 60 U/kg (maximum 4000 U) and maintenance of 12 U/kg/h (maximum 1000 U/kg/h [800 U/kg/h in elderly]). The goal is to maintain an activated partial thromboplastin time 1.5 to 2.0 times that of control times (or between 50 and 70 seconds). An alternative to unfractionated heparin is low molecular weight heparin (LMWH, 30 mg IV bolus and 1 mg/kg every 12 hours). Recent investigations have supported the use of LMWH over unfractionated heparin for the reduction of recurrent ischemic events in patients receiving fibrinolysis and those undergoing primary PCI [16,17]. However, LMWH should only be used in patients younger than 75 without renal dysfunction receiving fibrinolytic therapy. The role of LMWH in patients undergoing primary PCI is less clear. Fondaparinux, a novel factor Xa inhibitor, has been shown to significantly reduce mortality and reinfarction in patients with STEMI, particularly those not undergoing primary PCI and may be considered as an antithrombotic agent for those receiving fibrinolytic therapy [18].

Glycoprotein IIb/IIIa inhibitors

The American College of Cardiology/American Heart Association (ACC/AHA) guideline recommends that it is reasonable to start abciximab (a glycoprotein GP IIbIIIa receptor antagonist) as soon as possible in the emergency department once a decision for primary PCI is made (Class IIa recommendation, [2]). This treatment has been shown to be associated with increased infarct artery patency before primary PCI and reduction in recurrent ischemic events needing urgent target vessel revascularization in these patients [2]. Similarly, the guidelines recommend that the use of abciximab with half-dose reteplase or tenecteplase may be considered for preventing reinfarction in selected patients with STEMI (anterior infarction, age younger than 75 and low risk of bleeding, Class IIa recommendation). The role of eptifibatide and tirofiban is less well defined in patients with STEMI.

Beta-blockers, calcium antagonists, angiotensin converting enzyme (ACE) inhibitors, angiotension receptor blockers, lipid lowering agents, warfarin, and modulation of glucose-insulin axis

All STEMI patients without contraindications should receive beta-blocker therapy upon arrival. Contraindications to beta-blocker therapy include heart rate less than 50 beats per minute (bpm), peripheral hypoperfusion, decompensated congestive heart failure, shock, advanced AV block, asthma, or reactive airway disease [2]. The use of these agents has been shown to decrease the risks of mortality, recurrent ischemic events, reinfarction, ventricular fibrillation, sudden cardiac death, cardiac rupture, and intracranial hemorrhage. Oral over intravenous beta-blockers should be preferred unless patients have significant hypertension and tachyarrhythmias at presentation. Calcium channel blockers should be avoided in STEMI patients. However, verapamil or diltiazem may be prescribed to patients with STEMI and recurrent ischemic events or atrial tachyarrhythmias who are intolerant to beta-blocking agents and who do not have hypotension, advanced AV block, heart failure, shock, bradycardia, or left ventricular ejection fraction less than 40%.

An angiotensin converting enzyme (ACE) inhibitor should be started in the first 24 hours of admission in all patients with STEMI who have an left ventricular ejection fraction less than 40%, pulmonary congestion, anterior STEMI who do not have a systolic blood pressure less than 100 mm Hg or 30 mm Hg below baseline, or who have no contraindications to these agents (Class IA recommendation, [2]). In patients intolerant to ACE inhibitors, an angiotensin receptor blocker should be administered in this cohort

(Class IC recommendation). ACE inhibitors have been shown to decrease mortality, heart failure, and recurrent ischemic events in this high-risk cohort. ACE inhibitors (or angiotensin receptor blockers when ACE inhibitors are contraindicated) should also be used in all patients with STEMI with diabetes or hypertension. Intravenous ACE inhibitors have been shown to increase adverse events and should not be used in STEMI patients [2].

A lipid profile should be obtained within 24 hours of admission [2], since low density lipoproteins cholestrol levels begin decreasing immediately after the event. Aggressive lipid-lowering therapy in the acute phase has been shown to be associated with modest benefit. Nonetheless, aggressive lipid-lowering therapy has been unequivocally proven to be efficacious for secondary prevention of patients with coronary artery disease for reduction in mortality, recurrent ischemia or infarction, need for repeat revascularization, or stroke and should be prescribed at discharge unless contraindicated [19].

Long-term anticoagulation is indicated in patients with large anterior infarction, left ventricular aneurysm, or atrial fibrillation for prevention of intracardiac thrombus and its embolic complications. An insulin infusion should be given in the first 24 to 48 hours to normalize blood glucose in patients with STEMI, particularly those with complicated course. Finally, electrolyte abnormalities of potassium and magnesium should be closely monitored and treated appropriately to prevent arrhythmic events [2].

Other invasive management

Intraaortic balloon pump (IABP) use is indicated in all patients with cardiogenic shock, acute mitral regurgitation, ventricular septal rupture, refractory postinfarction angina, or recurrent intractable ventricular arrhythmias [2]. The need for temporary pacing has decreased significantly with the advent of reperfusion strategies but should be considered in patients with symptomatic bradyarrhythmias, bilateral alternating bundle branch block, new trifascicular block, or Mobitz type II block [2]. The use of pulmonary artery catheter may be considered in patients with severe progressive heart failure, progressive hypotension, shock, ventricular septal rupture, mitral regurgitation, or cardiac tamponade [2]. Similarly, invasive arterial monitoring is recommended for patients with systolic blood pressure less than 80 mm Hg, cardiogenic shock, and use of intravenous vasopressors or nitroprusside [2].

Complications of STEMI

Mitral regurgitation

Acute mitral regurgitation is a life-threatening complication that can occur with or without papillary muscle rupture. It is more common with inferior STEMI, usually because of occlusions of the right coronary or left circumflex arteries. Medical management carries a very high mortality (70%). Surgical mortality, although high, is still lower (40%) than medical treatment alone [20]. Diagnosis can be established rapidly by transthoracic and if required transesophageal echocardiography. All patients should be considered for emergent surgery while stabilization is achieved by IABP, inotropes, and vasodilators. Delay in operation increases the risk of myocardial and other organ injury and subsequent death [2]. Five-year survival is excellent and reported to be between 60% and 70% in patients who survive surgery [2]. Mitral regurgitation in absence of papillary muscle rupture indicates extensive infarct and severe left ventricular dysfunction. Medical treatment may sometimes lead to reduction in mitral regurgitation severity in this cohort. However, when surgery is required for ongoing ischemia or critical coronary anatomy, mitral valve surgery should be undertaken in patients with mitral regurgitation > grade 2 on transesophageal echocardiography [2].

Ventricular septal rupture

The frequency of acute ventricular septal rupture (VSR) has decreased in the reperfusion era and occurs in fewer than 1% of patients with STEMI. Emergency surgical repair is necessary not only in patients with pulmonary edema or cardiogenic shock, but also in hemodynamically stable patients, as sudden hemodynamic collapse occurs even in these patients. Initial stabilization with IABP, invasive monitoring, inotropes, and vasodilators and prompt surgical referral is recommended for almost every patient with an acute VSR. Surgical mortality remains high and has been reported to be 20% to 50% and is much higher in patients with cardiogenic shock [21]; however, surgical mortality is significantly less than medical management alone. Too few patients with postinfarction VSR have been treated by transcatheter closure with a septal occluding device to make any definitive recommendations.

Left ventricular free wall rupture

Cardiac rupture occurs in up to 2% of all patients admitted with STEMI and is typically manifested by chest pain and EKG changes, with rapid progression to hemodynamic collapse and electromechanical dissociation. Cardiac rupture is observed most frequently in patients with their first myocardial infarction, those with anterior infarction, the elderly, women, hypertension during the acute phase of STEMI, lack of previous angina and myocardial infarction, lack of collateral blood flow, Q waves on the EKG, use of corticosteroids or nonsteroidal anti-inflammatory drugs, and use of fibrinolytic therapy more than14 hours after onset [2]. Reperfusion therapy decreases risk of cardiac rupture [22]. Pseudoaneurysm is a serious complication after rupture of the free ventricular wall. Clot forms in the pericardial space, and an aneurysmal wall containing clot and pericardium prevents exsanguination. Prompt surgical correction is indicated for pseudoaneurysm to prevent rupture. Pericardiocentesis, preferably in the operating room, for relief of tamponade and emergency surgical repair may be life saving with repair of rupture undertaken soon. Surgical mortality in studies with small number of patients with this complication has been reported to be as high as 60% [2].

Left ventricular aneurysm

Left ventricular aneurysm after STEMI usually occurs in patients with anterior wall infarction with total left anterior descending artery occlusion. Clinical consequences include angina pectoris, heart failure, thromboembolism, and ventricular arrhythmias. Like all other complications of STEMI, reperfusion therapy is associated with a significantly reduced incidence of LV aneurysm formation. Oral anticoagulation is recommended in patients with mural thrombus and for 3 months after acute anterior STEMI. Surgery for ventricular aneurysm early after STEMI is recommended for control of heart failure or intractable ventricular arrhythmias unresponsive to conventional therapy. Patients with severe left ventricular dysfunction have an increase in mortality as high as 19% in those with left ventricular ejection fraction less than 20%. Operative survivors have clear improvement in New York Heart Association class and a 60% 5-year survival rate [2].

Right ventricular infarction

Right ventricular infarction (RVI) commonly occurs in patients with an inferior myocardial infarction (and very rarely with anterior myocardial infarction). Although RVI is evident in approximately 25% of an inferior STEMI patients, hemodynamic compromise is evident in fewer than 10% of these patients. Consequently, EKGs with right-sided precordial leads should be monitored in all patients with an inferior STEMI [2]. A triad of hypotension, jugular venous distention, and clear lungs is very specific but has poor sensitivity for RVI. In the ED, RVI can be diagnosed by ST elevation in lead V_{4R}, and suspected in hypotension induced by nitroglycerin. A right atrial pressure higher than 10 mm Hg and a right atrial/pulmonary capillary wedge pressure ratio of 0.8 or higher are strongly suggestive of RVI. Besides hypotension and shock, other concomitant findings include advanced atrioventricular block and atrial tachyarrhythmias. Treatment of RVI includes volume loading, inotropic support with dobutamine, and maintenance of atrioventricular synchrony. Immediate reperfusion with primary PCI (or fibrinolytic therapy when timely primary PCI not available) have shown to improve right ventricular function and decrease 30-day mortality [2].

Left ventricular failure and cardiogenic shock

Heart failure is present in 15% to 25% of patients with acute myocardial infarction with an in-hospital mortality rate of 15% to 40%. The severity of left ventricular dysfunction is proportional to the extent of myocardial injury. Mortality has been reported to vary from 6% in patients with clear lung fields and no third heart sound to up to 60% in patients with cardiogenic shock in reperfusion era. Low output, or cardiogenic shock can occur in patients with severe left or right ventricular dysfunction, acute papillary muscle, ventricular septal or left ventricular free wall rupture, or tachy- or bradyarrhythmias [2]. Those at high risk for cardiogenic shock are elderly, female, hypertensive, diabetic, and with prior myocardial infarction. Fibrinolysis is not an effective reperfusion strategy in this cohort, but emergency revascularization (percutaneous or surgical) is associated with significant reduction in mortality [23]. Medical stabilization with IABP, invasive monitoring, inotropes, and vasodilators should be achieved with a goal for emergent revascularization.

Arrhythmias in patients with STEMI

Detailed description and management of all arrhythmias complicating STEMI is beyond the scope of this review and some of these are discussed in detail in other sections of this monograph. The two important arrhythmic complications reviewed here are ventricular and atrial tachyarrhythmias.

Atrial fibrillation/flutter

Atrial fibrillation (and flutter) in STEMI is an independent predictor of 30-day mortality. While it may be related to atrial infarction, pericarditis, or excessive sympathetic stimulation from pain, distress, or anxiety, another important cause is left ventricular failure with elevated left atrial pressure [24]. Atrial fibrillation leads to increased oxygen demand, decreased left ventricular filling, loss of atrial contribution to left ventricular filling, and diminished forward cardiac output. Thus, all efforts should be directed at reducing ventricular rate (beta-blockers, verapamil, diltiazem, digitalis, anticongestive measures) and preferably toward restoration of sinus rhythm (cardioversion, procainamide, amiodarone, and rapid atrial overdrive pacing). Prevention of thromboembolic events with long-term warfarin should be an important goal if sinus rhythm is not restored [2].

Ventricular fibrillation and tachycardia

Ventricular tachycardia (VT) is defined as more than 100 bpm, with sustained VT for longer than 30 seconds and nonsustained VT for less than 30 seconds. VT occurs more frequently within the first 48 hours of symptom onset and, in the past, was generally believed to be unrelated to prognosis. Newer studies indicate that nonsustained VT and sustained monomorphic VT even within the first few hours of symptom onset indicate poorer in-hospital and long-term outcomes. VT that occurs more than 48 hours after STEMI may denote an arrhythmic substrate deserving of further evaluation by an electrophysiology study [2].

Sustained VT should be managed by immediate cardioversion if the patient is hemodynamically unstable. If angina, pulmonary edema, or hypotension are not present, patients may be treated with intravenous amiodarone, lidocaine, or procainamide. Replacement of potassium and magnesium, treatment with beta-blockers, and reperfusion with relief of ischemia may help decrease the incidence of VT.

Primary ventricular fibrillation (VF) must be distinguished from secondary ventricular fibrillation that occurs in patients with congestive heart failure or cardiogenic shock [25]. Late VF occurs more than 48 hours after onset of STEMI. Secondary and late VF is associated with significantly higher mortality than primary VF. VF should be treated immediately with unsynchronized monophasic electric shock. Other measures, such as correction of electrolytes, reperfusion, and beta-blockers, may help reduce the incidence of VF. Prophylactic use of lidocaine has no role in prevention of ventricular arrhythmias and may increase incidence of asystolic arrest and should be avoided in all patients with STEMI.

Finally, an implantable cardioverter defibrillator (ICD) is indicated for patients with VF or hemodyanamically significant sustained VT more than 2 days after STEMI, provided the arrhythmia is not judged to be due to transient or reversible ischemia or reinfarction. Additionally, patients without spontaneous VF or sustained VT more than 48 hours after STEMI whose STEMI occurred at least 1 month previously, who have a left ventricular ejection fraction between 31% and 40%, demonstrate additional evidence of electrical instability (eg, nonsustained VT), and have inducible VF or sustained VT on EP testing may also benefit from ICD for prevention of sudden cardiac death. In patients with left ventricular ejection fraction less than 30% at 1 month post-STEMI, ICD is also indicated for secondary prevention of sudden cardiac death even in the absence of any ventricular arrhythmias [2].

Recurrent ischemic events

Infarct extension may occur as extension of infarction in the same territory as subendocardial or transmural myocardial necrosis or involving adjacent territories. Postinfarct angina occurs in 23% to 60% of patients and is higher among patients receiving fibrinolysis compared with primary PCI [12]. Postinfarct angina is associated with increased incidence of sudden death, reinfarction, and other acute cardiac events. Definitive treatment is achieved with percutaneous or surgical revascularization of ischemic coronary arteries.

Pericarditis

Pericarditis occurs in about 10% of patients, usually within first 24 to 96 hours. This event is heralded by progressive, severe chest pain that increases with inspiration, swallowing, and body movements and is postural, being alleviated when the patient sits up. The incidence has decreased significantly in the era of reperfusion therapies. Treatment consists of high-dose aspirin (650 mg every 4 to 6 hours). Nonsteroidal anti-inflammatory agents and steroids should be avoided as they impair myocardial healing and promote infarct expansion. Colchicine may be beneficial in patients with recurrent pericarditis. Finally, Dressler's or post–myocardial infarction syndrome occurs in 1% to 3% of patients about 1 to 8 weeks after STEMI. Patients present with chest pain suggestive of pericarditis, fever, arthralgia, malaise, elevated leukocyte count, and elevated erythrocyte sedimentation rate [2]. Treatment is similar for acute pericarditis, and occasionally long-term corticosteroids with slow taper is needed.

Prognosis

Many risk prediction models have been developed for estimating the risk of patients presenting with STEMI. The Thrombolysis in Myocardial Infarction (TIMI) risk score for patients with STEMI is shown in Fig. 4 and has been validated in several trials [26]. The TIMI risk score is useful in discriminating patient risk across a wide spectrum with a score of 0 associated with less than 1% to that which is more than 30-fold higher when the total score is more than 8 (35.9%). It should be recognized that risk stratification is a continuous process and requires incorporation of information over time after initial assessments that includes indicators of failed reperfusion (eg, recurrence of chest pain, persistence of EKG findings indicating infarction), left ventricular systolic function, mechanical complications,

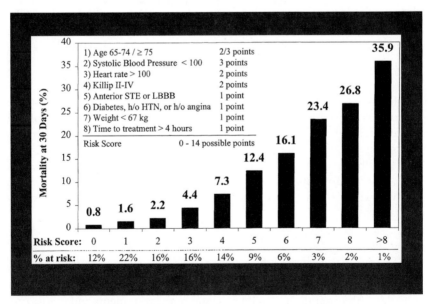

Fig. 4. Prediction of 30-day mortality using Thrombolysis in Myocardial Infarction (TIMI) risk score for ST-elevation myocardial infarction. (Adapted from Morrow DA, Antman EM, Charlesworth A, et al. TIMI risk score for ST-elevation myocardial infarction: a convenient, bedside, clinical score for risk assessment at presentation: An Intravenous nPA for Treatment of Infarcting Myocardium Early II trial substudy. Circulation 2000;102:2031–7; with permission.)

arrhythmic events after 48 hours, new-onset heart failure or shock, and lack of secondary prevention therapies or intolerance to these treatments, all of which increase subsequent risks. Risk stratification allows for early discharge of low-risk patients and aggressive invasive management and closure surveillance of the high-risk group.

Other in-hospital and discharge care of STEMI patients

Evidence-based approaches of the need for invasive procedures (cardiac catheterization and revascularization) and noninvasive tests are outlined in Fig. 2. This strategy is helpful in deciding the type of exercise test and the cohort who should undergo invasive procedures. Ejection fraction should be estimated by echocardiography in patients managed medically.

Finally, all secondary prevention strategies should be instituted before discharge and continued after discharge. Education regarding patient's disease and methods to prevent recurrent ischemic events should be an important part of discharge planning. All patients should be considered for long-term therapy with aspirin, beta-blockers, lipid-lowering agents, and ACE inhibitors. Clopidogrel is indicated in patients with aspirin allergy and in those who had coronary stent(s) implanted before discharge. Warfarin anticoagulation is indicated for patients with large anterior STEMI, left ventricular thrombus, atrial fibrillation, and those unable to take long-term aspirin or clopidogrel. All patients should be considered for a cardiac rehabilitation program and should follow diet and exercise prescriptions. Smoking cessation and control of hypertension, dyslipidemia, diabetes, and weight to target values should be vigorously pursued [2].

References

[1] American Heart Association. Heart disease and stroke statistics—2005 update. Dallas (TX): American Heart Association; 2005. Available at: http://www.americanheart.org/downloadable/heart/1105390918119HDSStats2005Update.pdf. Accessed August 12 2006.

[2] Antman EM, Anbe DT, Armstrong PW, et al. ACC/AHA guidelines for the management of patients with ST-elevation myocardial infarction. A report of the American College of Cardiology/American Heart Association Task Force on Practice Guidelines (Committee to Revise the 1999 Guidelines for the Management of patients with acute myocardial infarction). 2004. Available at: www.acc.org/clinical/guidelines/stemi/index.pdf. Accessed July 4, 2006.

[3] Cheitlin MD, McAllister HA, de Castro CM. Myocardial infarction without atherosclerosis. JAMA 1975;231:951–9.

[4] Sgarbossa EB, Pinsky SL, Barbagelata A, et al. Electrocardiographic diagnosis of evolving acute myocardial infarction in presence of left bundle branch block. N Engl J Med 1996;334: 481–7.

[5] Newby LK, Goldmann BU. Troponin: an important prognostic marker and risk-stratification tool in non-ST-segment elevation acute coronary syndromes. J Am Coll Cardiol 2003; 41(4 Suppl S):31S–6S.

[6] Ohman EM, Armstrong PW, Christenson RH, et al. Cardiac troponin T levels for risk stratification in acute myocardial ischemia. GUSTO IIA Investigators. N Engl J Med 1996;335: 1333–41.

[7] Ryan TJ, Anderson JL, Antman EM, et al. ACC/AHA guidelines for management of patients with acute myocardial infarction. A report of the American College of Cardiology/American Heart Association Task Force on Practice Guidelines (Committee on Management of Acute Myocardial Infarction). J Am Coll Cardiol 1999;34:890–911.

[8] National Heart Attack Alert Program Coordinating Committee. Emergency department: rapid identification and treatment of patients with acute myocardial infarction. Ann Emerg Med 1994;23:311–29.

[9] Fibrinolytic Therapy Trialists' (FTT) Collaborative Group. Indications for fibrinolytic therapy in suspected acute myocardial infarction: collaborative overview of early mortality and major morbidity results from all randomised trials of more than 1000 patients. Lancet 1994; 343(8893):311–22.

[10] Brass LM, Lichtman JH, Wang Y, et al. Intracranial hemorrhage associated with thrombolytic therapy for elderly patients with acute myocardial infarction: results from the Cooperative Cardiovascular Project. Stroke 2000;31:1802–11.

[11] Simoons ML, Maggioni AP, Knatterud G, et al. Individual risk assessment for intracranial haemorrhage during thrombolytic therapy. Lancet 1993;342:1523–8.

[12] Keeley EC, Boura JA, Grines CL. Primary angioplasty versus intravenous thrombolytic therapy for acute myocardial infarction: a quantitative review of 23 randomised trials. Lancet 2003;361:13 20.

[13] Baigent C, Sudlow C, Collins R, et al. Antithrombotic Trialists' Collaboration. Collaborative metaanalysis of randomised trials of antiplatelet therapy for prevention of death, myocardial infarction, and stroke in high-risk patients. BMJ 2002;324:71–86.

[14] Chen ZM, Pan HC, Chen YP, et al. The ClOpidogrel and Metoprolol in Myocardial Infarction Trial (COMMIT) Collaborative Group. Addition of clopidogrel to aspirin in 45 852 patients with acute myocardial infarction: randomised placebo-controlled trial. Lancet 2005; 366:1607–21.

[15] Sabatine MS, Cannon CP, Gibson CM, et al. Clopidogrel as adjunctive reperfusion therapy (CLARITY)-thrombolysis in myocardial infarction (TIMI) 28 investigators. Addition of clopidogrel to aspirin and fibrinolytic therapy for myocardial infarction with ST-segment elevation. JAMA 2005;294:1224–32.

[16] Antman EM, Morrow DA, McCabe CH, et al. Enoxaparin versus unfractionated heparin with fibrinolysis for ST-elevation myocardial infarction. N Engl J Med 2006;354:1477–88.

[17] Petersen JL, Mahaffey KW, Hasselblad V, et al. Efficacy and bleeding complications among patients randomized to enoxaparin or unfractionated heparin for antithrombin therapy in non–ST-segment elevation acute coronary syndromes: a systematic overview. JAMA 2004;292:89–96.

[18] Yusuf S, Mehta SR, Chrolavicius S, et al. OASIS 6 trial group Effects of Fondaparinux on mortality and reinfarction in patients with acute ST-segment elevation myocardial infarction: the OASIS-6 randomized trial. JAMA 2000;283:247–53.

[19] Randomised trial of cholesterol lowering in 4444 patients with coronary heart disease: the Scandinavian Simvastatin Survival Study (4S). Lancet 1994;344:1383–9.

[20] Thompson CR, Buller CE, Sleeper LA, et al. Cardiogenic shock due to acute severe mitral regurgitation complicating acute myocardial infarction: a report from the SHOCK Trial Registry. SHould we use emergently revascularize Occluded Coronaries in cardiogenic shocK? J Am Coll Cardiol 2000;36:1104–9.

[21] Menon V, Webb JG, Hillis LD, et al. Outcome and profile of ventricular septal rupture with cardiogenic shock after myocardial infarction: a report from the SHOCK Trial Registry. SHould we emergently revascularize Occluded Coronaries in cardiogenic shocK? J Am Coll Cardiol 2000;36:1110–6.

[22] Becker RC, Gore JM, Lambrew C, et al. A composite view of cardiac rupture in the United States National Registry of Myocardial Infarction. J Am Coll Cardiol 1996;27:1321–6.

[23] Hochman JS, Sleeper LA, Webb JG, et al. Early revascularization in acute myocardial infarction complicated by cardiogenic shock. N Engl J Med 1999;341:625–34.

[24] Crenshaw BS, Ward SR, Granger CB, et al. Atrial fibrillation in the setting of acute myocardial infarction: the GUSTO-I experience. Global Utilization of Streptokinase and TPA for Occluded Coronary Arteries. J Am Coll Cardiol 1997;30:406–13.

[25] Volpi A, Cavalli A, Santoro E, et al. GISSI Investigators. Incidence and prognosis of secondary ventricular fibrillation in acute myocardial infarction. Evidence for a protective effect of thrombolytic therapy. Circulation 1990;82:1279–88.

[26] Morrow DA, Antman EM, Charlesworth A, et al. TIMI risk score for ST-elevation myocardial infarction: a convenient, bedside, clinical score for risk assessment at presentation: an Intravenous nPA for treatment of infarcting myocardium early II trial substudy. Circulation 2000;102:2031–7.

ELSEVIER
SAUNDERS

CRITICAL
CARE
CLINICS

Crit Care Clin 23 (2007) 709–735

Acute Coronary Syndromes: Unstable Angina/Non-ST Elevation Myocardial Infarction

Rohit Bhatheja, MD[a,b],
Debabrata Mukherjee, MD, MS[a,b],*

[a]Gill Heart Institute, Division of Cardiovascular Medicine, University of Kentucky,
900 South Limestone Street, 326 Wethington Building, Lexington, KY 40536-0200, USA
[b]Department of Medicine, Division of Cardiovascular Medicine, University of Kentucky,
900 South Limestone Street, 326 Wethington Building, Lexington, KY 40536-0200, USA

Coronary artery disease (CAD) affects 13.2 million Americans, including 7.2 million individuals who have had a prior myocardial infarction (MI). In 2003, the estimated direct and indirect health care cost of CAD was an astounding $142.5 billion [1]. The data are sobering, in that every 26 seconds an American suffers a coronary event; or every minute, someone dies from CAD. More than 80% of those who die from CAD are more than 65 years of age [1]. Among patients who have CAD, acute coronary syndrome (ACS) is a major health problem affecting approximately 1.5 million individuals a year [1].

Patients who have CAD may present as having stable angina or ACS. The spectrum of ACS includes ST-segment elevation MI, unstable angina (UA), and non–ST-segment elevation MI (NSTEMI). UA is characterized by the clinical presentation of angina with or without ischemic ECG changes (ST segment depression or new T-wave inversion). NSTEMI is similar to UA but is characterized by positive biomarkers (troponin or creatine kinase-MB [CK-MB]) in the setting of angina or ECG changes. The presence of myonecrosis as evident by positive cardiac markers portends a higher risk than those presenting with just UA. UA and NSTEMI pathophysiologically and clinically are related and initially may be indistinguishable, as biomarkers may not be elevated at presentation.

* Corresponding author. Gill Heart Institute, Division of Cardiovascular Medicine, University of Kentucky, 900 South Limestone Street, 326 Wethington Building, Lexington, KY 40536-0200.
    E-mail address: mukherjee@uky.edu (D. Mukherjee).

Pathogenesis of unstable angina/non–ST-segment elevation myocardial infarction

Myocardial ischemia is the result of a mismatch between oxygen supply and demand and, when prolonged, may lead to myocardial necrosis and infarction. Patients who have UA/NSTEMI typically have obstructive coronary disease; however, ACS may occur in the absence of significant coronary obstruction due to rupture of a nonobstructive plaque, coronary vasospasm, or increased myocardial oxygen demand. Rupture of an atherosclerotic plaque and subsequent formation of a thrombus usually is the triggering event in the pathogenesis of most cases of ACS. Some other causes may lead to coronary ischemia but are relatively rare (Table 1).

Plaque rupture is precipitated by two main mechanisms—physical shear stress to the plaque or inflammatory mediators. Plaques that are prone to rupture have a large lipid core, high macrophage and activated T-lymphocyte density, low smooth muscle cell density, and a thin fibrous cap characterized by disorganized collagen. Rupture of the plaque shoulder, at its junction with the arterial wall, which is mechanically the weakest point, exposes the highly thrombogenic necrotic lipid core to platelets and circulating inflammatory cells, stimulating the formation of acute thrombi [2,3].

With the breakdown of the atherosclerotic plaque, the local milieu becomes prothrombotic because of the exposure of subendothelial matrix to the circulating blood. Platelet surface receptors recognize the vascular matrix components (collagen, von Willebrand factor [vWF], vitronectin, and fibronectin), stimulating platelet adhesion via the glycoprotein (GP) Ib receptor and vWF. After this, there is platelet activation leading to a change in platelet morphology and degranulation of the alpha and dense granules, which release substrates, thromboxane A2 [4], platelet factor 4, factor V [5], P-selectin, vWF, plasminogen activator inhibitor-1, fibrinogen, serotonin, and ADP [6]. These chemotactic and vasoactive substances lead to the recruitment and activation of GP IIb/IIIa receptors on the platelet surface. The activated GP IIb/IIIa receptors are cross-linked by fibrinogen (or vWF), leading to platelet aggregation and formation of the white

Table 1

Causes of unstable angina and non–ST-segment elevation myocardial infarction[a]

1. Nonocclusive thrombus on pre-existing plaque
2. Dynamic obstruction (coronary artery spasm or vasoconstriction)
3. Progressive mechanical obstruction
4. Inflammation or infection
5. Secondary UA

[a] These causes are not mutually exclusive; some patients have ≥ 2 causes.

From Braunwald E. Unstable angina: an etiologic approach to management. Circulation 1998;98:2220; with permission.

thrombus on the surface of the plaque [7]. Myocardial ischemia ensues, as there is transient reduction in coronary blood flow. Further, temporary arterial occlusion or microembolization of platelet-thrombus aggregates and plaque material into the microcirculation leads to myocardial necrosis.

Less common causes of an ACS include dynamic obstruction, progressive atherosclerosis or restenosis, and inflammation. Noncardiac surgery or stressful events can cause a mismatch in myocardial oxygen demand and supply, resulting in UA/NSTEMI. This may be caused by (1) increased myocardial oxygen demand (fever or thyrotoxicosis), (2) reduced myocardial oxygen delivery (anemia or hypoxemia), or (3) reduced coronary blood flow (arrhythmia or hypotension). Although there may be coexisting CAD, it usually is stable and management should focus on the precipitating condition.

Presenting symptoms and signs

Typical angina is defined as a deep, poorly localized chest or arm discomfort that is reproducible with physical exertion or emotional stress and is relieved within 5 minutes with rest or use of sublingual nitroglycerine. This characteristic association may be lacking in UA/NSTEMI. The discomfort usually is more severe and longer lasting, may occur at rest or at a lower level of physical exertion [8], and classically presents in one of the three ways (Table 2) [9].

Associated with the chest pain, in varying frequencies, are the symptoms of diaphoresis, dyspnea, nausea, and vomiting. Occasionally, patients (especially elderly and female) may have no discernable chest pain but may present solely with varying components of jaw, arm or neck pain, and epigastric discomfort. Fatigue or, more commonly, a decrease in exercise threshold with worsening dyspnea on exertion, also may be the presenting feature. When these nonchest pain symptoms clearly are related to physical or emotional stress and are relieved by nitroglycerin, they are considered anginal equivalents. Progression in frequency and intensity

Table 2
Three types of presentations of unstable angina

Rest angina	Angina occurring at rest and prolonged, usually > 20 minutes
New-onset angina	New-onset angina of at least CCS[a] class III severity
Increasing angina	Previously diagnosed angina that has become distinctly more frequent, longer in duration, or lower in threshold (ie, increased by ≥1 CCS class to at least CCS class III severity)

[a] Canadian Cardiac Society classification.

Data from Savonitto S, Cohen MG, Politi A, et al. Extent of ST-segment depression and cardiac events in non-ST-segment elevation acute coronary syndromes. Eur Heart J 2005;26:2106–13.

should warrant the same degree of concern as chest pain. Constant pain that lasts for many hours or days, or only a few seconds, and easily is reproducible with palpation of the chest wall is less likely to be ischemic in origin. Pain that clearly is pleuritic or positional or located with the tip of one finger also is unlikely to be cardiac in origin. A history and ECG aid physicians in classifying the presentation as high, intermediate, or low likelihood of acute ischemia caused by CAD (Table 3) [8].

Presence of hypotension, mitral regurgitation murmur, unequal pulses, tachycardia, pulmonary rales, bruits, and gallop aid not only in diagnosing

Table 3
Likelihood that signs and symptoms represent an acute coronary syndrome secondary to coronary disease

Feature	High likelihood	Intermediate likelihood	Low likelihood
	Any of the following:	Absence of high-likelihood features and presence of any of the following:	Absence of high- or intermediate-likelihood features but may have:
History	Chest or left arm pain or discomfort as chief symptom reproducing prior documented angina	Chest or left arm pain or discomfort as chief symptom	Probable ischemic symptoms in absence of any of the intermediate likelihood characteristics
	Known history of CAD, including MI	Age >70 years Male gender Diabetes mellitus	Recent cocaine use
Examination	Transient mitral regurgitation, hypotension, diaphoresis, pulmonary edema, or rales	Extracardiac vascular disease	Chest discomfort reproduced by palpation
ECG	New, or presumably new, transient ST-segment deviation (≥ 0.5 mm) or T-wave inversion (≥ 2 mm) with symptoms	Fixed Q waves	T-wave flattening or inversion in leads with dominant R waves
		Abnormal ST segments or T waves not documented to be new	Normal ECG
Cardiac markers	Elevated cardiac troponin I, troponin T, or CK-MB	Normal	Normal

From Braunwald E, Mark DB, Jones RH, et al. Unstable angina: diagnosis and management. Rockville, MD: Agency for Health Care Policy and Research and the National Heart, Lung, and Blood Institute, US Public Health Service, US Department of Health and Human Services; 1994; AHCPR Publication No. 94-0602.

ACS but also in providing prognostic information. Cardiogenic shock and ensuing organ hypoperfusion as a consequence of NSTEMI portends a poor prognosis and demands a more aggressive management [10].

Diagnostic evaluation

Electrocardiography

Most patients who have UA/NSTEMI have some ECG changes. The ECG is important for diagnostic and risk stratification purposes. Specific characteristics and the magnitude of pattern abnormalities increase the likelihood of CAD. ST–T-segment depression portends a poorer prognosis than T-wave inversion alone or no ECG changes [11]. New or dynamic ST-segment depression is suggestive of acute ischemia with an increase in thrombin activity associated with elevated fibrinopeptides [12]. Inverted T waves also may suggest ischemia or NSTEMI, although the risk is less than that with ST-segment depression. Nonspecific ST-segment changes (≤ 0.5 mm) and T-wave changes (≤ 2 mm) are not uncommon and may be related to drugs (phenothiazines, digitalis, and so forth), hyperventilation, or repolarization abnormalities in association with left ventricular (LV) hypertrophy or conduction disturbances. Conversely, the ECG may be normal in 1% to 6% of patients who have NSTEMI and in approximately 4% of patients who have UA [13].

The Global Use of Strategies to Open Occluded Coronary Arteries in Acute Coronary Syndromes (GUSTO-IIb) trial demonstrated that the 30-day incidence of death or MI was 10.5% in those who had ST-segment depression versus 5.5% in patients who had T-wave inversion, and a higher mortality also was seen at 6-month follow-up [14]. The sum of ST depression is a strong independent predictor of short-term mortality and the risk increases with the magnitude of depression [15].

Biochemical markers

Although many markers and assays that detect myocardial necrosis are available, the cardiac troponins T and I and the creatinine kinase–MB (CK-MB) isoform are those used most commonly, with the troponins gaining acceptance as the markers of choice in ACS. These have achieved an important role in diagnostic, prognostic, and treatment pathways by virtue of their high degree of sensitivity and specificity and their relative ease of use and interpretation. The joint statement of the European Society of Cardiology and the American College of Cardiology (ACC) defines myonecrosis as when the peak concentration of troponin T or I exceeds the decision limit (99th percentile for a reference group) on at least one occasion in a 24-hour period [16]. This new definition has increased the frequency of the diagnosis of NSTEMI in patients who have ACS by 30%. Troponin I may be more accurate in patients who have renal insufficiency compared with troponin T. The troponins are detectable approximately 6 hours after myocardial injury and are measurable for up to 2 weeks. Mortality risk is directly proportional to troponin levels and the prognostic information is independent of other clinical and ECG risk factors (Fig. 1) [17,18]. CK-MB is less specific because of its presence in skeletal muscle and in low levels in the blood of healthy persons. Unlike troponins, it is useful in detecting recurrent myocardial necrosis early after an initial event as levels tend to return to normal within 36 to 48 hours after initial release.

Noninvasive testing

Noninvasive stress testing is recommended for risk stratification (Table 4) in patients who are at low to intermediate risk and are free of angina at rest or minimal activity and heart failure for at least 24 hours. Although exercise ECG is the most appropriate testing modality, choice of stress test is based on the resting ECG, ability to exercise, and local expertise. Treadmill testing is suitable in patients who have good exercise tolerance in whom the ECG is free of ST-segment abnormalities, bundle branch block, LV hypertophy, intraventricular conduction delay, paced rhythm, pre-excitation, and digoxin effect. Echocardiography has the advantage of allowing for bedside and rapid determination of LV function. Imaging modalities, such as echocardiography or nuclear imaging, should be added in patients who have ECG abnormalities that prevent accurate interpretation and also in those

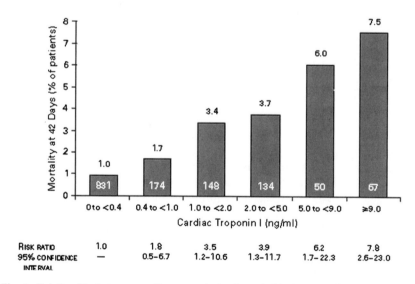

Fig. 1. Relationship between cardiac troponin levels and risk for mortality at 42 days in patients who have ACS. (*Reproduced from* Antman EM, Tanasijevic MJ, Thompson B, et al. Cardiac-specific troponin I levels to predict the risk of mortality in patients with acute coronary syndromes. N Engl J Med 1996;335:1342–9; with permission. Copyright © 1996, Massachusetts Medical Society.)

Table 4
Risk stratification based on noninvasive testing

High risk (>3% annual mortality rate)
1. Severe resting LV dysfunction (LVEF <35%)
2. High-risk treadmill score (score ≤ −11)
3. Severe exercise LV dysfunction (exercise LVEF <35%)
4. Stress-induced large perfusion defect (particularly if anterior)
5. Stress-induced multiple perfusion defects of moderate size
6. Large, fixed perfusion defect with LV dilation or increased lung uptake (thallium-201)
7. Stress-induced moderate perfusion defect with LV dilation or increased lung uptake (thallium-201)
8. Echocardiographic wall motion abnormality (involving >2 segments) developing at a low dose of dobutamine ($\leq$10 mg kg^{-1} · min^{-1}) or at a low heart rate (<120 bpm)
9. Stress echocardiographic evidence of extensive ischemia.
Intermediate risk (1%–3% annual mortality rate)
1. Mild/moderate resting LV dysfunction (LVEF 35%–49%)
2. Intermediate-risk treadmill score (−11 < score <5)
3. Stress-induced moderate perfusion defect without LV dilation or increased lung intake (thallium-201)
4. Limited stress echocardiographic ischemia with a wall motion abnormality only at higher doses of dobutamine involving ≤2 segments.
Low risk (<1% annual mortality rate)
1. Low-risk treadmill score (score ≥5)
2. Normal or small myocardial perfusion defect at rest or with stress
3. Normal stress echocardiographic wall motion or no change of limited resting wall motion abnormalities during stress

Abbreviation: LVEF, left ventricular ejection fraction.
From Gibbons RJ, Chatterjee K, Daley J, et al. ACC/AHA/ACP-ASIM guidelines for the management of patients with chronic stable angina. J Am Coll Cardiol 1999;33:2092–197; with permission. Copyright © 1999 American College of Cardiology.

who have a history of coronary revascularization. Pharmacologic stress testing can be performed in patients who cannot achieve an adequate exercise stress on the treadmill [8].

Cardiac catheterization and coronary angiography

Coronary angiography is an invasive approach to risk stratification that gives detailed structural information about the coronary tree and allows percutaneous coronary revascularization if appropriate. Immediate angiography usually is reserved for those presenting with high-risk features, such as cardiogenic shock, sustained ventricular tachycardia, mechanical complications (eg, acute mitral regurgitation or ventricular septal defect), severe cardiac dysfunction, or heart failure or for those having persistent chest pain despite adequate medical therapy. Routine early invasive strategy (ie, coronary angiography) in all patients followed by revascularization in those who have suitable coronary anatomy is recommended in those who have elevated troponins, LV dysfunction (ejection fraction <40%), heart failure, high-risk stress findings, history of percutaneous coronary intervention

(PCI) within the past 6 months or a prior coronary artery bypass graft (CABG), or new ST-segment depression on ECG [8]. This approach, specifically in those who are troponin positive, has proved to reduce rehosopitalization, severe angina, and long-term major cardiovascular events. The goal of early invasive therapy is not only to visualize the coronary vasculature, the extent and nature of the coronary obstruction, and the feasability of revascularization but also to assess the ventricular function and associated valvular disease.

Those who do not have the high-risk features described previously may not necessarily benefit from an invasive approach, and a conservative approach with medical therapy and risk stratification with an noninvasive imaging may be a reasonable strategy. Fig. 2 is a simplified algorithm for management of patients who have ACS based on American College of Cardiology/American Heart Association guidelines.

Complications

If left untreated, 5% to 10% of patients who have UA die and 10% to 20% suffer nonfatal MI within 30 days. One quarter of patients who have NSTEMI develop Q-wave MI, with the remaining having non–Q-wave MI. Arrhythmia, congestive heart failure, and cardiogenic shock are life-threatening complications. Recurrent ischemia may result in need for urgent coronary artery revascularization. The Thrombolysis in Myocardial Infarction (TIMI) risk score (Fig. 3) [19] has been shown to predict death, MI, and need for urgent revascularization. Another risk score that has been studied is the Global Registry of Acute Coronary Events (GRACE) risk score, which predicts 6-month postdischarge death (Fig. 4) [20].

Early invasive management may be associated with a shorter hospital stay, less in-hospital mortality, and other adverse outcomes. Those who have the highest risk derive the maximum benefit. There is a higher risk for blood transfusions, however, with this approach [21].

Therapy

Once the diagnosis of ACS is made, resources should be mobilized for effective and immediate management of this condition. The strategy should be relief of ischemia and prevention of the serious adverse outcomes of reinfarction and death. This may be achieved by prompt initiation of appropriate therapy, ongoing risk stratification, and, in selected cases, coronary artery revascularization. Coronary angiography performed after NSETMI has shown that in most patients, the infarction is associated with incomplete occlusion of the infarct-related artery; 37% of patients have no identifiable culprit lesion; and only 13% have a single occlusion of the infarct-related artery [22]. As UA and NSTEMI are distinguishable mainly by the rise in

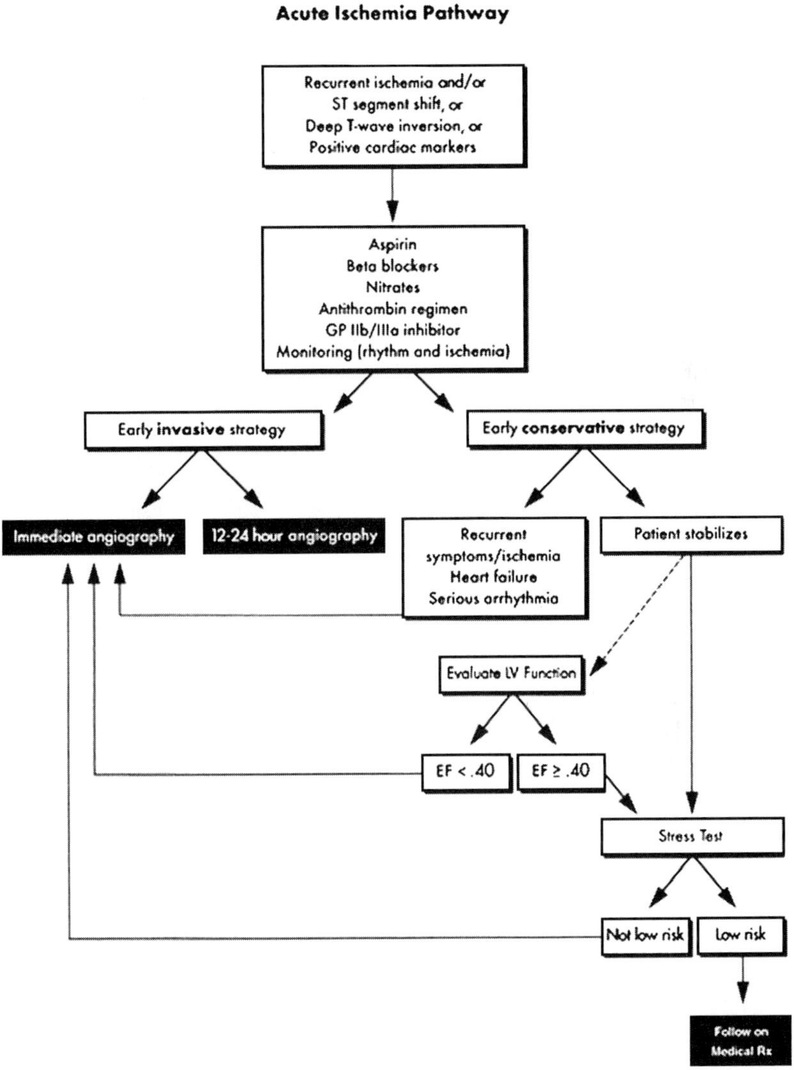

Acute Ischemia Pathway

Fig. 2. Approach to patients who have ACS. (*From* ACC/AHA Guidelines for the Management of Patients with Unstable Angina and Non-ST-Segment Elevation Myocardial Infarction. J Am Coll Cardiol 2000;36:970–1062; with permission. Copyright © 2002 American College of Cardiology.)

cardiac biomarkers, which may not be detectable for few hours after presentation, the initial management is the same.

General measures

Bed rest is recommended strongly in the presence of ongoing ischemia. When symptom free, mobility to a chair or bedside commode may be

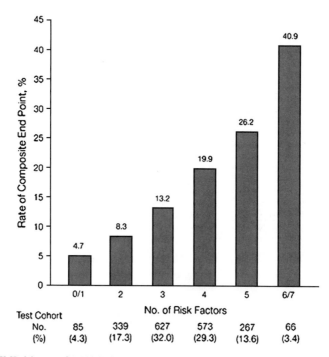

Fig. 3. TIMI risk score for UA/NSTEMI. The rates of composite endpoints (ie, all-cause mortality, MI, and recurrent ischemia) through day 14 in the TIMI 11B trial depending on the level of risk factors. The seven risk factors are age ≥65 years, presence of ≥3 risk factors for CAD, prior coronary stenosis of ≥50%, ST deviation, aspirin use in the last 7 days, severe angina, and elevated cardiac biomarkers. (*Reproduced from* Antman EM, Cohen M, Bernink PJ, et al. The TIMI risk score for unstable angina/non-ST elevation MI: a method for prognostication and therapeutic decision making. JAMA 2000;284:835–42; with permission.)

allowed. Supplemental oxygen should be administered to maintain oxygen saturation over 90% in those who have cyanosis, respiratory distress, and high-risk features. Continuous ECG monitoring for arrhythmias gives an opportunity to detect and treat potentially fatal rhythm disorders. In addition, ST-segment monitoring may have a role in detecting ongoing ischemia that otherwise may go undetected.

Anti-ischemic agents

Nitrates

Nitroglycerine has a potent endothelium-independent vasodilator effect on the coronary and peripheral vascular beds. Nitrates dilate venous capacitance vessels and peripheral arterioles, with a predominant decrease in preload and a lesser effect on afterload, thereby decreasing myocardial wall stress and oxygen demand. These drugs also may increase myocardial oxygen delivery by dilating epicardial coronary arteries and increasing collateral flow. Although there are no randomized placebo-controlled trials

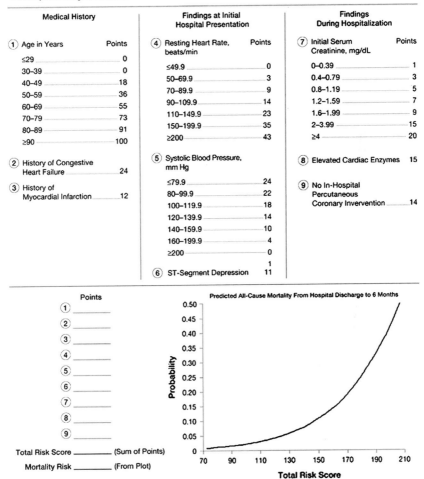

Risk Calculator for 6-Month Postdischarge Mortality After Hospitalization for Acute Coronary Syndrome

Record the points for each variable at the bottom left and sum the points to calculate the total risk score. Find the total score on the x-axis of the nomogram plot. The corresponding probability on the y-axis is the estimated probability of all-cause mortality from hospital discharge to 6 months.

Medical History		Findings at Initial Hospital Presentation		Findings During Hospitalization	
① Age in Years	Points	④ Resting Heart Rate, beats/min	Points	⑦ Initial Serum Creatinine, mg/dL	Points
≤29	0	≤49.9	0	0–0.39	1
30–39	0	50–69.9	3	0.4–0.79	3
40–49	18	70–89.9	9	0.8–1.19	5
50–59	36	90–109.9	14	1.2–1.59	7
60–69	55	110–149.9	23	1.6–1.99	9
70–79	73	150–199.9	35	2–3.99	15
80–89	91	≥200	43	≥4	20
≥90	100				
② History of Congestive Heart Failure	24	⑤ Systolic Blood Pressure, mm Hg		⑧ Elevated Cardiac Enzymes	15
③ History of Myocardial Infarction	12	≤79.9	24	⑨ No In-Hospital Percutaneous Coronary Invervention	14
		80–99.9	22		
		100–119.9	18		
		120–139.9	14		
		140–159.9	10		
		160–199.9	4		
		≥200	0		
		⑥ ST-Segment Depression	1 11		

Points
① ____
② ____
③ ____
④ ____
⑤ ____
⑥ ____
⑦ ____
⑧ ____
⑨ ____

Total Risk Score ____ (Sum of Points)

Mortality Risk ____ (From Plot)

Predicted All-Cause Mortality From Hospital Discharge to 6 Months

Probability (y-axis): 0, 0.05, 0.10, 0.15, 0.20, 0.25, 0.30, 0.35, 0.40, 0.45, 0.50

Total Risk Score (x-axis): 70, 90, 110, 130, 150, 170, 190, 210

Fig. 4. GRACE prediction scorecard and nomogram for all-cause mortality from discharge to 6 months. (*Reproduced from* Eagle KA, Lim MJ, Dabbous OH, et al. A validated prediction model for all forms of acute coronary syndrome: estimating the risk of 6-month postdischarge death in an international registry. JAMA 2004;291:2727–33; with permission.)

that address the effect of nitrates on symptom relief or reduction in cardiac events, its use is based on observational studies that have demonstrated safety and efficacy in ACS [23]. In the absence of relief of symptoms of ongoing ischemia after sublingual nitroglycerin tablet, intravenous nitroglycerin may be started and increased every 3 to 5 minutes until ischemia is relieved or there is a significant drop in blood pressure (systolic blood pressure [BP] <110 mm Hg or >25% decrease from starting). Because of the phenomenon of nitrate tolerance, the dose may have to be increased periodically. In patients who do not have refractory symptoms, intravenous nitroglycerin should be converted to an oral or topical form within 24 hours, with nitrate-free periods to avoid tolerance. Use of sildenafil in the preceding 24-hour period is a contraindication to the use of nitrates, as it promotes a prolonged and exaggerated hypotension, which may lead to MI and even death [24].

β-Blockers

β-Blockers are recommended for all patients who have UA/NSTEMI, unless contraindicated. If there is ongoing ischemia or chest pain, they initially are given intravenously followed by oral delivery. Inhibition of β1 receptors in the myocardium decreases myocardial contractility, systolic blood pressure, sinus node rate, and atrioventricular (AV) node conduction velocity. By reducing contractility and slowing the heat rate, they decrease myocardial oxygen demand, shifting the oxygen supply-demand ratio in favor of the ischemic myocardium. Although, there are limited clinical trial data on the use of β-blockers in UA and non–Q-wave MI, its use is associated with a 13% relative reduction in the risk for progression to MI [25]. There is no evidence of superiority of any member of this class over the others, but β1 selective blockers (metoprolol or atenolol) are preferred over those with intrinsic sympathomimetic activity. Caution should be exercised in patients who have active asthma, and therapy should not be initiated in those presenting with severe conduction disturbances, congestive heart failure, bradycardia, or hypotension [26]. In patients who have LV systolic dysfunction after an acute MI, long-term use of carvedilol is associated with reduction of all-cause and cardiovascular mortality and recurrent, nonfatal MIs.

Calcium channel blockers

These agents are not used routinely because of lack of convincing evidence in favor of reducing mortality. They variably produce vasodilation, decrease myocardial contractility and AV block, and slow the sinus node. They may be useful especially in those who have no heart failure symptoms [27] in reducing death or nonfatal MI and anginal symptoms [28]. These agents may have added benefit in patients who have coronary spasm, recurrent ischemia on nitrates and β-blockers, β-blocker intolerance, or hypertension. Calcium channel blockers may be used as a third-line antianginal medication after β-blockers and nitrates.

Antiplatelet therapy

Aspirin. Platelet activation and aggregation is the core to pathophysiology of ACS, as platelets play a major role in the thrombotic response to a ruptured coronary plaque. Aspirin inhibits platelet aggregation by inhibiting thromboxane A2 pathway and it has additive anti-inflammatory effects [29]. In doses ranging from 75 mg to 1300 mg, it reduces the risk for angina, death, or MI by more than 50% [30–32]. Consequently, aspirin should be initiated as soon as possible after presentation in all patients who have ACS and should be continued indefinitely. The long-term clinical benefit from aspirin is relatively independent of the dose. An initial dose of 160 mg/day is an appropriate starting dose for at least a month [33] and subsequently the dose may be reduced to 81 mg/day. It is prudent to continue it lifelong, unless contraindications, such as allergy, active bleeding, or hemophilia, develop. For those who have true allergy, clopidogrel is an effective alternative.

Thienopyridines. The thienopyridines, ticlopidine and clopidogrel, inhibit binding of ADP to P2Y12 receptor on platelet receptor, thereby inhibiting adenyl cyclase and platelet aggregation. These drugs take longer time than aspirin to cause irreversible antiplatelet effects and a loading dose usually is used.

In the Clopidogrel in Unstable Angina to Prevent Recurrent Events (CURE) trial, 12,562 patients who had UA/NSTEMI were randomized to aspirin alone or aspirin plus clopidogrel. There was a 20% reduction in the composite endpoint of cardiovascular death, MI, or stroke, although there was an increase in the risk for bleeding with combination antiplatelet therapy [34]. Those undergoing invasive strategy derive maximum benefit when pretreated with clopidogrel (300 mg) in addition to aspirin, and this benefit was observed even in those patients who did not undergo revascularization procedures [35]. When clopidogrel is given for approximately a year after PCI, there is a 27% risk reduction in the combined risk for death, stroke, or MI without a significant increase in risk for major bleeding [36]. It now is suggested that a 600-mg loading dose be used in patients undergoing same day PCI, as this seems to produce a maximum antiplatelet activity quicker (within 2–3 hours) and decreases the likelihood of clopidogrel resistance [37].

Ticlopidine has similar mechanism of action to clopidogrel and is associated with reduction in the rate of vascular death and MI by 46% in patients who have NSTEMI [38]. Lack of randomized trials of dual therapy, with ticlopidine and aspirin, and the risk for neutropenia, thrombocytopenia, and gastrointestinal side effects have limited its use to short duration and in patients who have aspirin or clopidogrel intolerance. Clopidogrel has a faster onset of action, fewer side effects, and has become the preferred thienopyridine. It usually is stopped for 5 days in patients before CABG to reduce the risk for bleeding. Several newer ADP antagonists currently are being tested in clinical trials.

Glycoprotein IIb/IIIa inhibitors. The platelet GP IIb/IIIa receptor is a part of the integrin family of receptors that is composed of α and β subunits (α_{IIb} and β_{III}) that is key to platelet aggregation. After platelet activation,

GP IIb/IIIa receptor undergoes a conformational change and leads to fibrinogen-mediated cross-linking of platelets. By preventing this final common pathway of platelet aggregation, GP IIb/IIIa inhibitors are potent inhibitors of platelet aggregation from all types of stimuli (eg, ADP, serotonin, collagen, and thrombin).

There currently are three intravenous agents approved for clinical use: abciximab is a monoclonal antibody; and eptifibatide and tirofiban are small molecule IIb/IIIa receptor inhibitors, the former a cyclic heptapeptide and the latter a nonpeptide mimetic. These agents are used as medical therapy and as adjuncts to PCI. Abciximab is the most studied clinically and was the first GP IIb/IIIa inhibitor to be used in patients. It has a rapid onset of action, short plasma half-life, but a long platelet bound half-life. Within 2 hours, almost 80% of platelet GP IIb/IIIa receptors are occupied by this drug, leading to complete inhibition of platelet aggregation. Typically, bleeding time returns to normal within 12 hours after the standard 12-hour infusion [39]. Platelet function recovers gradually to baseline in 48 hours in most patients and its antiplatelet effects may be reversed with platelet transfusion. Tirofiban and eptifibatide, alternatively, potentially are less immunogenic, smaller in size, and much more specific to the GP IIb/IIIa receptor, and their effects on platelet aggregation are dissipated rapidly once the infusion is terminated [40]. As they are excreted via the kidneys, their dose needs to be adjusted in those who have reduced creatinine clearance.

The benefit of platelet GP IIb/IIIa inhibitors in patients who have ACS has been demonstrated in many randomized clinical trials, both in the conservative treatment strategy group and in those who undergo revascularization (Fig. 5). Recent meta-analysis of six major randomized clinical trials involving 31,402 patients from the "five P" trials (Platelet Glycoprotein IIb-IIIa in Unstable Angina: Receptor Suppression Using Integrilin Therapy [PURSUIT], Platelet Receptor Inhibition in Ischemic Syndrome Management [PRISM], Platelet Receptor Inhibition in Ischemic Syndrome Management in Patients Limited by Unstable Signs and Symptoms [PRISM-PLUS], and Platelet IIb/IIIa Antagonism for the Reduction of Acute Coronary Syndrome Events in a Global Organization Network [PARAGON] A and B) and GUSTO IV ACS reported a 9% reduction in the risk reduction in the odds of death or MI at 30 days. This benefit was largest in the subset of patients who had positive troponin, in whom there was a 15% reduction in the odds of death or MI, whereas no reduction was seen in those who had negative troponin. In those who underwent PCI within 5 days of randomization, there was a 23% reduction in the combined endpoint of 30-day death or MI. This is not surprising, as those who had positive troponin have a threefold to eightfold increase in the risk for death in NSTEMI ACS [41]. Moreover, the TACTICS-TIMI 18 showed that an invasive approach is preferable in patients who had UA/NSTEMI patients in the presence of GP IIb/IIIa inhibitors [42]. There is emerging evidence that the upstream use of tirofiban in high-risk patients

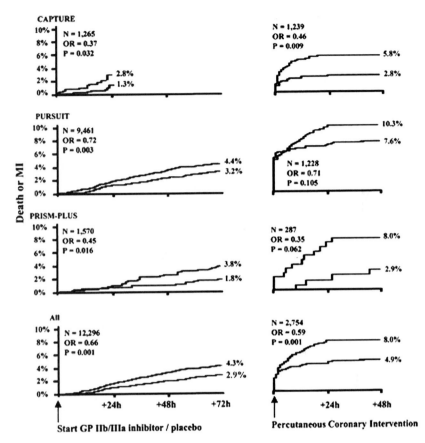

Fig. 5. Kaplan-Meier curves showing cumulative incidence of death or MI in patients randomly assigned to platelet GP IIb/IIIa receptor antagonist (*bold line*) or placebo. Data are derived from the *c* 7E3 *A*nti *P*latelet *T*herapy in *U*nstable *R*efractory angina [CAPTURE], PURSUIT, and PRISM-PLUS trials. (*Left*) Events during the initial period of medical treatment until the moment of PCI or CABG. In the CAPTURE trial, abciximab was administered for 18 to 24 hours before the PCI was performed in almost all patients as per study design; abciximab was discontinued 1 hour after the intervention. In PURSUIT, a PCI was performed in 11.2% of patients during a period of medical therapy with eptifibatide that lasted 72 hours and for 24 hours after the intervention. In PRISM-PLUS, an intervention was performed in 30.2% of patients after a 48-hour period of medical therapy with tirofiban, and the drug infusion was maintained for 12 to 24 hours after an intervention. (*Right*) Events occurring at the time of PCI and the next 48 hours, with the event rates reset to 0% before the intervention. CK or CK-MB elevations exceeding 2 times the upper limit of normal were considered as infarction during medical management and exceeding 3 times the upper limit of normal for PCI-related events (*From* Braunwald E, Antman EM, Beasley JW, et al. ACC/AHA 2002 guideline update for the management of patients with unstable angina and non-ST-segment elevation myocardial infarction—summary article: a report of the American College of Cardiology/American Heart Association task force on practice guidelines [Committee on the Management of Patients With Unstable Angina]. J Am Coll Cardiol 2002;40:136–74; with permission. Copyright © 2002 American College of Cardiology.)

with an early invasive strategy is associated with improved tissue-level perfusion and less postprocedural troponin release [43]. These drugs are administered in addition to ASA and heparin in those whom catheterization and PCI is planned or in patients who have continuing ischemia, an elevated troponin, or other high-risk features. Even on a background of a 600-mg loading dose of clopidogrel (at least 2 hours before PCI), administration of abciximab in high-risk ACS patients undergoing PCI is associated with a reduction in death, MI, or urgent target vessel revascularization by 30 days compared with placebo [44].

In regard to safety, patients receiving GP IIb/IIIa inhibitors have a slight but significantly increased risk for major bleeding compared with controls, but with no increase in the risk for intracranial hemorrhage [45]. Thrombocytopenia is unusual, and severe thrombocytopenia (platelet count less than 50,000/mL) is seen in only 0.5% of patients.

Anticoagulants or antithrombin agents

Unfractionated heparin. Unfractionated heparin (UFH) has been used in the management of ACS for more than 3 decades and its use has been more robust with the increase in number of PCIs being done.

Heparin is a glycosaminoglycan made up of multiple different polysaccharide chain lengths with different anticoagulant activity. Antithrombin (AT), a proteolytic enzyme, undergoes a conformational change when bound to heparin that accelerates its inhibition of thrombin (factor IIa) and factor Xa. This prevents further thrombus formation and propagation without lysing the existing thrombi. Heparin also binds competitively to other plasma proteins (acute phase reactants), blood cells, and endothelial cells, which have varying concentrations, thus affecting its bioavailability. The variability in the response of heparin may be in part the result of the binding of these other proteins to the AT binding site on heparin. The so-called "heparin resistance" also may be the result of its degradation by platelet factor 4 released by activated platelets, increased heparin clearance, AT deficiency, and increased levels of factor VIII and fibrinogen levels. Another limitation of heparin is its lack of effect against clot-bound or platelet-rich thrombus because of its inability to inactivate thrombin bound to fibrin (clot) or factor Xa bound to the platelet rich thrombus. Because of variable protein binding and bioavailability, heparin therapy requires frequent monitoring to assure that a safe therapeutic range is maintained as recommended by a standard nomogram. A dose of 60-U/kg intravenous bolus followed by 12-U/kg/hour infusion to maintain a target activated partial thromboplastin time (aPTT) between 50 and 70 seconds is the optimal dose for ACS [46]. Serial platelet counts also are recommended to monitor for heparin-induced thrombocytopenia.

The incremental benefit of heparin in combination with aspirin in UA and NSTEMI has been studied in several trials. Although these trials were small and inconclusive regarding the benefit of UFH plus aspirin versus aspirin alone, a meta-analysis of six trials showed that the addition of UFH to aspirin reduced risk for death or MI by 33% compared with aspirin alone [47]. Most of these benefits are short term and do not seem sustained, which may be the result of reactivation of the thrombotic milieu after its discontinuation. Although there is no defined duration of therapy, it usually is administered for 2 to 5 days. With the concomitant use of GP IIb/IIIa inhibitors, caution needs to be observed with regard to bleeding and a lower dose of UFH usually is recommended.

Low-molecular-weight heparin. Low-molecular-weight heparin (LMWH) is prepared by depolymerization of the polysaccharide chains of heparin [48]. This yields fragments that have a mean molecular weight of 4000 to 5000 daltons. The majority of chains contain less than 18 saccharide units and inactivate factor Xa more than factor IIa in contrast to the longer chains of UFH, which inhibit factor Xa and factor IIa (thrombin) equally. Thus, the PTT usually is not affected by LMWH; however, this specificity results in more potent inhibition of thrombin generation (anti-Xa:anti-IIa activity of UFH is 1:1 versus 2–4:1 for LMWH). Moreover, this inhibition of factor Xa may be a more important step in ACS, as factor Xa is shown to contribute more to the procoagulant activity than thrombin [49].

Compared with UFH, LMWH has many favorable pharmacologic properties. It has lower plasma protein binding with a more predictable anticoagulant effect, greater bioavailability even when given subcutaneously (thus permitting once- or twice-daily dosing), greater resistance to neutralization by platelet factor 4, greater release of tissue factor pathway inhibitor, and a lower incidence of heparin-induced thrombocytopenia. In addition, a fixed weight-base dose and no mandatory monitoring of Xa levels are attractive features.

Currently, enoxaparin and dalteparin are approved by the United States Food and Drug Administration for the treatment of UA/NSTEMI. The Efficacy and Safety of Subcutaneous Enoxaparin in Non-Q-wave Coronary Events (ESSENCE) trial randomized patients who had UA/NSTEMI to enoxaparin (1 mg/kg twice daily) or standard UFH (for 2 to 8 days). At 2 weeks, those treated with LMWH demonstrated a 16.2% risk reduction in the composite endpoint of death, MI, or recurrent angina [50] and this was sustained at 1-year follow-up [51]. Similarly, the TIMI 11B trial randomized patients to enoxaparin or UFH for 3 to 8 days while hospitalized and then to placebo or enoxaparin as outpatients through day 43. There was a 14.6% risk reduction at 8 days and 12.3% risk reduction at 43 days in the composite endpoint of death, MI, or urgent revascularization in the enoxaparin-treated group [52]. In the Superior Yield of the New Strategy of Enoxaparin, Revascularization and Glycoprotein IIb/IIIa Inhibitors (SYNERGY) trial, the use of enoxaparin was noninferior to UFH, although it was associated with higher bleeding rate in high-risk ACS patients undergoing invasive strategy [53].

The Fast Revascularization During Instability in Coronary Artery Disease (FRISC) trial randomized patients to dalteparin (120 U/kg twice daily) or UFH during the first 5 to 7 days of hospitalization and then to dalteparin (7500 U subcutaneous daily) or aspirin alone as an outpatient for 35 to 45 days. During the first 6 days, dalteparin was associated with a 63% relative risk reduction in death or MI that was sustained, although not statistically significant at 40 days [54]. A meta-analysis of five LMWH trials suggested a 15% reduction of major adverse cardiovascular events with LMWH over UFH [55].

It is recommended that anticoagulation with subcutaneous LMWH or intravenous heparin (UFH) be added to antiplatelet therapy for ACS. Enoxaparin is preferable to UFH unless CABG is planned in 24 hours. Therapy should be tailored to each patient and it is preferable to use triple antithrombotic therapy with aspirin, heparin, and GP IIb/IIIa inhibitor in patients who have high-risk features or those who have ongoing ischemia and planned early invasive strategy.

Direct thrombin and factor X inhibitors. Direct thrombin inhibitors have the mechanistic advantage over heparin of inhibiting clot-bound thrombin and not being inhibited by circulating plasma proteins and platelet factor 4 [56]. The aPTT can be used to monitor anticoagulation activity but usually is not necessary. Hirudin is an irreversible inhibitor of thrombin and is excreted primarily from kidneys. Its use is associated with a reduction in death, MI, and refractory angina but there is an increased risk for bleeding [57]. Bivalirudin is a synthetic polypeptide that is akin to hirudin in being able to form a bivalent complex with thrombin leading to a potent and selective inhibition of thrombin. In contrast to hirudin, it has a shorter plasma half-life of less than 30 minutes that gives it a potential advantage of minimizing bleeding risk. The use of bivalirudin alone in patients presenting with UA/NSTEMI and high-risk features is associated with improved net clinical benefit compared with the UFH/enoxaparin plus GP IIb/IIIa inhibitor, primarily driven by a reduction in bleeding (3% versus 5.7%, $P < .001$ for superiority). Additionally, the use of bivalirudin plus a GP IIb/IIIa inhibitor is noninferior compared with UFH/enoxaparin plus GP IIb/IIIa inhibitor [58]. Even long-term clinical outcomes at 6 months to 1 year with bivalirudin and provisional GP IIb/IIIa inhibitor are comparable to that of UFH with GP IIb/IIa inhibitor in patients undergoing PCI. Reduced bleeding complications, ease of use, reduced cost, and the ability to permit selective rather than universal use of GP IIb/IIIa inhibitor substantiates the benefit of this drug in PCI and ACS. Moreover, the effect of bivalirudin was greatest in those who had high-risk features and independent of the choice of GP IIb/IIIa inhibitor used or pretreatment with thienopyridine [59]. In addition to this, bivalirudin can be used in patients who have heparin-induced thrombocytopenia.

Fondaparinux is a synthetic pentasaccharide that is a novel factor Xa inhibitor. It acts early in the coagulation cascade by binding to AT, thus inhibiting factor Xa. In the Organization to Assess Strategies for Ischemic Syndromes (OASIS)-5 trial, the primary efficacy outcome (death, MI, or refractory ischemia at 9 days) occurred in 579 of the 10,057 patients assigned to receive fondaparinux (5.8%) compared with 573 of the 10,021 patients assigned to receive enoxaparin (5.7%) (hazard ratio 1.01; 95% CI, 0.90 to 1.13). The composite of death, MI, refractory ischemia, or major bleeding occurred in 7.3% of the patients in the fondaparinux group compared with 9.0% of the patients in the enoxaparin group (hazard ratio 0.81; 95% CI, 0.73 to 0.89; $P < .001$) at 9 days. Fondaparinux (at a dose of 2.5 mg daily) seems similar to enoxaparin in the short term in preventing ischemic events among patients who have ACS without ST-segment elevation but may be associated with substantially less bleeding [60]. There was an increase in the rate of guiding-catheter thrombus formation with fondaparinux (29 episodes [0.9%] versus 8 episodes with enoxaparin [0.3%]), which is of concern. Head-to-head trials comparing bivalirudin and fondaparinux are indicated to determine superiority or equivalence.

Coronary revascularization

Coronary angiography helps define the extent and location of CAD, ventricular function, and presence of any other significant valvular problems. Those who have left main- or three-vessel disease, especially with LV dysfunction or diabetes, or those who have two-vessel disease involving the left anterior descending artery with reduced ejection fraction often are managed by surgical revascularization (CABG). Almost 30% to 40% of patients have multivessel stenosis, and significant left main stenosis is seen in 4% to 10% of patients. Thus, these patients may undergo CABG, as seen in the 33% to 42% of patients in the trials with "early revascularization" strategy (FRISC II [61]; Treat Angina with aggrastat and determine Cost of Therapy with an Invasive or Conservative Strategy [TACTICS]-TIMI 18 [42]; and Randomized Intervention Trial of unstable Angina [RITA] 3 [62]). The number of patients who have ACS requiring surgical revascularization has diminished in the contemporary era.

With the advent of drug-eluting stents, the restenosis rate has been reduced to single digits and, along with low complication rates, PCI seems the preferred revascularization strategy—particularly in patients who have preserved LV function, one- or two-vessel disease, or contraindications for surgery. The decision to pursue an early conservative strategy versus an early invasive strategy aimed toward revascularization has been evaluated [42,61,62]. Although similar in scope, these trials differed in design and level of patient acuity. In FRISC II [61] and TIMI 18 [42], an early invasive strategy was preceded by standard anti-ischemic and antithrombotic medications and was associated with a reduced risk for death, MI, and rehospitalization. The benefits were most significant in high- or intermediate-risk subsets (age > 65 years, troponin positive, or ST-segment depression). Importantly, early invasive strategy is associated with reduced duration of hospital stay without any increased overall costs [63].

As the contemporary invasive strategy involves revascularization by stenting (PCI) or, in selective cases, CABG, the inclusion of studies done in the prestent era (TIMI 3B [64]; Veterans Affairs Non-Q-Wave Infarction Strategies in Hospital VANQWISH [65]) may underestimate the value of early invasive approach. Also, the use of more potent antiplatelet drugs, such as GP IIb/IIIa inhibitors, may affect the outcomes independently. The Invasive versus Conservative Treatment in Unstable Coronary Syndromes (ICTUS) study did not demonstrate that an early invasive strategy was superior to a selectively invasive strategy if patients received contemporary medical therapy that included LMWH, GP IIb/IIIa inhibition at the time of percutaneous procedures, clopidogrel, and intensive lipid-lowering therapy [66]. A recent meta-analysis of 7618 patients looked specifically at the trials that compared early invasive versus conservative strategy for patients who had UA/NSTEMI, including the ICTUS trial. A total of five randomized trials, of which two used a GP IIb/IIIa inhibitor routinely (TACTICS-TIMI 18 [42] and ICTUS [66]) and three used it only provisionally (FRISC II [67]; RITA-3 [62]; and Value of First Day Angiography/ Angioplasty in Evolving Non-ST Segment Elevation Myocardial Infarction: An Open Multicenter Randomized Trial [VINO] [68]), when pooled, suggested that a conservative approach may be better than early invasive strategy in regards to reduction in early death, as mortality benefit appeared late (2–5 years follow-up). There was a 33% risk reduction in early and intermediate refractory angina and rehospitalizations with an invasive strategy. The routine use of GP IIb/IIIa inhibitor combined with an early invasive strategy was associated with a reduction in MI and in the combined endpoint of MI and death but only in those who had high-risk features (ie, troponin-positive patients). Excess access site bleeding but no increase in stroke risk was seen with an invasive approach [69].

Statins. Regardless of the baseline low-density lipoprotein (LDL) cholesterol levels, statin therapy should be instituted and continued long term in patients who have ACS. The early and sustained benefit of statin therapy goes beyond the LDL lowering effect. Plaque stabilization [70], reduction of endothelial dysfunction [71], reduced thrombogenicity [72], and reduced inflammation [73] are some of the postulated mechanisms.

In the Pravastatin or Atorvastatin Evaluation and Infection Therapy (PROVE IT)-TIMI 22 study, patients hospitalized for an ACS were assigned randomly to pravastatin (40 mg/d) (considered standard therapy) or atorvastatin (80 mg/d) (intensive therapy) and followed up for a mean of 24 months. The median LDLcholesterol reduced from pretreatment level of 106 mg/dL to 95 mg/dL and 62 mg/dL in the respective treatment groups. Primary endpoint (ie, death from any cause, MI, documented UA requiring rehospitalization, revascularization [performed at least 30 days after randomization], and stroke) was lower in the intensively (atorvastatin) treated group versus that with standard (pravastatin) therapy (22.4% versus 26%) [74].

There does not seem to be a lower limit on the LDL level and it is recommended that statins be initiated and continued in all patients presenting with AC, as there are improved clinical efficacy and no adverse affects with safety with lower LDL levels (even <40 mg/dL) [75].

In the A to Z trial, subjects were randomized to an early intensive statin treatment strategy (40 mg/d of simvastatin for 30 days and then 80 mg/d of simvastatin thereafter) or a less aggressive strategy (placebo for 4 months and then 20 mg/d of simvastatin thereafter) and followed up for 24 months. The study did not reach the primary endpoint (composite of cardiovascular death, nonfatal MI, readmission for ACS, and stroke) and the 11% relative (2.3% absolute) reduction in the rate of the primary endpoint in the early intensive statin group was not statistically significant. This may be because of the delayed initiation of high-dose statin (80 mg/d), as the period of maximum benefit could be early on with greatest clinical instability, which may achieve a more rapid clinical benefit. The early intensive statin regimen was associated, however, with a reduction in cardiovascular mortality of 25% (absolute reduction, 1.3%; $P = .05$) and congestive heart failure of 28% (absolute reduction, 1.3%; $P = .04$) [76].

Follow-up and long-term therapy

After an acute coronary event, ongoing plaque instability and endothelial dysfunction persist for weeks as the healing process is taking place. There also is evidence of continued inflammation and a prothrombotic state. Many clinical and ECG features are shown to increase the risk for death at 1 year and they include persistent ST-segment depression, heart failure, advanced age, ST-segment elevation, severe chronic obstructive pulmonary disease, positive troponin, prior CABG, renal insufficiency, and diabetes. Of paramount importance is that the aggressive and intensive risk reduction strategies that are initiated in hospitals be continued for outpatients. These include lifestyle and pharmacologic strategies to control BP, lipid reduction with statins (target LDL <70), smoking cessation, and maintenance of adequate weight [8]. Women in particular are under treated and special attention should be paid toward achieving these goals in them.

Long-term use of medications, such as statins, antiplatelet agents, β-blockers, and angiotensin-converting enzyme (ACE) inhibitors, is associated with significantly improved outcomes in patients presenting with ACS. These agents seem to be even more effective when used in combination with significant synergistic effects and should be prescribed to all patients who have ACS whenever appropriate (Fig. 6) [77].

Patients presenting with ACS represent an important high-risk cohort, where secondary vascular disease prevention likely is particularly effective

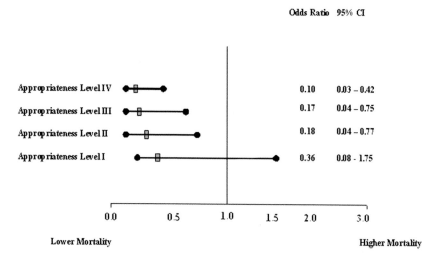

Fig. 6. Effect of combined use of evidence-based medical therapies (aspirin, β-blocker, statin, angiotensin converting enzyme) on 6-month mortality in patients who have ACS. Appropriateness levels (I–IV) are compared with level 0 (nonuse of any of the indicated medications) and show a gradient of survival benefit in this cohort. Level 4 means all four medications were used; level 3 means three out of four medications were used; level 2 means two out of four medications were used; and level 1 means only one out of four medications was used. (*Reproduced from* Mukherjee D, Fang J, Chetcuti S, et al. Impact of combination evidence-based medical therapy on mortality in patients with acute coronary syndromes. Circulation 2004;109:745–9; with permission.)

and cost effective. Clinicians have an opportunity to provide high-quality and appropriate evidence-based care to this high-risk cohort and to seize this opportunity in aggressively treating the underlying atherosclerotic process through lifestyle modifications and effective pharmacologic therapies (Box 1). Attention to these disease management opportunities has significant survival advantage in this high-risk cohort and should be pursued aggressively.

Summary

ACS remains associated with high rates of adverse cardiovascular events despite recent advances. Clinical studies have shown that early diagnosis and appropriate evidence-based therapies improve outcomes. The clinical history, physical examination, ECG, and biomarkers (such as troponin) provide critical information for early risk stratification. Most patients in the United States undergo an early invasive strategy where patients are taken to a cardiac catheterization laboratory within 48 hours and revascularization is performed if indicated. Such a strategy seems particularly beneficial in high-risk patients and is recommended in such individuals by

---

Box 1. Long-term therapy in patients after an acute coronary syndrome

- Smoking cessation
- Regular exercise
- Low-fat diet
- Appropriate follow-up
- Statin therapy for LDL >100 mg/dL
- BP medications if >130/85
- Optimal therapy for diabetes (target glycosylated haemoglobin (HbAlc) <6.0)
- Aspirin
- Clopidogrel for 1–12 months
- β-Blockers
- ACE inhibitors, in particular those who have LV systolic dysfunction, hypertension, and diabetes

---

current guidelines. The use of dual antiplatelet therapy, potent antithrombotic drugs, and drug-eluting stents continues to improve clinical outcomes with percutaneous revascularization. Newer antithrombotic drugs, such as bivalirudin and fondaparinux, seem effective and associated with lower bleeding rates making them clinically attractive agents.

It is important to have a team effort to continue posthospital discharge risk reduction measure and to emphasize medication and dietary compliance. Long-term pharmacotherapy should include aspirin, β-blocker, clopidogrel (for at least 1 year), statins, and an ACE inhibitor if indicated.

References

[1] American Heart Association/American Stroke Association-Heart Disease and Stroke Statistics. 2006.
[2] Fernandez-Ortiz A, Badimon JJ, Falk E, et al. Characterization of the relative thrombogenicity of atherosclerotic plaque components: implications for consequences of plaque rupture. J Am Coll Cardiol 1994;23:1562–9.
[3] van der Wal AC, Becker AE, van der Loos CM, et al. Site of intimal rupture or erosion of thrombosed coronary atherosclerotic plaques is characterized by an inflammatory process irrespective of the dominant plaque morphology. Circulation 1994;89:36–44.
[4] Fitzgerald DJ, Roy L, Catella F, et al. Platelet activation in unstable coronary disease. N Engl J Med 1986;315:983–9.
[5] Holt JC, Harris ME, Holt AM, et al. Characterization of human platelet basic protein, a precursor form of low-affinity platelet factor 4 and beta-thromboglobulin. Biochemistry 1986; 25:1988–96.
[6] Baumgartner HR, Born GV. Effects of 5-hydroxytryptamine on platelet aggregation. Nature 1968;218:137–41.

[7] Coller BS. The role of platelets in arterial thrombosis and the rationale for blockade of plate-
    let GPIIb/IIIa receptors as antithrombotic therapy. Eur Heart J 1995;16(Suppl L):11–5.
[8] Braunwald E, Antman EM, Beasley JW, et al. ACC/AHA 2002 guideline update for the
    management of patients with unstable angina and non-ST-segment elevation myocardial
    infarction—summary article: a report of the American College of Cardiology/American
    Heart Association task force on practice guidelines (Committee on the Management of
    Patients With Unstable Angina). J Am Coll Cardiol 2002;40:1366–74.
[9] Braunwald E. Unstable angina. A classification. Circulation 1989;80:410–4.
[10] Holmes DR Jr, Berger PB, Hochman JS, et al. Cardiogenic shock in patients with acute
    ischemic syndromes with and without ST-segment elevation. Circulation 1999;100:
    2067–73.
[11] Cannon CP, McCabe CH, Stone PH, et al. The electrocardiogram predicts one-year
    outcome of patients with unstable angina and non-Q wave myocardial infarction: results
    of the TIMI III Registry ECG Ancillary Study. Thrombolysis in Myocardial Ischemia.
    J Am Coll Cardiol 1997;30:133–40.
[12] Eisenberg PR, Kenzora JL, Sobel BE, et al. Relation between ST segment shifts during
    ischemia and thrombin activity in patients with unstable angina. J Am Coll Cardiol 1991;
    18:898–903.
[13] Slater DK, Hlatky MA, Mark DB, et al. Outcome in suspected acute myocardial infarction
    with normal or minimally abnormal admission electrocardiographic findings. Am J Cardiol
    1987;60:766–70.
[14] Savonitto S, Ardissino D, Granger CB, et al. Prognostic value of the admission
    electrocardiogram in acute coronary syndromes. JAMA 1999;281:707–13.
[15] Savonitto S, Cohen MG, Politi A, et al. Extent of ST-segment depression and cardiac events
    in non-ST-segment elevation acute coronary syndromes. Eur Heart J 2005;26:2106–13.
[16] Alpert JS, Thygesen K, Antman E, et al. Myocardial infarction redefined—a consensus
    document of The Joint European Society of Cardiology/American College of Cardiology
    Committee for the redefinition of myocardial infarction. J Am Coll Cardiol 2000;36:959–69.
[17] Lindahl B, Venge P, Wallentin L. Relation between troponin T and the risk of subsequent
    cardiac events in unstable coronary artery disease. The FRISC study group. Circulation
    1996;93:1651–7.
[18] Antman EM, Tanasijevic MJ, Thompson B, et al. Cardiac-specific troponin I levels to
    predict the risk of mortality in patients with acute coronary syndromes. N Engl J Med
    1996;335:1342–9.
[19] Antman EM, Cohen M, Bernink PJ, et al. The TIMI risk score for unstable angina/non-ST
    elevation MI: a method for prognostication and therapeutic decision making. JAMA 2000;
    284:835–42.
[20] Eagle KA, Lim MJ, Dabbous OH, et al. A validated prediction model for all forms of acute
    coronary syndrome: estimating the risk of 6-month postdischarge death in an international
    registry. JAMA 2004;291:2727–33.
[21] Bhatt DL, Roe MT, Peterson ED, et al. Utilization of early invasive management strategies
    for high-risk patients with non-ST-segment elevation acute coronary syndromes: results
    from the CRUSADE Quality Improvement Initiative. JAMA 2004;292:2096–104.
[22] Kerensky RA, Wade M, Deedwania P, et al. Revisiting the culprit lesion in non-Q-wave
    myocardial infarction. Results from the VANQWISH trial angiographic core laboratory.
    J Am Coll Cardiol 2002;39:1456–63.
[23] ISIS-4 (Fourth International Study of Infarct Survival) Collaborative Group. ISIS-4: a rand-
    omised factorial trial assessing early oral captopril, oral mononitrate, and intravenous mag-
    nesium sulphate in 58,050 patients with suspected acute myocardial infarction. Lancet 1995;
    345:669–85.
[24] Cheitlin MD, Hutter AM Jr, Brindis RG, et al. ACC/AHA expert consensus document. Use
    of sildenafil (Viagra) in patients with cardiovascular disease. American College of
    Cardiology/American Heart Association. J Am Coll Cardiol 1999;33:273–82.

[25] Yusuf S, Wittes J, Friedman L. Overview of results of randomized clinical trials in heart disease. II. Unstable angina, heart failure, primary prevention with aspirin, and risk factor modification. JAMA 1988;260:2259–63.

[26] Chen ZM, Pan HC, Chen YP, et al. Early intravenous then oral metoprolol in 45,852 patients with acute myocardial infarction: randomised placebo-controlled trial. Lancet 2005;366: 1622–32.

[27] Gibson RS, Hansen JF, Miserly F, et al. Long-term effects of diltiazem and verapamil on mortality and cardiac events in non-Q-wave acute myocardial infarction without pulmonary congestion: post hoc subset analysis of the multicenter diltiazem postinfarction trial and the second Danish verapamil infarction trial studies. Am J Cardiol 2000;86:275–9.

[28] Pepine CJ, Faich G, Makuch R. Verapamil use in patients with cardiovascular disease: an overview of randomized trials. Clin Cardiol 1998;21:633–41.

[29] Ridker PM, Cushman M, Stampfer MJ, et al. Inflammation, aspirin, and the risk of cardiovascular disease in apparently healthy men. N Engl J Med 1997;336:973–9.

[30] Theroux P, Ouimet H, McCans J, et al. Aspirin, heparin, or both to treat acute unstable angina. N Engl J Med 1988;319:1105–11.

[31] Lewis HD Jr, Davis JW, Archibald DG, et al. Protective effects of aspirin against acute myocardial infarction and death in men with unstable angina. Results of a Veterans Administration Cooperative Study. N Engl J Med 1983;309:396–403.

[32] The RISC Group. Risk of myocardial infarction and death during treatment with low dose aspirin and intravenous heparin in men with unstable coronary artery disease. Lancet 1990; 336:827–30.

[33] ISIS-2 (Second International Study of Infarct Survival) Collaborative Group. Randomised trial of intravenous streptokinase, oral aspirin, both, or neither among 17,187 cases of suspected acute myocardial infarction: ISIS-2. Lancet 1988;2:349–60.

[34] Yusuf S, Zhao F, Mehta SR, et al. Effects of clopidogrel in addition to aspirin in patients with acute coronary syndromes without ST-segment elevation. N Engl J Med 2001;345:494–502.

[35] Mehta SR, Yusuf S, Peters RJ, et al. Effects of pretreatment with clopidogrel and aspirin followed by long-term therapy in patients undergoing percutaneous coronary intervention: the PCI-CURE study. Lancet 2001;358:527–33.

[36] Steinhubl SR, Berger PB, Mann JT 3rd, et al. Early and sustained dual oral antiplatelet therapy following percutaneous coronary intervention: a randomized controlled trial. JAMA 2002;288:2411–20.

[37] Patti G, Colonna G, Pasceri V, et al. Randomized trial of high loading dose of clopidogrel for reduction of periprocedural myocardial infarction in patients undergoing coronary intervention: results from the ARMYDA-2 (Antiplatelet therapy for Reduction of MYocardial Damage during Angioplasty) study. Circulation 2005;111:2099–106.

[38] Balsano F, Rizzon P, Violi F, et al. Antiplatelet treatment with ticlopidine in unstable angina. A controlled multicenter clinical trial. The Studio della Ticlopidina nell'Angina Instabile Group. Circulation 1990;82:17–26.

[39] Tcheng JE, Ellis SG, George BS, et al. Pharmacodynamics of chimeric glycoprotein IIb/IIIa integrin antiplatelet antibody Fab 7E3 in high-risk coronary angioplasty. Circulation 1994; 90:1757–64.

[40] Kleiman NS. Pharmacokinetics and pharmacodynamics of glycoprotein IIb-IIIa inhibitors. Am Heart J 1999;138:263–75.

[41] Heidenreich PA, Alloggiamento T, Melsop K, et al. The prognostic value of troponin in patients with non-ST elevation acute coronary syndromes: a meta-analysis. J Am Coll Cardiol 2001;38:478–85.

[42] Cannon CP, Weintraub WS, Demopoulos LA, et al. Comparison of early invasive and conservative strategies in patients with unstable coronary syndromes treated with the glycoprotein IIb/IIIa inhibitor tirofiban. N Engl J Med 2001;344:1879–87.

[43] Bolognese L, Falsini G, Liistro F, et al. Randomized comparison of upstream tirofiban versus downstream high bolus dose tirofiban or abciximab on tissue-level perfusion and

troponin release in high-risk acute coronary syndromes treated with percutaneous coronary interventions: the EVEREST trial. J Am Coll Cardiol 2006;47:522–8.

[44] Kastrati A, Mehilli J, Neumann FJ, et al. Abciximab in patients with acute coronary syndromes undergoing percutaneous coronary intervention after clopidogrel pretreatment: the ISAR-REACT 2 randomized trial. JAMA 2006;295:1531–8.

[45] Peterson ED, Pollack CV Jr, Roe MT, et al. Early use of glycoprotein IIb/IIIa inhibitors in non-ST-elevation acute myocardial infarction: observations from the National Registry of Myocardial Infarction 4. J Am Coll Cardiol 2003;42:45–53.

[46] Becker RC, Ball SP, Eisenberg P, et al. A randomized, multicenter trial of weight-adjusted intravenous heparin dose titration and point-of-care coagulation monitoring in hospitalized patients with active thromboembolic disease. Antithrombotic Therapy Consortium Investigators. Am Heart J 1999;137:59–71.

[47] Oler A, Whooley MA, Oler J, et al. Adding heparin to aspirin reduces the incidence of myocardial infarction and death in patients with unstable angina. A meta-analysis. JAMA 1996;276:811–5.

[48] Weitz JI. Low-molecular-weight heparins. N Engl J Med 1997;337:688–98.

[49] Prager NA, Abendschein DR, McKenzie CR, et al. Role of thrombin compared with factor Xa in the procoagulant activity of whole blood clots. Circulation 1995;92:962–7.

[50] Cohen M, Demers C, Gurfinkel EP, et al. A comparison of low-molecular-weight heparin with unfractionated heparin for unstable coronary artery disease. Efficacy and Safety of Subcutaneous Enoxaparin in Non-Q-Wave Coronary Events Study Group. N Engl J Med 1997;337:447–52.

[51] Goodman SG, Cohen M, Bigonzi F, et al. Randomized trial of low molecular weight heparin (enoxaparin) versus unfractionated heparin for unstable coronary artery disease: one-year results of the ESSENCE Study. Efficacy and Safety of Subcutaneous Enoxaparin in Non-Q Wave Coronary Events. J Am Coll Cardiol 2000;36:693–8.

[52] Antman EM, McCabe CH, Gurfinkel EP, et al. Enoxaparin prevents death and cardiac ischemic events in unstable angina/non-Q-wave myocardial infarction. Results of the thrombolysis in myocardial infarction (TIMI) 11B trial. Circulation 1999;100:1593–601.

[53] Ferguson JJ, Califf RM, Antman EM, et al. Enoxaparin vs unfractionated heparin in high-risk patients with non-ST-segment elevation acute coronary syndromes managed with an intended early invasive strategy: primary results of the SYNERGY randomized trial. JAMA 2004;292:45–54.

[54] Swahn E, Wallentin L. Low-molecular-weight heparin (Fragmin) during instability in coronary artery disease (FRISC). FRISC Study Group. Am J Cardiol 1997;80:25E–9E.

[55] Mukherjee D, Topol EJ. The role of low-molecular-weight heparin in cardiovascular diseases. Prog Cardiovasc Dis 2002;45:139–56.

[56] Bates ER. Bivalirudin for percutaneous coronary intervention and in acute coronary syndromes. Curr Cardiol Rep 2001;3:348–54.

[57] Organisation to Assess Strategies for Ischemic Syndromes (OASIS-2) Investigators. Effects of recombinant hirudin (lepirudin) compared with heparin on death, myocardial infarction, refractory angina, and revascularisation procedures in patients with acute myocardial ischaemia without ST elevation: a randomised trial. Lancet 1999;353:429–38.

[58] Stone GW, McLaurin BT, Cox DA, et al. Bivalirudin for patients with acute coronary syndromes. N Engl J Med 2006;355:2203–16.

[59] Lincoff AM, Kleiman NS, Kereiakes DJ, et al. Long-term efficacy of bivalirudin and provisional glycoprotein IIb/IIIa blockade vs heparin and planned glycoprotein IIb/IIIa blockade during percutaneous coronary revascularization: REPLACE-2 randomized trial. JAMA 2004;292:696–703.

[60] Yusuf S, Mehta SR, Chrolavicius S, et al. Comparison of fondaparinux and enoxaparin in acute coronary syndromes. N Engl J Med 2006;354:1464–76.

[61] Invasive compared with non-invasive treatment in unstable coronary-artery disease: FRISC II prospective randomised multicentre study. FRagmin and Fast Revascularisation during InStability in Coronary artery disease Investigators. Lancet 1999;354:708–15.

[62] Fox KA, Poole-Wilson PA, Henderson RA, et al. Interventional versus conservative treatment for patients with unstable angina or non-ST-elevation myocardial infarction: the British Heart Foundation RITA 3 randomised trial. Randomized Intervention Trial of unstable Angina. Lancet 2002;360:743–51.

[63] Mahoney EM, Jurkovitz CT, Chu H, et al. Cost and cost-effectiveness of an early invasive vs conservative strategy for the treatment of unstable angina and non-ST-segment elevation myocardial infarction. JAMA 2002;288:1851–8.

[64] Anderson HV, Cannon CP, Stone PH, et al. One-year results of the Thrombolysis in Myocardial Infarction (TIMI) IIIB clinical trial. A randomized comparison of tissue-type plasminogen activator versus placebo and early invasive versus early conservative strategies in unstable angina and non-Q wave myocardial infarction. J Am Coll Cardiol 1995;26: 1643–50.

[65] Boden WE, O'Rourke RA, Crawford MH, et al. Outcomes in patients with acute non-Q-wave myocardial infarction randomly assigned to an invasive as compared with a conservative management strategy. Veterans Affairs Non-Q-Wave Infarction Strategies in Hospital (VANQWISH) Trial Investigators. N Engl J Med 1998;338:1785–92.

[66] de Winter RJ, Windhausen F, Cornel JH, et al. Early invasive versus selectively invasive management for acute coronary syndromes. N Engl J Med 2005;353:1095–104.

[67] Lagerqvist B, Husted S, Kontny F, et al. A long-term perspective on the protective effects of an early invasive strategy in unstable coronary artery disease: two-year follow-up of the FRISC-II invasive study. J Am Coll Cardiol 2002;40:1902–14.

[68] Spacek R, Widimsky P, Straka Z, et al. Value of first day angiography/angioplasty in evolving Non-ST segment elevation myocardial infarction: an open multicenter randomized trial. The VINO Study. Eur Heart J 2002;23:230–8.

[69] Hoenig M, Doust J, Aroney C, et al. Early invasive versus conservative strategies for unstable angina & non-ST-elevation myocardial infarction in the stent era. Cochrane Database Syst Rev 2006;3:CD004815.

[70] Schartl M, Bocksch W, Koschyk DH, et al. Use of intravascular ultrasound to compare effects of different strategies of lipid-lowering therapy on plaque volume and composition in patients with coronary artery disease. Circulation 2001;104:387–92.

[71] Dupuis J, Tardif JC, Cernacek P, et al. Cholesterol reduction rapidly improves endothelial function after acute coronary syndromes. The RECIFE (reduction of cholesterol in ischemia and function of the endothelium) trial. Circulation 1999;99:3227–33.

[72] Rosenson RS, Tangney CC. Antiatherothrombotic properties of statins: implications for cardiovascular event reduction. JAMA 1998;279:1643–50.

[73] Jialal I, Stein D, Balis D, et al. Effect of hydroxymethyl glutaryl coenzyme a reductase inhibitor therapy on high sensitive C-reactive protein levels. Circulation 2001;103:1933–5.

[74] Cannon CP, Braunwald E, McCabe CH, et al. Intensive versus moderate lipid lowering with statins after acute coronary syndromes. N Engl J Med 2004;350:1495–504.

[75] Wiviott SD, Cannon CP, Morrow DA, et al. Can low-density lipoprotein be too low? The safety and efficacy of achieving very low low-density lipoprotein with intensive statin therapy: a PROVE IT-TIMI 22 substudy. J Am Coll Cardiol 2005;46:1411–6.

[76] de Lemos JA, Blazing MA, Wiviott SD, et al. Early intensive vs a delayed conservative simvastatin strategy in patients with acute coronary syndromes: phase Z of the A to Z trial. JAMA 2004;292:1307–16.

[77] Mukherjee D, Fang J, Chetcuti S, et al. Impact of combination evidence-based medical therapy on mortality in patients with acute coronary syndromes. Circulation 2004;109: 745–9.

ELSEVIER
SAUNDERS

CRITICAL
CARE
CLINICS

Crit Care Clin 23 (2007) 737–758

Acute Decompensated Heart Failure

James F. Neuenschwander II, MD, FACEP[a],
Ragavendra R. Baliga, MD, MBA, FRCP, FACC[b,c],*

[a]*Emergency Department, The Ohio State University Medical Center,*
1492 E. Broad Street, #1104, Columbus, OH 43205, USA
[b]*Cardiovascular Medicine, University Hospitals East, The Ohio State University,*
1492 E. Broad Street, #1104, Columbus, OH 43205, USA
[c]*The Ohio State University, 1492 E. Broad Street, #1104, Columbus, OH 43205, USA*

Acute decompensated heart failure (ADHF) is the direct cause of approximately one million hospital admissions and contributes to an additional 2.4 million hospitalizations in the United States. It accounts for over 50% of the total annual direct costs for heart failure (HF) [1,2]. The in-hospital mortality is in the range of 3% to 4%, and more significantly, the 60- to 90-day mortality rates approach 10% [3]. The burden becomes even more significant when one considers that almost 50% of all patients admitted with this diagnosis are readmitted within 90 days after they are discharged. Although as many as 60% of all patients hospitalized for HF die within 1 year, only about 5% to 8% actually die in the hospital [3]. This clearly places the responsibility of HF management in the hands of emergency department (ED) physicians, internists, cardiologists, family practice physicians, and nurses, who rapidly must diagnose and treat the symptoms of HF both acutely and in the long-term outpatient setting.

Definition

ADHF refers broadly to new or worsening of signs and symptoms of HF that is progressing rapidly, whereby unscheduled medical care or hospital evaluation is necessary. The mode of presentation of acute HF depends on the etiology and accompanying comorbidities. Common etiologies of ADHF include ischemic cardiomyopathy (60%), hypertension (70%), nonischemic cardiomyopathy, valvular disease, pericardial disease, and acute

---

* Corresponding author. The Ohio State University, 1492 E. Broad Street, #1104, OH 43205.

E-mail address: ragavendra.baliga@osumc.edu (R.R. Baliga).

doi:10.1016/j.ccc.2007.08.003   *criticalcare.theclinics.com*

myocarditis (Box 1). Typically ADHF is a consequence of impaired left ventricular (LV) function, either systolic or diastolic, with diastolic dysfunction and hypertension contributing to as much as 50% of all HF-related hospitalizations. Also, about 50% of the patients who have ADHF have reactive hypertension that tends to return to normal within 6 hours of appropriate treatment.

Common clinical presentations include ADHF, acute HF accompanying elevation of systemic blood pressure, pulmonary edema, cardiogenic shock with or without low-output syndrome, high-output cardiac failure, and right-sided failure (Table 1) [4].

The management of ADHF is urgent to reduce mortality, decrease length of stay, and avoid need for therapies such as mechanical ventilatory support. The management of ADHF is complicated, however, because many disease processes present with similar symptoms. For example, shortness of breath can be the chief complaint of many other illnesses such as, pneumonia, pulmonary embolism, myocardial infarction, chronic obstructive pulmonary disease (COPD) exacerbation, and asthma. Specifically, differential diagnoses include:

- Myocardial infarction
- Congestive HF
- Pneumonia
- COPD exacerbation
- Cardiac tamponade
- Anxiety
- Pulmonary embolism
- Asthma

Box 1. Common precipitating factors in decompensated heart failure

Medicine and dietary noncompliance
Cardiac causes
    Ischemia
    Arrhythmia
    Uncontrolled hypertension
Noncardiac causes
    Infection (pneumonia with or without hypoxia)
    Exacerbation of comorbidity (chronic obstructive pulmonary disease)
    Pulmonary embolus

Toxins (nonsteroidal anti-inflammatory drugs)
Volume overload

Table 1
Modes of presentation of ADHF [4]

Clinical status	Heart rate	Systolic blood pressure mm Hg	CI L/min/m²	Pulmonary capillary wedge pressure mm Hg	Congestion Killip/ Forrester	Diuresis	Hypoperfusion	End organ hypoperfusion
I Acute decompensated congestive heart failure	+/-	Low normal/ high	Low normal/ high	Mild elevation	K II/F II	+	+/-	-
II Acute heart failure with hypertension/ hypertensive crisis	Usually increased	High	+/-	>18	K II-IV/ FII-III	+/-	+/-	+, with central nervous system symptoms
III Acute heart failure with pulmonary edema	+	Low normal	Low	Elevated	KIII/FII	+	+/-	-
IVa Cardiogenic shock[a]/low-output syndrome	+	Low normal	Low, <2.2	>16	K III-IV/ F I-III	Low	+	+
IVb Severe cardiogenic shock	>90	<90	<1.8	>18	K IV/F IV	Very low	++	+
V High-output failure	+	+/-	+	+/-	KII/FI-II	+	-	-
VI Right-sided acute heart failure	Usually low	Low	Low	Low	F I	+/-	+/-, acute onset	+/-

There are exceptions; the values in Table 1 are general rules.

[a] The differentiation from low cardiac output syndrome is subjective, and the clinical presentation may overlap these classifications.

From Nieminen MS, Bohm M, Cowie MR, et al. Executive summary of the guidelines on the diagnosis and treatment of acute heart failure: the Task Force on Acute Heart Failure of the European Society of Cardiology. Eur Hear J 2005;26(4):384-416; with permission.

Making the correct diagnosis is therefore a challenge and selecting the best therapy is even more challenging, requiring a methodical clinical evaluation [5].

Clinical evaluation

Patients who have ADHF often complain of shortness of breath and other symptoms depending on their hemodynamic status. The clinician must be diligent in gathering a history from the patient and other sources to arrive at the correct diagnosis. Incorporating family members can be helpful in determining how compliant the patient is with medications and diet, and aid in a more rapid realization of what precipitated the episode of HF (Box 2). Patients may complain of dyspnea on exertion or at rest, paroxysmal nocturnal dyspnea orthopnea, peripheral edema, fatigue, or cough. In the ADHERE Registry (Acute Decompensated Heart Failure National Registry), which enrolled over 190,000 patient episodes, dyspnea occurred in about 89% of all patients presenting with HF [6]. Dyspnea on exertion is the most sensitive symptom (negative likelihood ratio .45 with 95% confidence interval [CI], .35 to .67), and paroxysmal nocturnal dyspnea is the most specific (positive likelihood ratio 2.6, 95% CI, 1.5 to 4.5 [7]. Peripheral edema was less common, at only 66% [6].

Rapid clinical examination of the patient requires assessment for congestion and signs of low perfusion. Assessment of congestion includes estimation of the jugular venous pressure (JVP) and examination of the lung for crackles. Although the JVP often is evaluated inaccurately, in one study it was found to be the best indicator of ADHF (positive likelihood ratio 5.1, 95% CI, 3.2 to 7.9; negative likelihood ratio 0.66, 95% CI, .57 to .77) [7]. Jugular venous distention above 10 cm corresponds to a pulmonary capillary wedge pressure of above 22 mm Hg, with an accuracy of 80% [8]. It

---

Box 2. Clinical presentation of patients hospitalized with heart failure

Presenting feature
Any dyspnea (89%)
Dyspnea at rest (36%)
Fatigue (33%)
Peripheral edema (66%)
Radiographic pulmonary congestion (76%)

Adapted from Fonarow GC, ADHERE. Scientific Advisory Committee. The Acute Decompensated Heart Failure National Registry (ADHERE): opportunities to improve care of patients hospitalized with acute decompensated heart failure. Rev Cardiovasc Medicine 2003;4(Suppl 7):S21–30. Copyright © 2002 MedReviews, LLC.

must be remembered, however, that the JVP provides closer estimations of right atrial and right ventricular (RV) end–diastolic pressures, and in the absence of lung pathology, provides only a general estimation of left-sided filling pressures. To synthesize the findings of congestion and signs of low perfusion the 2 × 2 table has been recommended (Fig. 1) [9], in which the clinician can determine in which quadrant the patient currently resides and then select the appropriate therapy [10]. Most patients presenting with HF are in the right upper quadrant, which is the warm-and- wet sector. This means they have adequate perfusion and are volume overloaded. A few patients who have HF are cold and wet, meaning they are volume overloaded and not perfusing well, as marked by their hypotension. Cold and dry (left lower quadrant) is much more uncommon and is often the result of patients being over diuresed from a group that includes patients who were cold and wet (see Fig. 1). Patients in the left upper quadrant are not congested and have normal cardiac output and have been admitted to the hospital because of a reason other than HF. A more recent study has emphasized the importance of an elevated JVP and third heart sound in evaluating the prognosis of HF [11]. An elevated JVP is associated with an increased risk of hospitalization for HF (relative risk, 1.32; 95% CI, 1.08 to 1.62; $P < .01$), death or hospitalization for HF (relative risk, 1.30; 95%

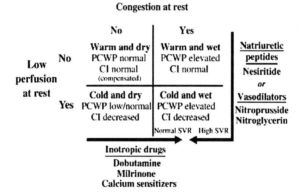

Fig. 1. Patient selection and treatment. Diagram indicating 2 × 2 table of hemodynamic profiles for patients presenting with heart failure. Most patients can be classified in a 2-minute bedside assessment according to the signs and symptoms shown, although in practice, some patients may be on the border between the warm-and-wet and cold-and-wet profiles. This classification helps guide initial therapy and prognosis for patients presenting with advanced heart failure. Although most patients presenting with hypoperfusion also have elevated filling pressures (cold-and-wet profile), many patients present with elevated filling pressures without major reduction in perfusion (warm-and-wet profile). Patients presenting with symptoms of heart failure at rest or minimal exertion without clinical evidence of elevated filling pressures or hypoperfusion (warm-and-dry profile) should be evaluated carefully to determine whether their symptoms result from heart failure [9,10]. *Abbreviations:* CI, cardiac index; PCWP, pulmonary capillary wedge pressure. (*From* Nohria A, Lewis E, Stevenson LW. Medical management of advanced heart failure. JAMA 2002;287(5):628–40; with permission).

CI, 1.11 to 1.53; $P<.005$), and death from pump failure (relative risk, 1.37; 95% CI, 1.07 to 1.75; $P<.05$). The presence of a third heart sound is associated with similar increased risks of these outcomes.

Ancillary evaluation

Several tests may be performed to determine the etiology and support the clinical evaluation of ADHF.

Chest radiographs can be obtained quickly, but findings from the ADHERE registry showed that confirmatory evidence of HF occurs in only about 75% of patients [6]. Consistent chest radiograph findings in left side HF is descending order: dilated upper lobe vessels, cardiomegaly, interstitial edema, enlarged pulmonary arteries, pleural effusion, alveolar edema, prominent superior vena cava, and Kerley B lines [12]. This means that 25% of all patients presenting with HF have no findings, and one must consider that acute abnormalities may not appear for up to 6 hours after clinical symptoms are present [13]. Thus although chest radiographs are helpful, they are not definitive. The presence of interstitial edema on a chest radiograph suggests that the LV end–diastolic pressure or the left atrial pressure is at least 25 mm Hg and increases the likelihood of ADHF about 12-fold [7]. An important caveat is that symptoms and signs (orthopnea, edema, rales, third heart sound and elevated JVP) or radiologic features (cardiomegaly, vascular redistribution, interstitial or alveolar edema) have a poor predictive value in identifying an elevated LV diastolic pressure greater than 30 mm Hg [14].

An EKG is helpful to detect acute myocardial infarction, ischemia, LV hypertrophy, and arrhythmias. Atrial fibrillation, which is present in about 31% of patients presenting with ADHF or heart block also can contribute to HF symptoms [15]. Additionally, pacemaker malfunction can be detected and is becoming more important with the increasing prevalence of cardiac resynchronization therapy.

Laboratory evaluation should include a complete blood count, basic metabolic panel, cardiac biomarkers, and international normalized ratio (INR), particularly if the patient is on warfarin. Liver function and thyroid studies should be screened when the situation warrants. The results from some of these tests can lead to useful risk stratification, as recently demonstrated by the classification and regression tree (CART) analysis derived from the ADHERE registry. It showed that a serum urea nitrogen (BUN) of greater than 43 mg/dL was the single best predictor for in hospital mortality, with a systolic blood pressure of less than 115 mm HG being second, and a creatinine of 2.75 mg/dL being third [16]. A combination of two or more of these risk factors increases the likelihood of mortality (Fig. 2). Hyponatremia in an HF patient is a sign of failing circulatory homeostasis and is associated with longer length of stay and higher in-hospital and early postdischarge mortality [17]. In both OPTIMIZE-CHF, and in Evaluation Study of Congestive Heart Failure and Pulmonary Artery Catheter Effectiveness (ESCAPE),

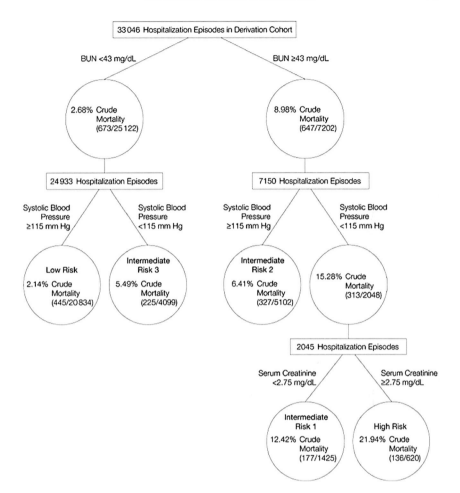

Fig. 2. Predictors of in-hospital mortality and risk stratification for the derivation cohort. Each node is based on available data from registry patient hospitalizations for each predictive variable presented. *Abbreviation:* BUN, blood (serum) urea nitrogen. To convert BUN to mmol/L, multiply by 0.357; to convert creatinine to μmol/L, multiply by 88.4. (*From* Fonarow GC, Adams KF, Abraham WT, et al. Risk stratification for in-hospital mortality in acutely decompensated heart failure: classification and regression tree analysis. JAMA 2005;293(5):576; with permission.)

25% of patients had hyponatremia on admission and discharge. Tolvaptan has been shown to ameliorate hyponatremia, but it does not improve long-term mortality [18,19]. Anemia is a well- recognized poor prognostic indicator in HF [20,21] and has been attributed to iron deficiency in HF patients because of malabsorption, nutritional deficiencies, and impaired metabolism. Hemodilution (excess fluid retention) also may contribute to anemia in patients who have HF. A higher red cell distribution width (RDW) also has been shown to be associated with morbidity and mortality (adjusted hazard

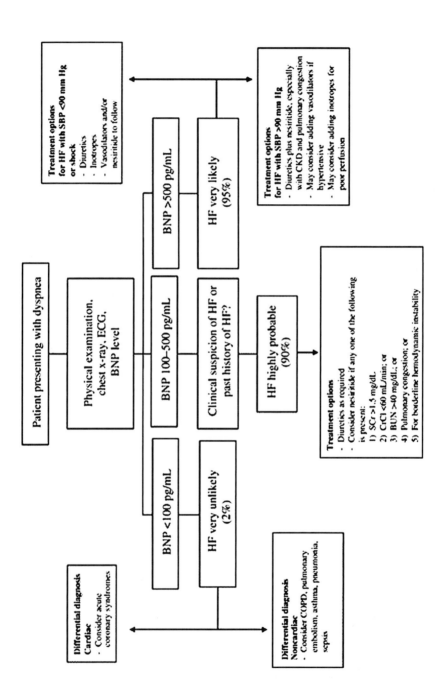

ratio 1.17 per 1-SD increase, $P < .001$) among 36 laboratory values considered in the CHARM program [22]. In fact, higher RDW was among the most powerful overall predictors, with only age and cardiomegaly showing a stronger independent association with outcome. This finding was replicated in the Duke databank, in which higher RDW was associated strongly with all-cause mortality (adjusted hazard ratio 1.29 per 1 SD, $P < .001$), second only to age as a predictor of outcome. Further studies are needed regarding the management of anemia and high RDW in heart failure.

B-type natriuretic peptide (BNP): At least three types of natriuretic peptides have been identified, with the B type being the only one commercially available for testing. The release of the B-type natriuretic peptide is from ventricular stretch or volume overload and can aid in the diagnosis of HF. In patients not experiencing HF, BNP levels averaged 38 pg/mL compared with those with HF, whose average was 1076 pg/mL [23]. BNP levels also can be used to risk stratify patients for future events. When patients presented to an ED with a BNP greater than 480 pg/mL, their likelihood of death or HR rehospitalization within 6 months was almost 40%, as compared with a level of 230 pg/mL, in which the likelihood was only 3% [24]. In patients who had stable coronary heart disease (CHD) and no history of heart failure, NT-proBNP levels lower than 100 pg/mL effectively rule out ventricular dysfunction, with a negative likelihood ratio of 0.28 [25]. So far two forms of testing for this peptide are available in the form of BNP and NT pro-BNP, which is the precursor form. Only BNP has point-of-care capability at this time, but both show great promise in helping determine the presence or absence of HF. The diagnosis of HF should not be made with BNP or NT pro-BNP alone, but should be used in conjunction with history, physical examination, chest radiograph, echocardiography, other laboratory tests, and EKG. Special consideration should be made, because conditions exist in which BNP levels can be affected. The levels may be increased with age, female sex, and decreased renal function. Morbid obesity has the potential to decrease the level of BNP, making it appear low compared with the true hemodynamic status. Among the greatest values of BNP are its negative predictive value of 89% (95% CI, 87% to 91% when the results are low, less than 100 pg/mL) and the ability to use it as a bedside test to rule in or rule out HF. Among the frustrating aspects of this test are the midrange values between 100 pg/mL and 500 pg/mL in which the

---

Fig. 3. Evaluation and treatment algorithm for patients presenting with acute dyspnea integrating BNP-based diagnosis and therapy. (Note that this figure is not intended to recommend that nesiritide is the only therapeutic agent of choice in the clinical scenarios presented. Other vasodilators can be used interchangeably) Close attention to renal function is recommended while on BNP therapy. *Abbreviations*: CKD, chronic kidney disease; COPD, chronic obstructive pulmonary disease; CrCl, creatinine clearance. (*From* Maisel A. B-type natriuretic peptide measurements in diagnosing congestive heart failure in the dyspneic emergency department patient. Rev Cardiovasc Med 2002;3(Suppl 4):S10–7; with permission. Copyright © 2002 MedReviews, LLC.)

diagnosis of HF may be present. This is when clinical acumen and further testing may be necessary. A chart is provided to help clinicians navigate through the numerous causes of dyspnea and how BNP can help (Fig. 3) [26]. An elevated BNP, together with elevated troponins (an indicator of myocardial necrosis), is reported to be associated with a 12-fold increase in mortality [27], and serial measurements of both biomarkers can add substantially to risk assessment [28]. The results from the IMPROVE-CHF study indicate that N-terminal pro-B type natriuretic peptide testing also improves the management of patients who have suspected acute HF [29].

Echocardiography is extremely useful in determining LV ejection fraction, volume, and dimensions, wall motion abnormalities, valvular function, and the presence or absence of endocarditis is invaluable. Any patient who has newly diagnosed HF should have an echocardiogram performed as part of his or her initial work-up. The Joint Commission recommends assessment of LV systolic function in all patients who have suspected HF [30]. With the widespread availability of tissue Doppler, it is possible to obtain an estimate of the LV end–diastolic pressure by determining the E:E ratio. When the diagnosis of ADHF is in doubt a markedly elevated E:E' ratio suggests elevated LV end–diastolic pressure [31]. To improve prescription of angiotensin-converting enzyme (ACE) inhibitors and beta-blockers, it has been suggested that reminders be attached to echocardiograms reporting impaired LV systolic function [32].

Hemodynamic monitoring

The role of the flow-directed thermodilution pulmonary artery catheter (Swan-Ganz catheter) for managing patients who have not responded to initial management and are hypotensive, in shock or a preshock state, has been shown to be of value in experienced centers [33]. This type of monitoring rarely is needed in the routine management of ADHF [34]. When indicated, hemodynamic monitoring can help guide pharmacologic and nonpharmacologic therapy and if there is a need for mechanical support or other interventions. The parameters of greatest interest include: cardiac output, pulmonary capillary wedge pressure, systemic arterial pressure, heart rate, and the calculated systemic vascular resistance (SVR, mean arterial pressure minus mean right atrial pressure, divided by cardiac output). It is important to recognize that metabolic demand may vary significantly among patients; some individuals are able to tolerate a much lower cardiac output, so attention to perfusion, urine output, and mental status must be followed closely. The role of lactate in managing critically ill patients is becoming more important and should be considered in this circumstance [35].

Hemodynamic monitoring in HF has come under close scrutiny, and its value has been questioned, especially after the advent of the ESCAPE trial. This study showed no significant differences in 30-day mortality or clinical outcomes or adverse events at 6 months between patients who received a Swan-Ganz catheter and those who did not, begging the question whether this form of monitoring has utility [34]. Although invasive hemodynamic monitoring is not ideal, noninvasive hemodynamic monitoring such as tissue Doppler [31] or thoracic bioimpedance [36] should continue to play a role in guiding management. In the ESCAPE trial, lower pulmonary capillary wedge pressures achieved during therapy independently predicted lower 6-month event rates [34].

Treatment

In-hospital treatment of ADHF involves both rapid relief of symptoms and congestion, hemodynamic stabilization, initiation of long-term therapy, and management of comorbidities. Postdischarge management includes maintenance of euvolemia and promoting adherence to dietary and medical therapy. The immediate goals of treatment are based on the severity of the presentation. Because dyspnea is present in almost all of these patients, symptom relief, stabilization of patients' hemodynamic status, relief of congestion, and improving low output states, are the focal points of the acute presentation.

Starting with oxygen, pulse oximetry should be used to guide management. Hypoxia seems to carry a greater burden than concern of CO_2 retention. Therefore, it seems more reasonable to give oxygen rather than to withhold it. If the concern for CO_2 retention exists, a blood gas should be obtained to help guide management.

Biphasic positive airway pressure (Bi PAP), which delivers inspiratory and expiratory pressures by means of a facemask, and continuous positive airway pressure (CPAP), which delivers constant pressure throughout the respiratory cycle, are being used more commonly to treat HF. Benefits have been shown for patients who have COPD, but the data are controversial surrounding pulmonary edema. Although CPAP and BiPAP appear to decrease emergent intubations, there are no randomized studies to show improvement in mortality. The major obstacle to this therapy seems to be the patient's inability to tolerate the face mask, which in the authors' clinical practice is not infrequent.

Morphine sulfate is a venodilator and can be helpful in decreasing anxiety. It also reduces preload by causing venodilatation and is used often when there is severe pulmonary edema accompanied by anxiety. It can be started in dose of 2 to 5 mg provided adequate blood pressures are present. It should be used with caution in patients who have decreased mental status and or diminished respiratory drive. Naloxone can be used if the effects are greater than desired.

Diuretics have long been a mainstay of HF treatment. Oral diuretics are postulated to lose their effectiveness because of bowel wall edema, which prevents proper gastrointestinal absorption. Therefore the intravenous form of loop diuretics is indicated, because it reduces congestive symptoms through the reduction of volume overload, reduction of mesenteric edema, and improving perfusion across renal vascular beds by means of a decrease in venous pressures without dropping arterial pressure [37]. Because no improvement in mortality has been shown with the use of furosemide, it is not indicated as monotherapy for heart failure [38]. Some form of renal impairment can occur because of increasingly higher doses of oral diuretics. Studies have shown that intravenous furosemide can decrease glomerular filtration rate [39]. The mechanism of loop diuretics is to promote water and sodium excretion. If the patient has not used furosemide previously, a starting dose of 40 mg intravenously should be instituted. If the patient is on chronic furosemide one can start by giving his or her usual oral dose intravenously (range, 20 to 180 mg). Bumetanide can be given instead, and 1 mg equals 40 mg of furosemide. A thiazide diuretic can be added and used because of its action at a different site of the nephron. In the event of a true sulfa allergy, ethacrynic acid can be used as a loop diuretic. No major trials have compared the bolus intravenous loop diuretics with continuous infusion, making definitive recommendations unlikely until such trials are conducted.

Diuretics are considered standard care for managing HF, largely based on clinical and anecdotal experience. Because of this widespread acceptance, it is unlikely a large multicenter randomized trial ever will be conducted. Important questions, however, remain, including optimal dosage, route of administration, and potential long-term adverse effects [40,41], and are worthy of further investigation.

The ADHERE study reported that 89% of patients presented with symptoms of volume overload; 88% received intravenous diuretics. Despite this, only 50% of patients were asymptomatic at the time of discharge, and 51% had little or no weight loss (less than 5 lbs) during their hospitalization [15]. This report suggests that too many patients are being discharged prematurely. The IMPACT-HF study found that 60% of patients are being discharged with continuing symptoms of fatigue or dyspnea, resulting in a 25% rehospitalization rate within 60 days after discharge [42]. Although diuretics seem to be helpful in patients who have HF [43], Wuerz and Meador [44] showed that when patients experiencing dyspnea were given diuretics in the absence of HF, they had increased mortality. This emphasizes that diuretics are not benign and underscores the importance of making the correct diagnosis and providing proper treatment. Among promising agents are A1-adenosine antagonists, which have shown to increase sodium excretion without causing hypokalemia or azotemia, but large randomized trials of efficacy and safety are needed [45].

Vasodilators

Vasodilators are important for managing HF due to the hyperadrenergic state and the activation of the renin-angiotensin-aldosterone axis. The most common three agents are nitroglycerin, nitroprusside, and nesiritide. They are not recommended when patients are hypotensive. If a patient becomes hypotensive after a vasodilator has been administered, the clinician should consider the presence of aortic stenosis, volume depletion, RV infarct, or excessive dosing of the drug.

Nitroglycerin

Nitroglycerin's effects are mediated through the relaxation of vascular smooth muscle, and it reduces preload and afterload. It can be given orally, topically, or intravenously, as long as blood pressure is maintained. The oral/sublingual form is fast- acting and is given in form that is 10 times greater than the intravenous form, 0.4 mg, versus the starting intravenous dose of .2 μg/kg/min. The coronary artery dilation is thought to help with coronary artery perfusion and decrease ischemia.

The dosing of nitroglycerin is often suboptimal and may need to reach doses of about 160 μg/kg/min to achieve measurable decreases in pulmonary capillary wedge pressure [46]. Headache is a common adverse effect but is generally ameliorated with acetaminophen, while tachyphylaxis poses a more difficult management issue. Tachyphylaxis is the tolerance level the body develops to a medication. Therefore the body needs increasing amounts to achieve the desired affects. The clinician is left titrating the medication in higher doses and in an unpredictable fashion.

Nitroprusside

Nitroprusside is very effective in reducing preload and afterload. It should be started at doses of .3 μg/kg/min and titrated every 5 to 10 minutes according to the change in blood pressure. It no longer is used frequently in HF because of its adverse effect profile and cumbersome requirements for administration. Nitroprusside often requires arterial line monitoring. Its theoretical coronary steal effect, where arteriolar dilation in nonischemic areas shunts blood from areas of ischemia, and accompanying thiocyanate toxicity make it less desirable for managing ADHF [47,48].

Nesiritide

Nesiritide is identical to the endogenous BNP produced by the body. It acts as a vasodilator on veins and arteries and has some effect on increasing coronary blood flow. antagonizing the renin-angiotensin-aldosterone system and dampening the sympathetic nervous system cause its vasodilator effects. Its starting dose is 2 μg/kg bolus, then infusion of .01 μg/kg/min.

Although nesiritide is more expensive, its use has been accompanied by clinical improvement in symptoms, greater decreases in pulmonary capillary wedge pressures, and less dyspnea at 24 hours than nitroglycerin [49]. It has a similar effect profile as nitroglycerin except with headache, in which case it is less frequent. The occurrence of symptomatic hypotension in the first

3 hours is about 0.5% [50]. Its use also has been associated with shorter ICU and hospital stays and improvements in heart failure outcomes. Analysis of the ADHERE reported the inpatient survival equivalence between nitroglycerin and nesiritide and increased risk of mortality in patients requiring inotropes [51].

Recent pooled analyses have raised concerns about nesiritide being linked to decreasing renal function and mortality [52,53], resulting in a rapid decline in its use in the United States [54]. These studies have been criticized for not controlling qualitative heterogeneity among patient cohorts and the inability to control for baseline inotrope use. More recent data have shown favorable safety [55,56], but reports of larger studies that are underway, such as the ASCEND-HF, NAPA, FUSION-II, and BRain NatrIuretic Peptide Versus the Clinical CongesTion ScorE (STARBRITE) trials, will be needed to definitively answer these questions [55,57,58].

Inotropes

Inotropes are useful for low-output failure and their role is limited in patients who have normal LV systolic function. The adverse effects of arrhythmias, myocardial infarction, and adverse LV remodeling narrow their therapeutic window to one of bridging until a more definitive therapy can be used. Inotropes improve cardiac output and renal blood flow.

Dobutamine

Dobutamine may be employed when hypoperfusion is present with HF [59]. It is a catecholamine that has inotropic properties. It is used best to treat pulmonary congestion and low cardiac output. It is a racemic mixture of levo and dextroisomers of potent beta and alpha adrenergic agonists. Dobutamine's mechanism of action is through stimulation of the myocardial beta-1 and to some extent the alpha-1 receptors, which are balanced by opposing alpha-1 and beta-2 stimulation, resulting in minimal vascular resistance, but producing positive inotropic effects.

Dobutamine should be used with caution in patients where myocardial ischemia may be present. The effects of dobutamine can increase myocardial oxygen consumption and make ischemia worse, while other properties of the drug actually improve myocardial perfusion in proportion to the increase in oxygen consumption [59]. Ideally, the drug should be monitored carefully, and when a heart rate increase above 10% of baseline occurs, many clinicians will consider stopping it. Problems in patients who are receiving beta blocker therapy and concurrent dobutamine therapy have been reported and should be considered when difficulties with titration are encountered. In addition, a retrospective analysis suggested increased mortality associated with the use of dobutamine [60], but it may be useful in selected patients.

Milrinone

Milrinone works by inhibiting the phosphodiesterase III isoenzyme, which leads to increased cyclic adenosine monophosphate (cAMP) and enhanced inotropy. It differs from dobutamine, because it elevates cAMP by preventing its degradation as opposed to dobutamine, which increases cAMP production. Milrinone's effect is achieved by reducing RV and LV filling pressures and increasing cardiac output without significant changes to heart rate and blood pressure. Because it has the potential to decrease blood pressure, it should be used cautiously with hypotension.

The pharmacokinetic properties of milrinone make it a less desirable first-line agent because of its slow onset and long half-life [61]. It is for this reason that hypotension can become such a problem in the management of a HF patient with milrinone. Milrinone seems to have some advantage over dobutamine in patients on chronic beta-blocker therapy. It acts beyond the beta receptor level, and therefore its inotropic effects should be unchanged. This is an important consideration, in that so many HF patients are on chronic beta-blocker therapy. If the patient who has HF is on milrinone, the beta-blocker dosage can remain the same or slightly decreased depending on the status of the patient. If the inotropic support becomes prolonged, the beta-blocker should be stopped.

Serious concerns about the safety and efficacy of milrinone were raised in the OPTIME study, where patients were found to have about the same mortality rates compared with placebo and a greater incidence of arrhythmias [62].

The typical patient in acute compensated HF does not benefit from vasopressor therapy in most circumstances. This class of agents is indicated only for the support of blood pressure and to maintain organ perfusion when shock exists. The prognosis is very poor when vasopressor therapy is instituted, especially for an extended duration. Therefore, its role in HF should be minimized, except in conditions of extreme hemodynamic instability [63].

Device therapy

In selected cases of ADHF, device therapy may be considered. Indirect unloading and stabilization of the heart can be achieved with intra-aortic balloon pulsation, extracorporeal membrane oxygenation (ECMO) [64], or TandemHeart [65,66]. In emergent cases, mechanical unloading of the heart has been used as rescue therapy. The strengths and limitations of each device need to be known, and cardiologists will have to work closely with cardiothoracic surgeons to determine the best device and most appropriate patients [67].

Ultrafiltration

Ultrafiltration has emerged as a new therapy to assist in patients who are volume-overloaded and have some element of diuretic resistance. The mechanism of action is to draw fluid off through hydrostatic pressures across a semipermeable membrane. The advantages to this process are small swings in electrolyte balance, while a large volume of fluid can be pulled off. The patient also seems to experience fewer hemodynamic imbalances compared with hemodialysis, even when taking off up to 500 mL per hour. The recent advent of using peripheral venous access has made this modality a possibility in several clinical settings [68,69]. In the UNLOAD trial, at 48 hours into treatment, the ultrafiltration group demonstrated a 38% greater weight loss and a 28% greater net fluid loss over standard care. Ninety days following discharge, the ultrafiltration group, when compared with standard care, showed a 43% reduction in HF rehospitalizations, 52% reduction in ED or clinic visits for HF, and 63% reduction in days rehospitalized for HF during the study period. Researchers found that although ultrafiltration was efficient at removing fluid, it did not alleviate dyspnea better than diuretics. There were no significant changes in serum creatinine or potassium in the ultrafiltration group.

Long-term treatment

ACE inhibitors have been shown to decrease mortality and hospitalizations [70]. It is recommended that all patients with HF be on an ACE inhibitor before hospital discharge unless there is a contraindication. A decrease of 31% in mortality was shown for patients receiving enalapril who had class IV HF, and a decrease of 16% was shown for patients who had class II and class III HF [71]. Although the role of ACE inhibitors for managing chronic HF is established, their role in ADHF remains unclear.

The adverse effects of ACE inhibitors can include angioedema, which results from increased bradykinin; anaphylaxis is rare. Cough also is reported as an adverse effect of ACE inhibitors, but should prompt a clinician to search for other causes such as a upper respiratory tract infection or worsening HF before stopping the ACE inhibitor. In general, the cough will go away within 1 to 2 weeks after stopping the drug.

Mild azotemia can be encountered when ACE inhibitors are started, and this is tolerated well by patients; rapid rises in azotemia should prompt a consideration of bilateral renal artery stenosis. Oliguria and serum creatinine levels above 3 mg/dL are also contraindications to the use of ACE inhibitors; avoid starting an ACE inhibitor/angiotensin receptor blocker (ARB) when the patient is intravascularly dry.

Patients should be started on low doses and titrated up to target levels. Even lower than target doses have been shown to decrease mortality, although higher doses are more cost-effective [72]. It may take several weeks to months to exert the full symptomatic benefit, but ACE inhibitors should be instituted for their long-term effects on LV remodeling and mortality.

ARBs block the angiotensin II receptors, thereby reducing LV remodeling, arterial vasoconstriction, and renal damage. They seem to have a more favorable adverse effect profile with less cough and angioedema, but they are reserved for patients who are intolerant to ACE inhibitors.

Beta-blocker therapy is effective in reducing sympathetic nervous system activity, symptoms, and mortality in patients who have HF. The hyperadrenergic state of HF, as measured by increases in norepinephrine levels, leads to myocardial hypertrophy, increases in afterload, coronary vasoconstriction, and mortality. Both carvedilol and long-acting metoprolol have been shown to reduce mortality in HF [73,74]. Beta-blockers do not seem to have a role in the acute and or critical care setting, except to decrease heart rate if needed; avoid starting a beta-blocker when the patient is wet. This therapy generally is reserved for stable patients. Patients on beta-blocker therapy offer an interesting challenge during an acute decompensated episode. Withdrawing beta-blocker therapy may cause deterioration in the patient's condition; however, the dose may compromise any tenuous hemodynamics. When dobutamine therapy (a beta-agonist) is being used, beta-blockers may need to be stopped, and in some instances milrinone used instead of dobutamine to help improve the patient's condition.

Digoxin inhibits the Na+K+ATPase of the myocardial cellular membrane and has been used for years to control ventricular response in atrial fibrillation. Digoxin should be avoided as monotherapy in HF. Levels need to be monitored closely, particularly in the elderly and those who have renal insufficiency. Because digoxin does not improve survival [75], there is a tendency to avoid using it in HF patients with sinus rhythm.

Spironolactone has been shown to decrease mortality in class III and IV HF patients by about 30% [76]. It also has been shown to be beneficial in mild-to-moderate HF [77,78]. Aldosterone receptor blockade, therefore, should be considered in all patients who have HF. Spironolactone should be avoided in patients who have a creatinine level over 2.5 mg/dL or a potassium level over 5 mEq/L.

Postdischarge management

As mentioned earlier, although as many as 60% of all patients who are hospitalized for HF die within 1 year, only about 5% to 8% actually die in the hospital [3]. Thirty percent to 50% of recurrent episodes of HF are caused by noncompliance, which also contributes to one third to one half of all patients readmitted for HF within 6 months of initial hospital discharge [79]. Discharge planning is, therefore, important and should include the prescription of ACE inhibitors and beta-blockers at discharge, and education regarding diet, exercise, compliance with medications, the importance of monitoring daily weights, and smoking cessation. Patients often do not comply with these recommendations because of socio–economic factors and presence of comorbidities including stroke dementia, anemia, diabetes mellitus, hypertension, atrial fibrillation, hyperlipidemia, COPD, and orthostatic hypotension, making a multidisciplinary approach necessary. An approach including the patient as the key member of a team, the HF specialist [80], a specialist nurse [81], a pharmacist [82], a social worker, and a dietician, is required to ensure successful postdischarge management of ADHF [83]. With the Centers for Medicare and Medicaid Services decision to publish 30-day mortality of patients following discharge from hospital, it is inevitable most hospitals will be compelled to set-up such multidisciplinary teams to ensure a low 30-day mortality.

Summary

Temporal trends suggest that over a 3-year period, demographics and clinical characteristics of ADHF are relatively similar, but advances in therapeutics, improved adherence to quality-of-care measures, increased application of evidence-based HF medications, and substantial improvements in in-hospital morbidity and mortality have occurred [84]. These findings are heartening, because they indicate rapid translation of data from clinical trials to day-to-day medical practice. The diagnosis and management of HF remain a challenge, and until robust data from randomized trials are available, the treatment will remain empirical. The practicing clinician will have to continue to make choices with the present therapies available, and clinicians are advised to follow two important tenets:

- The Hippocratic principle of primum non nocere (first do no harm)
- William Peabody's teaching regarding patient care: "To Cure Sometimes, to Relieve Often, and to Comfort Always"

References

[1] Kozak LJ, Owings MF, Hall MJ. National Hospital Discharge Survey: 2002 annual summary with detailed diagnosis and procedure data. Vital Health Stat 13, 2005;(158):1–199.

[2] Rosamond W, et al. Heart disease and stroke statistics–2007 update: a report from the American Heart Association Statistics Committee and Stroke Statistics Subcommittee. Circulation 2007;115(5):e69–171.

[3] Francis GS. Acute heart failure: patient management of a growing epidemic. Am Heart Hosp J 2004;2(4 Suppl 1):10–4.

[4] Nieminen MS, et al. Executive summary of the guidelines on the diagnosis and treatment of acute heart failure: the Task Force on Acute Heart Failure of the European Society of Cardiology. Eur Heart J 2005;26(4):384–416.

[5] Badgett RG, Lucey CR, Mulrow CD. Can the clinical examination diagnose left-sided heart failure in adults? Jama 1997;277(21):1712–9.

[6] Fonarow GC. The Acute Decompensated Heart Failure National Registry (ADHERE): opportunities to improve care of patients hospitalized with acute decompensated heart failure. Rev Cardiovasc Med 2003;(4 Suppl 7):S21–30.

[7] Wang CS, et al. Does this dyspneic patient in the emergency department have congestive heart failure? Jama 2005;294(15):1944–56.

[8] Stevenson LW, Perloff JK. The limited reliability of physical signs for estimating hemodynamics in chronic heart failure. Jama 1989;261(6):884–8.

[9] Stevenson LW. Tailored therapy to hemodynamic goals for advanced heart failure. Eur J Heart Fail 1999;1(3):251–7.

[10] Drazner MH, et al. Prognostic importance of elevated jugular venous pressure and a third heart sound in patients with heart failure. N Engl J Med 2001;345(8):574–81.

[11] Chait A, et al. The bedside chest radiograph in the evaluation of incipient heart failure. Radiology 1972;105(3):563–6.

[12] Peacock WF. Using the emergency department clinical decision unit for acute decompensated heart failure. Cardiol Clin 2005;23(4):569–88, viii.

[13] Chakko S, et al. Clinical, radiographic, and hemodynamic correlations in chronic congestive heart failure: conflicting results may lead to inappropriate care. Am J Med 1991;90(3): 353–9.

[14] Adams KF Jr, et al. Characteristics and outcomes of patients hospitalized for heart failure in the United States: rationale, design, and preliminary observations from the first 100,000 cases in the Acute Decompensated Heart Failure National Registry (ADHERE). Am Heart J 2005;149(2):209–16.

[15] Fonarow GC, et al. Risk stratification for in-hospital mortality in acutely decompensated heart failure: classification and regression tree analysis. Jama 2005;293(5):572–80.

[16] Gheorghiade M, et al. Relationship between admission serum sodium concentration and clinical outcomes in patients hospitalized for heart failure: an analysis from the OPTIMIZE-HF registry. Eur Heart J 2007;28(8):980–8.

[17] Gheorghiade M, et al. Short-term clinical effects of tolvaptan, an oral vasopressin antagonist, in patients hospitalized for heart failure: the EVEREST Clinical Status Trials. Jama 2007;297(12):1332–43.

[18] Konstam MA, et al. Effects of oral tolvaptan in patients hospitalized for worsening heart failure: the EVEREST Outcome Trial. Jama 2007;297(12):1319–31.

[19] Nanas JN, et al. Etiology of anemia in patients with advanced heart failure. J Am Coll Cardiol 2006;48(12):2485–9.

[20] Dec GW. Anemia in heart failure time to rethink its etiology and treatment? J Am Coll Cardiol 2006;48(12):2490–2.

[21] Felker GM, et al. Red cell distribution width as a novel prognostic marker in heart failure: data from the CHARM Program and the Duke Databank. J Am Coll Cardiol 2007;50(1): 40–7.

[22] Dao Q, et al. Utility of B-type natriuretic peptide in the diagnosis of congestive heart failure in an urgent-care setting. J Am Coll Cardiol 2001;37(2):379–85.

[23] Harrison A, et al. B-type natriuretic peptide predicts future cardiac events in patients presenting to the emergency department with dyspnea. Ann Emerg Med 2002;39(2):131–8.

[24] Corteville DC, et al. N-terminal pro-B-type natriuretic peptide as a diagnostic test for ventricular dysfunction in patients with coronary disease: data from the heart and soul study. Arch Intern Med 2007;167(5):483–9.

[25] Maisel A. B-type natriuretic peptide measurements in diagnosing congestive heart failure in the dyspneic emergency department patient. Rev Cardiovasc Med 2002;(3 Suppl 4): S10–7.

[26] Horwich TB, et al. Cardiac troponin I is associated with impaired hemodynamics, progressive left ventricular dysfunction, and increased mortality rates in advanced heart failure. Circulation 2003;108(7):833–8.

[27] Miller WL, et al. Serial biomarker measurements in ambulatory patients with chronic heart failure: the importance of change over time. Circulation 2007;116(3):249–57.

[28] Moe GW, et al. N-terminal pro-B-type natriuretic peptide testing improves the management of patients with suspected acute heart failure: primary results of the Canadian prospective randomized multicenter IMPROVE-CHF study. Circulation 2007;115(24):3103–10.

[29] Getting started with core measures. Jt Comm Perspect 2002;22(5):7–8.

[30] Huang CH, et al. Diagnostic accuracy of tissue Doppler echocardiography for patients with acute heart failure. Heart 2006;92(12):1790–4.

[31] Heidenreich PA, et al. ACE inhibitor reminders attached to echocardiography reports of patients with reduced left ventricular ejection fraction. Am J Med 2005;118(9):1034–7.

[32] Stevenson LW. Are hemodynamic goals viable in tailoring heart failure therapy? Hemodynamic goals are relevant. Circulation 2006;113(7):1020–7, discussion 1033.

[33] Binanay C, et al. Evaluation study of congestive heart failure and pulmonary artery catheterization effectiveness: the ESCAPE trial. Jama 2005;294(13):1625–33.

[34] Mavric Z, et al. Usefulness of blood lactate as a predictor of shock development in acute myocardial infarction. Am J Cardiol 1991;67(7):565–8.

[35] Rosenberg P, Yancy CW. Noninvasive assessment of hemodynamics: an emphasis on bioimpedance cardiography. Curr Opin Cardiol 2000;15(3):151–5.

[36] Heart Failure Society Of, A. Evaluation and management of patients with acute decompensated heart failure. J Card Fail 2006;12(1):e86–103.

[37] Packer M, Miller AB. Can physicians always explain the results of clinical trials? A case study of amlodipine in heart failure. Am J Cardiol 1999;84(4A):1L–2L.

[38] Iyengar S, Abraham WT. Diuretics for the treatment of acute decompensated heart failure. Heart Fail Rev 2007;12(2):125–30.

[39] Ahmed A, et al. Heart failure, chronic diuretic use, and increase in mortality and hospitalization: an observational study using propensity score methods. Eur Heart J 2006;27(12): 1431–9.

[40] Lopez B, et al. Effects of loop diuretics on myocardial fibrosis and collagen type I turnover in chronic heart failure. J Am Coll Cardiol 2004;43(11):2028–35.

[41] Gattis WA, et al. Predischarge initiation of carvedilol in patients hospitalized for decompensated heart failure: results of the Initiation Management Predischarge: Process for Assessment of Carvedilol Therapy in Heart Failure (IMPACT-HF) trial. J Am Coll Cardiol 2004;43(9):1534–41.

[42] Costanzo MR, et al. The safety of intravenous diuretics alone versus diuretics plus parenteral vasoactive therapies in hospitalized patients with acutely decompensated heart failure: a propensity score and instrumental variable analysis using the Acutely Decompensated Heart Failure National Registry (ADHERE) database. Am Heart J 2007;154(2):267–77.

[43] Wuerz RC, Meador SA. Effects of prehospital medications on mortality and length of stay in congestive heart failure. Ann Emerg Med 1992;21(6):669–74.

[44] Greenberg B, et al. Effects of multiple oral doses of an A1 adenosine antagonist, BG9928, in patients with heart failure: results of a placebo-controlled, dose-escalation study. J Am Coll Cardiol 2007;50(7):600–6.

[45] Elkayam U, et al. Comparison of effects on left ventricular filling pressure of intravenous nesiritide and high-dose nitroglycerin in patients with decompensated heart failure. Am J Cardiol 2004;93(2):237–40.

[46] Hasenfuss G, et al. Myocardial energetics in patients with dilated cardiomyopathy. Influence of nitroprusside and enoximone. Circulation 1989;80(1):51–64.

[47] Mann T, et al. Effect of nitroprusside on regional myocardial blood flow in coronary artery disease. Results in 25 patients and comparison with nitroglycerin. Circulation 1978;57(4): 732–8.

[48] Colucci WS, et al. Intravenous nesiritide, a natriuretic peptide, in the treatment of decompensated congestive heart failure. Nesiritide Study Group. N Engl J Med 2000;343(4): 246–53.

[49] Intravenous nesiritide vs nitroglycerin for treatment of decompensated congestive heart failure: a randomized controlled trial. Jama 2002;287(12):1531–40.

[50] Abraham WT, et al. In-hospital mortality in patients with acute decompensated heart failure requiring intravenous vasoactive medications: an analysis from the Acute Decompensated Heart Failure National Registry (ADHERE). J Am Coll Cardiol 2005;46(1):57–64.

[51] Sackner-Bernstein J, Aaronson KD. Nesiritide for acute decompensated heart failure: does the benefit justify the risk? Curr Cardiol Rep 2007;9(3):187–93.

[52] Sackner-Bernstein JD, et al. Short-term risk of death after treatment with nesiritide for de-compensated heart failure: a pooled analysis of randomized controlled trials. Jama 2005; 293(15):1900–5.

[53] Hauptman PJ, et al. Use of nesiritide before and after publications suggesting drug-related risks in patients with acute decompensated heart failure. Jama 2006;296(15):1877–84.

[54] Yancy CW, et al. The Second Follow-up Serial Infusions of Nesiritide (FUSION II) trial for advanced heart failure: study rationale and design. Am Heart J 2007;153(4):478–84.

[55] Yancy CW, et al. Safety and feasibility of using serial infusions of nesiritide for heart failure in an outpatient setting (from the FUSION I trial). Am J Cardiol 2004;94(5):595–601.

[56] Shah MR, et al. Testing new targets of therapy in advanced heart failure: the design and ra-tionale of the Strategies for Tailoring Advanced Heart Failure Regimens in the Outpatient Setting: BRain NatrIuretic Peptide Versus the Clinical CongesTion ScorE (STARBRITE) trial. Am Heart J 2005;150(5):893–8.

[57] Mentzer RM Jr, et al. Effects of perioperative nesiritide in patients with left ventricular dys-function undergoing cardiac surgery:the NAPA Trial. J Am Coll Cardiol 2007;49(6):716–26.

[58] Leier CV, Binkley PF. Parenteral inotropic support for advanced congestive heart failure. Prog Cardiovasc Dis 1998;41(3):207–24.

[59] Elkayam U, et al. Use and impact of inotropes and vasodilator therapy in hospitalized pa-tients with severe heart failure. Am Heart J 2007;153(1):98–104.

[60] Leier CV. Positive inotropic therapy: an update and new agents. Curr Probl Cardiol 1996; 21(8):521–81.

[61] Cuffe MS, et al. Short-term intravenous milrinone for acute exacerbation of chronic heart failure: a randomized controlled trial. Jama 2002;287(12):1541–7.

[62] Felker GM, et al. Heart failure etiology and response to milrinone in decompensated heart failure: results from the OPTIME-CHF study. J Am Coll Cardiol 2003;41(6):997–1003.

[63] Pagani FD, et al. Extracorporeal life support to left ventricular assist device bridge to heart transplant: A strategy to optimize survival and resource utilization. Circulation 1999; 100(19 Suppl):II206–10.

[64] Burkhoff D, et al. A randomized multicenter clinical study to evaluate the safety and efficacy of the TandemHeart percutaneous ventricular assist device versus conventional therapy with intraaortic balloon pumping for treatment of cardiogenic shock. Am Heart J 2006;152(3): 469, e1–8.

[65] Chandra D, et al. Usefulness of percutaneous left ventricular assist device as a bridge to re-covery from myocarditis. Am J Cardiol 2007;99(12):1755–6.

[66] Lietz K, et al. Outcomes of left ventricular assist device implantation as destination therapy in the post-REMATCH era: implications for patient selection. Circulation 2007;116(5): 497–505.

[67] Costanzo MR, et al. Ultrafiltration versus intravenous diuretics for patients hospitalized for acute decompensated heart failure. J Am Coll Cardiol 2007;49(6):675–83.

[68] Jaski BE, et al. Peripherally inserted veno-venous ultrafiltration for rapid treatment of vol-ume overloaded patients. J Card Fail 2003;9(3):227–31.

[69] Hunt SA. ACC/AHA 2005 guideline update for the diagnosis and management of chronic heart failure in the adult: a report of the American College of Cardiology/American Heart Association Task Force on Practice Guidelines (Writing Committee to Update the 2001 Guidelines for the Evaluation and Management of Heart Failure). J Am Coll Cardiol 2005;46(6):e1–82.

[70] Effect of enalapril on survival in patients with reduced left ventricular ejection fractions and congestive heart failure. The SOLVD Investigators. N Engl J Med 1991;325(5):293–302.

[71] Sculpher MJ, et al. Low doses vs. high doses of the angiotensin converting-enzyme inhibitor lisinopril in chronic heart failure: a cost-effectiveness analysis based on the Assessment of Treatment with Lisinopril and Survival (ATLAS) study. The ATLAS Study Group. Eur J Heart Fail 2000;2(4):447–54.

[72] Packer M, et al. The effect of carvedilol on morbidity and mortality in patients with chronic heart failure. U.S. Carvedilol Heart Failure Study Group. N Engl J Med 1996;334(21): 1349–55.

[73] Effect of metoprolol CR/XL in chronic heart failure: Metoprolol CR/XL Randomised Intervention Trial in Congestive Heart Failure (MERIT-HF). Lancet 1999;353(9169):2001–7.

[74] The effect of digoxin on mortality and morbidity in patients with heart failure. The Digitalis Investigation Group. N Engl J Med 1997;336(8):525–33.

[75] Pitt B, et al. The effect of spironolactone on morbidity and mortality in patients with severe heart failure. Randomized Aldactone Evaluation Study Investigators. N Engl J Med 1999; 341(10):709–17.

[76] Baliga RR, et al. Spironolactone treatment and clinical outcomes in patients with systolic dysfunction and mild heart failure symptoms: a retrospective analysis. J Card Fail 2006; 12(4):250–6.

[77] Pitt B, et al. Eplerenone, a selective aldosterone blocker, in patients with left ventricular dysfunction after myocardial infarction. N Engl J Med 2003;348(14):1309–21.

[78] Krumholz HM, et al. Readmission after hospitalization for congestive heart failure among Medicare beneficiaries. Arch Intern Med 1997;157(1):99–104.

[79] Koelling TM, et al. Discharge education improves clinical outcomes in patients with chronic heart failure. Circulation 2005;111(2):179–85.

[80] Inglis SC, et al. Extending the horizon in chronic heart failure: effects of multidisciplinary, home-based intervention relative to usual care. Circulation 2006;114(23):2466–73.

[81] Murray MD, et al. Pharmacist intervention to improve medication adherence in heart failure: a randomized trial. Ann Intern Med 2007;146(10):714–25.

[82] Holland R, et al. Systematic review of multidisciplinary interventions in heart failure. Heart 2005;91(7):899–906.

[83] Fonarow GC, et al. Temporal trends in clinical characteristics, treatments, and outcomes for heart failure hospitalizations, 2002 to 2004: findings from Acute Decompensated Heart Failure National Registry (ADHERE). Am Heart J 2007;153(6):1021–8.

[84] Nohria A, Lewis E, Stevenson LW. Medical management of advanced heart failure. Jama 2002;287(5):628–40.

ELSEVIER
SAUNDERS

Crit Care Clin 23 (2007) 759–777

CRITICAL
CARE
CLINICS

Cardiogenic Shock Complicating
Myocardial Infarction

Hitinder S. Gurm, MD, Eric R. Bates, MD*

*Division of Cardiovascular Medicine, Department of Internal Medicine, University
of Michigan, Cardiovascular Center, 1500 East Medical Center Drive,
Ann Arbor, MI 48109-5869, USA*

The organization of coronary care units in the 1960s to treat lethal arrhythmias and the development of reperfusion therapy in the 1980s to reduce infarct size were major breakthroughs in reducing the morbidity and mortality associated with acute myocardial infarction (MI). Unfortunately, the incidence of cardiogenic shock has remained unchanged over the past two decades, despite dramatic advances in MI treatment [1,2]. Cardiogenic shock, not arrhythmia, is now the primary cause of death in patients hospitalized with MI [3,4]. Reducing mortality rates as high as 80% to less than 50% requires excellent supportive care and an aggressive approach to infarct artery revascularization [5]. One-year outcome for hospital survivors is good with 80% alive and 80% in New York Heart Association congestive heart failure class I or II [6]; over 60% are alive at 6 years [7].

Definition

Cardiogenic shock is defined as a state of inadequate tissue perfusion resulting from severe impairment of ventricular pump function in the presence of adequate intravascular volume. It is important to separate the shock state, in which tissue blood flow and oxygen delivery are inadequate to meet metabolic demands, from hypotension, in which tissue metabolic demands may be met by increasing cardiac output or decreasing systemic resistance. Patients in cardiogenic shock generally must have:

---

* Corresponding author. Division of Cardiovascular Medicine, Department of Internal Medicine, University of Michigan, B1 238 Taubman Center, 1500 East Medical Center Drive, Ann Arbor, MI 48109-0022.

E-mail address: ebates@umich.edu (E.R. Bates).

0749-0704/07/$ - see front matter © 2007 Elsevier Inc. All rights reserved.
doi:10.1016/j.ccc.2007.06.004
criticalcare.theclinics.com

- A sustained systolic blood pressure less than 90 mm Hg (or 30 mm Hg below baseline mean arterial pressure) for at least 30 minutes (or the need for vasopressors or intra-aortic balloon pump [IABP] counterpulsation to maintain the systolic blood pressure above 90 mm Hg)
- A cardiac index less than 2.2 L/min/m^2 not related to hypovolemia (pulmonary artery wedge pressure less than 12 mm Hg), arrhythmia, hypoxemia, acidosis, or atrioventricular block
- Evidence of tissue hypoperfusion (oliguria, altered mental status, or peripheral vasoconstriction)

Most patients have left ventricular (LV) failure [8]; right ventricular (RV) failure is present in only 3% of patients [9]. Mechanical causes of cardiogenic shock, including acute mitral regurgitation, ventricular septal rupture, and ventricular free wall rupture, account for approximately 12% of cases [10–12].

Incidence

The incidence has remained unchanged over the past 25 years, with approximately 8% of patients with ST elevation MI [1,2] and 2.5% of patients with non-ST segment elevation MI developing cardiogenic shock [13,14]. The latter group is more likely to have circumflex artery occlusion, comorbid disease, and severe three-vessel disease or left main disease [14]. Risk factors for developing cardiogenic shock include older age, anterior MI location, hypertension, diabetes mellitus, multivessel coronary artery disease, prior MI, prior congestive heart failure, ST elevation MI, or left bundle branch block [4]. Cardiogenic shock usually develops early after onset of symptoms, with approximately half the patients developing shock within 6 hours and 72% within 24 hours [15]. Others first develop a preshock state manifested by systemic hypoperfusion without hypotension [16]. These patients benefit from aggressive supportive therapy and revascularization; early intervention may abort the onset of cardiogenic shock.

Pathogenesis

Most patients develop cardiogenic shock because of extensive myocardial ischemia or necrosis, which directly impairs myocardial contractility and results in diminished stroke volume and arterial pressure. A large first infarction can initiate cardiogenic shock, or it may result from reinfarction or infarct extension in the same territory or from cumulative smaller infarctions. Triple vessel disease (60%) or left main disease (20%) is often present [17]. The pathophysiology of cardiogenic shock, however, is more complicated than a reduction in myocardial contractility. In fact, LV ejection fraction may be only moderately depressed acutely and unchanged days later when functional status has improved. Contributing to the acute shock state is a series of neurohormonal responses, including activation of the sympathetic nervous system and the renin–angiotensin system because of a perceived reduction in circulating volume and pressure. These cause peripheral vasoconstriction and salt and water retention. A systemic inflammatory state with high plasma levels of cytokines (eg, tumor necrosis factor-alpha, interleukin-6) and inappropriate nitric oxide production additionally may depress myocardial function or impair catecholamine-induced vasoconstriction, respectively. All of these factors in turn lead to diminished coronary artery perfusion and thus trigger a vicious cycle of further myocardial ischemia and necrosis, resulting in even lower blood pressure, lactic acidosis, multiple organ failure, and ultimately death (Fig. 1).

Clinical presentation

Rapid assessment of patients presenting in shock is critical to determine subsequent therapy [18]. Aortic dissection, tension pneumothorax, massive pulmonary embolism, ruptured viscus, hemorrhage, and sepsis need to be excluded as etiologies for the shock state. A limited, relevant history should be obtained while resuscitative efforts are proceeding. Physical examination generally reveals an ashen or cyanotic patient who may be confused or

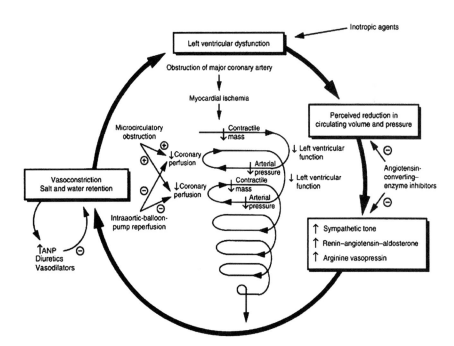

Fig. 1. The vicious cycle of mechanical and neurohormonal events that lead to progressive cardiogenic shock and death in MI. (*Adapted from* Pasternak RC, Braunwald E. Acute myocardial infarction. In: Wilson JD, Braunwald E, Isselbacher KJ, editors. Harrison's principles of internal medicine. 12th ed. Vol. 1. New York: McGraw-Hill, 1991:953–64; and Francis GS. Neuroendocrine manifestations of congestive heart failure. Am J Cardiol 1988;62:Suppl:9A–13A; with permission.)

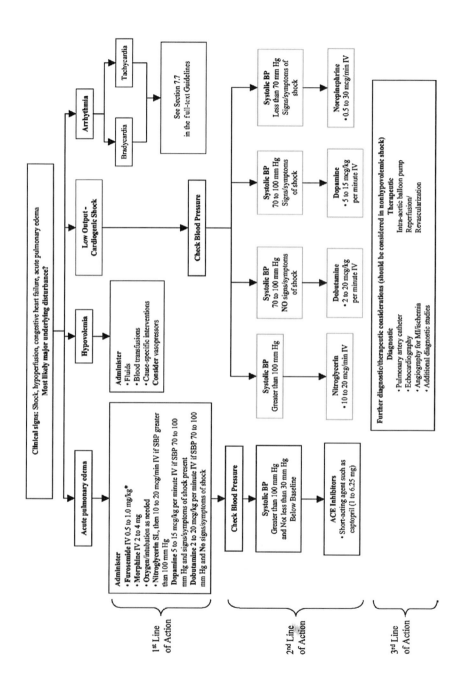

agitated secondary to inadequate cerebral perfusion. The pulses are rapid and faint, the pulse pressure is narrow, and arrhythmias are common. Jugular venous distention and pulmonary rales are usually present in LV shock, whereas jugular venous distention, Kussmaul's sign (a paradoxical increase in jugular venous pressure during inspiration), and absent rales usually are found in RV shock. The cardiovascular examination generally reveals distant heart sounds. Third and fourth heart sounds or a summation gallop may be auscultated. Although the presence of a systolic murmur may suggest ventricular septal rupture or acute mitral regurgitation, the absence of a murmur does not exclude these complications. The extremities usually are vasoconstricted.

Initial diagnostic strategies should include a 12-lead electrocardiogram, a chest radiograph, arterial blood gas measurement, electrolytes, complete blood count, coagulation values, and cardiac enzymes. Most patients will have ECG findings of acute ST elevation myocardial infarction. A large anterior or anterolateral infarction pattern is often present. In others, the ECG may show old Q waves or diffuse ST depression. A relatively normal ECG should alert one to other causes of shock such as cardiac tamponade, aortic dissection, or hemorrhage. Right precordial leads should be recorded in the setting of inferior MI to evaluate for right ventricular infarction. Third-degree atrioventricular block or left bundle branch block are ominous findings. Lactic acidosis, hypoxemia, and mixed venous oxygen desaturation are usually present.

Bedside echocardiography is a critical tool in determining the etiology of cardiogenic shock [19,20]. A dilated, hypokinetic left ventricle suggests LV shock, whereas a dilated right ventricle suggests RV involvement. Normal ventricular function, low cardiac output, and mitral regurgitation are consistent with acute severe mitral regurgitation. Pericardial tamponade from free wall rupture can be detected quickly. The Doppler evaluation can confirm the presence of significant mitral regurgitation or ventricular septal rupture easily. Transesophageal echo is helpful in patients where image quality is inadequate or when a flail mitral leaflet is suspected but not seen on transthoracic echocardiography.

Initial stabilization

Initial resuscitation is aimed at stabilizing oxygenation and perfusion while revascularization is contemplated. A careful fluid challenge should

←─────────────────────────────

Fig. 2. Emergency management of complicated ST-elevation myocardial infarction. *Abbreviations:* ACE, angiotensin converting enzyme; BP, blood pressure; IV, intravenous; MI, myocardial infarction; SBP, systolic blood pressure; SL, sublingual. (*Adapted from* Antman EM, Anbe DT, Armstrong PW, et al. ACC/AHA guidelines for the management of patients with ST-elevation myocardial infarction: a report of the American College of Cardiology/American Heart Association Task Force on Practice Guidelines (Committee to Revise the 1999 Guidelines for the Management of Patients with Acute Myocardial Infarction). Circulation 2004; 110:e82–92.)

be used to exclude hypovolemic shock, unless the patient is in obvious pulmonary edema (Fig. 2). Prespecified boluses should be administered and followed by careful assessment of clinical endpoints such as urine output, blood pressure, and heart rate. In RV shock, where preload is critical, fluid support and avoidance of nitrates and morphine are indicated.

Oxygenation and airway support usually require tracheal intubation and mechanical ventilation (Box 1). Positive end-expiratory pressure (PEEP) decreases preload and afterload. Muscular paralysis (in addition to sedation) improves procedural safety and decreases oxygen demand. Urine output needs to be monitored hourly through catheter drainage. An arterial catheter allows constant monitoring of blood pressure. Central hemodynamic monitoring using a pulmonary artery catheter can provide valuable information and aid in the titration of fluids and medications. Specific hemodynamic profiles include:

- Left ventricular shock: high pulmonary capillary wedge pressure (PCWP), low cardiac output (CO), high systemic vascular resistance (SVR)
- Right ventricular shock: high right atrial (RA), RA/PCWP greater than 0.8, exaggerated RA y descent, RV square root sign
- Mitral regurgitation: large PCWP v wave
- Ventricular septal defect: large PCWP v wave, oxygen saturation step-up (greater than 5%) from RA to RV
- Pericardial tamponade: equalization of diastolic pressures approximately 20 mm Hg

Cardiac power (mean arterial pressure times cardiac output/451) is the strongest hemodynamic predictor of hospital mortality [21]. Although use of the pulmonary artery catheter has not been associated with mortality benefit in patients without MI, it is very helpful in managing cardiogenic shock.

Box 1. Conventional therapy for cardiogenic shock

Maximize volume (right atrial pressure 10 to 14 mm Hg, PCWP 18 to 20 mm Hg)
Maximize oxygenation (eg, ventilator)
Control rhythm (eg, pacemaker, cardioversion)
Correct electrolyte and acid–base imbalances
Sympathomimetic amines (eg, dobutamine, dopamine, norepinephrine, phenylephrine)
Phosphodiesterase inhibitors (eg, milrinone)
Vasodilators (eg, nitroglycerin, nitroprusside)
Diuretics (eg, furosemide)
Antiarrhythmics (eg, amiodarone)
Intra-aortic balloon counterpulsation

Sustained atrial and ventricular tachyarrhythmias should be converted electrically to sinus rhythm to maximize cardiac output. Often, agents such as amiodarone are required to maintain sinus rhythm. Likewise, bradycardia and high-degree heart block should be treated with atropine or temporary pacing. Atrioventricular pacing is preferable, especially in the setting of RV failure [22].

Hypokalemia and hypomagnesemia predispose to ventricular arrhythmias and should be corrected. Hyperventilation may be required to correct metabolic acidosis, but sodium bicarbonate should be avoided, given a short half-life and the large sodium load. Aspirin and heparin should be administered to facilitate further invasive care and to prevent reinfarction, ventricular mural thrombus formation, or deep venous thrombosis. Clopidogrel is best withheld until cardiac catheterization has determined the need for emergency surgery because of its prolonged action and increased risk for perioperative bleeding. Morphine sulfate decreases pain, excessive sympathetic activity, preload, and afterload, but should only be administered in small increments. Diuretics decrease filling pressures and should be used to control volume. Beta-blockers and calcium channel blockers should be avoided, because they are negative inotropic agents.

Inotropic and vasopressor drugs are the major initial interventions for reversing hypotension and improving vital organ perfusion (Box 2). The choice of sympathomimetic agents should be dictated by hemodynamic parameters, which often change as the clinical condition evolves and complications develop. Beta agonists enhance contractility and can provide support until stunned and reperfused myocardium recovers. They also induce tachycardia, can worsen myocardial ischemia in the peri-infarct zone, and enhance arrhythmogenicity, however. The lowest dose needed to support the circulation should be used, and, as the patient's condition improves or as other means of support are instituted, the dose should be titrated down

---

Box 2. Pharmacologic treatment

Drugs and doses
Dobutamine: 2–20 mcg/kg/min IV
Dopamine: 5–15 mcg/kg/min IV
Norepinephrine: 0.5–30 mcg/min IV
Phenylephrine: 0.1–0.5 mcg/kg/min IV
Nitroglycerin: 10 mcg/min, increased by 10 mcg every 10 min
Nitroprusside: 10 mcg/min, increased by 5 mcg every 10 min
Milrinone: 50 mcg/kg over 10 min, then 0.375–0.75 mcg/kg/min
Furosemide: 20–160 mg IV
Bumetanide: 1–3 mg IV
Amiodarone: 150 mg over 10 min, 1 mg/min over 6 hours,
    0.5 mg/min over 18 hours

to the minimum dose required to provide circulatory support. Dobutamine increases myocardial contractility and induces peripheral vasodilation. It has less of a chronotropic response compared with dopamine, and its short half-life (2 minutes) makes it an ideal inotropic agent in patients who have systolic blood pressure greater than 70 mm Hg. Dopamine is the preferred initial pressor agent in hypotensive patients who have systolic blood pressure greater than 70 mm Hg. For refractory hypotension, norepinephrine or phenylephrine may be added to maintain perfusion to vital organs. Epinephrine is a powerful alpha and beta stimulant, and given its unselective nature, it is used only in setting of cardiac arrest. Milrinone has a longer half-life and rarely is used in patients with cardiogenic shock.

Intra-aortic balloon counterpulsation

When pharmacological therapy provides insufficient hemodynamic support, mechanical circulatory assistance can be instituted. The best use of intra-aortic balloon pump (IABP) counterpulsation is in patients who have ischemic, viable, but nonfunctioning myocardium that can be revascularized, or with mitral regurgitation or ventricular septal rupture amenable to surgical repair. IABP counterpulsation offers little support to shock patients with extensively scarred ventricles or after late presentation. Observational data show no mortality reduction benefit for IABP counterpulsation in the reperfusion era [23]. Therefore, IABP counterpulsation should be considered a stabilizing measure that facilitates reperfusion strategies. The pump is designed to inflate a balloon in the descending aorta during cardiac diastole, leading to an increase in diastolic blood pressure, and then to deflate it just before the onset of systole, creating a potential space in the aorta that then leads to decreased systemic vascular resistance, reductions in end-systolic and end-diastolic volumes, and reduced LV wall tension. Because of these effects, pulmonary capillary wedge pressure and myocardial oxygen demand decrease; subendocardial blood flow improves, and cardiac output increases. No improvement in coronary blood flow occurs in highly stenotic coronary arteries, however [24]. This likely explains why there is no improvement in infarct size reduction or survival with IABP use, despite hemodynamic improvement in 60% to 70% of patients [25,26].

Several reports have examined the use of the IABP counterpulsation in conjunction with fibrinolytic strategies [27–31]. There were some favorable trends, but significantly more bleeding episodes. There has been only one randomized controlled trial comparing IABP counterpulsation plus fibrinolytic therapy with fibrinolysis alone. The Thrombolysis and Counterpulsation to Improve Cardiogenic Shock Survival (TACTICS) trial [31] sought to enroll 500 patients with acute ST elevation MI complicated by shock. Unfortunately, only 57 patients were enrolled. Six-month follow-up showed a trend toward mortality reduction in the IABP group, but this was not significant because of small sample size. The strategy of early fibrinolytic therapy and IABP counterpulsation, followed by immediate transfer for percutaneous transluminal coronary angioplasty (PTCA) or coronary artery bypass graft (CABG,) may be appropriate for hospitals that do not have revascularization capability.

The use of IABP therapy in patients undergoing primary or rescue percutaneous coronary intervention (PCI) has been evaluated in a few studies. Early data suggested a reduction in infarct artery reocclusion rates and improvement in clinical outcome in patients without cardiogenic shock [32,33]. A more recent trial [34], however, failed to demonstrate any improvement in recovery of LV function or survival, and hence its use is best restricted to patients who have hemodynamic instability. In patients who have cardiogenic shock, the IABP catheter needs to be inserted before angiography to provide optimal hemodynamic support during the procedure.

The American College of Cardiology/American Heart Association ST elevation myocardial infarction (STEMI) guidelines have given a class I (general agreement that a procedure/treatment should be performed/administered) recommendation to IABP therapy for:

- Cardiogenic shock not quickly reversed with pharmacological therapy as a stabilizing measure for angiography and prompt revascularization
- Acute mitral regurgitation or ventricular septal defect complicating MI as a stabilizing therapy for angiography and repair/revascularization
- Refractory post-MI angina as a bridge to angiography and revascularization [35]

Contraindications for IABP counterpulsation include aortic regurgitation, aortic dissection, and peripheral vascular disease. Prolonged use of IABP counterpulsation is associated with complications in 10% to 30% of patients in cardiogenic shock. These include limb ischemia, femoral artery laceration, aortic dissection, infection, hemolysis, thrombocytopenia, thrombosis, and embolism.

Reperfusion strategies

Fibrinolytic therapy

Treatment of MI with fibrinolytic therapy saves lives, reduces infarct size, and preserves left ventricular function [35,36]. It also reduces the risk of subsequent cardiogenic shock in patients who initially present without shock [37–39]. Comparative trials of fibrinolytic agents have shown variable results. Those that show no difference in mortality between agents also do not show a reduction in the incidence of cardiogenic shock with any one agent [40–42]. In contrast, those comparative trials that show a mortality benefit in favor of one agent also show a significant reduction in the incidence of cardiogenic shock in favor of that agent [43–45]. Thus, one can conclude that therapy with fibrinolytic agents in acute MI significantly reduces the subsequent development of cardiogenic shock, and that those agents that are associated with higher patency rates and improved survival in comparative studies also lead to lower rates of shock.

Fibrinolytic therapy for patients presenting in manifest cardiogenic shock is associated with relatively low reperfusion rates and no clear-cut treatment benefit [46]. Mean arterial pressure must be above 65 mm Hg for coronary blood flow to be maintained; flow ceases when mean arterial pressure is below 30 mm Hg. Furthermore, vasoconstriction and passive collapse of the arterial wall are additional factors that may limit the ability of the fibrinolytic agent to penetrate an intracoronary thrombus [47]. Canine studies demonstrated that restoration of blood pressure to normal ranges with norepinephrine infusion improved reperfusion rates, suggesting that coronary perfusion pressure, not cardiac output, is the major determinant of fibrinolytic efficacy [48]. Interestingly, the trials that compared streptokinase with alteplase showed mortality benefit for shock patients randomized to streptokinase, despite the fact that patients treated with alteplase fared better [40,44]. Streptokinase may be beneficial in this subset of patients, because it causes a prolonged lytic state in the setting of low coronary blood flow (which may reduce the risk of reocclusion). Additionally, it is less fibrinspecific and therefore may penetrate the thrombus better, because it does not bind preferentially to the surface of the clot. Because of the limitations of fibrinolytic therapy for cardiogenic shock, it should be considered as a secondary treatment option when revascularization therapy with PCI or CABG is not rapidly available. Viable patients then should be transferred to a hospital with revascularization capability as soon as possible so that the potential benefits of revascularization therapy might still be obtained.

Percutaneous coronary intervention

Multiple observational reports suggest improved survival for patients with cardiogenic shock treated with PCI. Two small randomized trials have been performed. The Swiss Multicenter trial of Angioplasty SHock (SMASH)trial [49] randomized 55 patients to either undergo emergency angiography and revascularization when indicated or initial medical management, but was terminated prematurely because of poor enrollment. Mortality at 30 days was 69% in the invasive arm versus 78% in the medical arm (P = NS). At one year, the mortality figures were 74% and 83%, respectively. Although the study failed to reach statistical significance because of sample size, the trend was clinically important. The SHOCK trial [5–7] randomized 302 patients to emergent revascularization or immediate medical stabilization. Concurrently, the 30 participating sites collected registry data on 1190 patients presenting with cardiogenic shock who were not randomized [50]. Medical stabilization included fibrinolytic therapy in over half the patients as well as inotropic and vasopressor agents. IABP counterpulsation was used in 86% of the patients. In the revascularization arm, 97% of patients underwent early angiography; 64% underwent PCI and 36% had coronary artery bypass graft surgery. There was no statistically significant difference in 30-day mortality between the revascularization and medical therapy groups (46.7% versus 56.0%; $P = .11$), but by the 6-month endpoint, a significant survival advantage had emerged for patients randomized to revascularization (50.3% versus 63.1%, $P = .027$) that was maintained at one year (53.3% versus 66.4%). Patients surviving to hospital discharge had a 6-year survival rate of 62% with revascularization, compared with 44% for early medical stabilization, with an annualized death rate of 8.3% versus 14.3% (Fig. 3). Similar early improvement in survival was noted in the SHOCK registry population after exclusion of those patients presenting with mechanical complications. Of multiple pre-specified subgroup analyses performed in the SHOCK trial, only age ≥ 75 years fared significantly better in the medical stabilization arm of the study than in the revascularization group. The results of the SMASH trial and the SHOCK trial and registry have proven that appropriate candidates with cardiogenic shock complicating acute MI should be referred for coronary angiography and emergent revascularization unless contraindications exist (Fig. 4). Although CABG will be an option for some patients, most will be treated with PCI of the infarct artery.

Analysis of the elderly patient subgroup in the SHOCK Trial registry [51] was performed to gain further insight in patients > 75 yrs of age. Whereas the randomized trial included only 56 patients in that age group, the registry included 277 patients. They were significantly more likely to be women and to have prior history of MI, congestive heart failure, renal insufficiency, and other comorbidities. They were less likely to have therapeutic interventions such as pulmonary artery catheterization, IABP counterpulsation, coronary angiography, PCI, and coronary artery bypass surgery. Overall, in-hospital

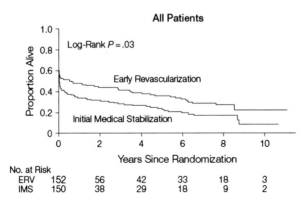

Fig. 3. Kaplan-Meier long-term survival of patients in the SHOCK trial. (*Adapted from* Hochman JS, Sleeper LA, Webb JG, et al. Early revascularization and long-term survival in cardiogenic shock complicating acute myocardial infarction. JAMA 2006;295:2511–5.)

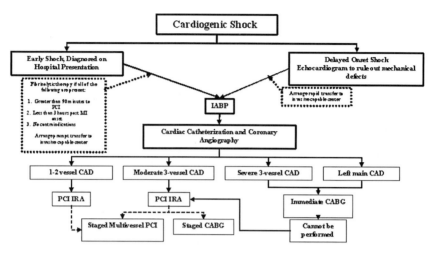

Fig. 4. Recommendations for initial reperfusion therapy. *Abbreviations:* CABG, coronary artery bypass graft surgery; CAD, coronary artery disease; IABP, intra-aortic balloon counterpulsation; IRA, infarct-related artery; LBBB, left bundle branch block; MI, myocardial infarction; PCI, percutaneous coronary intervention. (*Adapted from* Hochman JS. Cardiogenic shock complicating acute myocardial infarction: expanding the paradigm. Circulation 2003;107: 2998–3002.)

mortality in the elderly versus the younger age group was 76% versus 55% (*P* < .001). The 44 elderly patients selected for early revascularization, however, showed a significantly lower mortality rate than those who did not undergo revascularization (48% versus 81%; *P* = .0002). Other reports [52–54] also support the use of primary PCI in selected patients with cardiogenic shock complicating MI, so age alone should not be an exclusion for selecting patients for cardiac catheterization.

Coronary stents decrease restenosis rates by 50% in elective PCI compared with balloon angioplasty, but have not reduced mortality rates in primary PCI [35]. Some observational studies in cardiogenic shock that have not completely corrected for confounding variables suggest lower mortality rates with stents than PTCA [55–57], but others show no benefit [58] or higher mortality rates [59]. Randomized studies have not been performed. Most patients undergoing primary PCI for cardiogenic shock will receive stents because they improve the immediate angiographic result and decrease subsequent target vessel revascularization in survivors.

The use of platelet glycoprotein (GP) IIb/IIIa inhibitors has been demonstrated to improve outcome of patients with acute myocardial infarction undergoing primary PCI [60]. Observational studies suggest a benefit of abciximab in primary stenting for cardiogenic shock [56,57,59,61]. While there are no randomized controlled trials evaluating use of abciximab or other GP IIb/IIIa inhibitors in cardiogenic shock, they are commonly used as adjunctive therapy.

PCI should be performed only when maximal pharmacological and mechanical support has been achieved. Using nonionic contrast medium, two injections of the left coronary artery and one injection of the right coronary artery are made in an attempt to identify the infarct artery. Left ventriculography should usually be avoided because of the contrast medium load. If PCI is to be attempted, it should be performed as quickly and efficiently as possible with limited contrast injections. Although PCI for acute MI is usually limited to the infarct artery, patients in cardiogenic shock with multivessel disease may sometimes have the best survival chance with PCI of all proximal discrete lesions. Surviving patients with multivessel disease can subsequently be considered for additional PCI or CABG to achieve more complete revascularization.

A recent large registry evaluated the outcome of 1333 patients undergoing PCI for cardiogenic shock [62]. The in-hospital mortality in this cohort was 46%. Final TIMI flow was a major predictor of outcome with mortality rates of 78%, 66% and 37% for TIMI 0/1, TIMI 2 and TIMI 3 flow, respectively. The independent predictors of mortality were left main disease, TIMI flow <3 after PCI, older age, three-vessel disease, and longer time interval between symptom onset and PCI.

Surgical revascularization

Emergency coronary artery bypass surgery for patients in cardiogenic shock is associated with mortality rates ranging from 25% to 60% [3]. The SHOCK trial documented that revascularization improved outcomes when compared with medical therapy; one-third of the patients randomized to revascularization in that study were treated with a surgical approach [63]. Patients chosen for surgical revascularization were more likely to have left main disease and three-vessel disease than those treated with PCI. Thirty-day mortality for patients undergoing PCI was equivalent to surgical mortality (45% versus 42%). Those patients presenting with mechanical complications (acute mitral regurgitation due to papillary muscle rupture or LV free wall or septal rupture) require surgical intervention for survival, but carry a poorer prognosis than patients requiring revascularization only.

Various surgical strategies designed to optimize outcomes for patients in cardiogenic shock have been discussed in the literature. The use of warm blood cardioplegia enriched with glutamate and aspartate, grafting of large areas of viable myocardium first followed by treatment of the infarct artery last, and preferential or sole use of saphenous vein grafts that can be quickly harvested and provide high initial flow rates have all been advocated.

Other mechanical support devices

Devices that offer greater circulatory support than IABP counterpulsation are available and have been used in cardiogenic shock as a bridge to recovery or to transplantation. These devices may be classified into those that can be placed percutaneously and those that require surgical placement. It is critical to recognize which patients will require greater hemodynamic support than provided by IABP therapy.

Percutaneous cardiopulmonary bypass can be initiated at the bedside via the femoral artery and vein and can provide 3 to 5 L/min of nonpulsatile flow and a mean aortic pressure of 50 to 70 mm Hg despite cardiac standstill [64]. Support is limited to several hours because of blood cell destruction. A recent review of 42 studies (533 patients) suggested a mean survival to discharge of 51% (median 38%) among patients with cardiogenic shock treated with percutaneous bypass [65]. Extracorporeal life support (ECLS) also has been used in critically ill patients and 33% survival to discharge for adult cardiogenic shock patients has been reported [66]. These results are encouraging since ECLS in these cases has typically been placed percutaneously during arrest or near-arrest circumstances, when the expected mortality would be 100%. Left ventricular decompression is not possible with these devices.

Another strategy has been to use ventricular assist devices (VADs) as a bridge to recovery or to transplant. These devices can be placed percutaneously or surgically. The standard left heart support configuration of the percutaneous ventricular assist device (Tandem-Heart, Cardiac Assist, Pittsburgh, PA) uses a 21 F femoral cannula placed across the interatrial septum into the left atrium, while a shorter 15 or 17 F cannula is placed in the iliac artery, allowing left atrial to arterial assist pumping by an extracorporeal centrifugal pump [67,68]. This device has been successfully used in cardiogenic shock from LV failure [67] and RV failure (right atrial to pulmonary artery bypass) [69]. A small trial recently compared IABP counterpulsation and the percutaneous ventricular assist device (PVAD) in patients undergoing primary PCI for acute MI complicated by cardiogenic shock. While the PVAD provided better hemodynamic support, the risk of complications was higher and there was no difference in 30-day mortality [70]. Surgically implanted VADs have also been used in cardiogenic shock. These devices require placement via thoracotomy, but can be left in place long-term. In a recent single center series, the Thoratec biventricular assist device was used as a successful bridge to cardiac transplantation in 11/19 patients in cardiogenic shock [71]. Both percutaneous and surgical VADs are available only at select centers and early transfer of patients to these facilities should be considered for patients failing standard supportive measures.

New approaches

New approaches to cardiogenic shock have focused on mechanisms beyond mechanical support and revascularization. A significant proportion of patients in the SHOCK trial exhibited a systemic inflammatory response syndrome marked by fever, leukocytosis, and low systemic vascular resistance [72]. Complement activation, release of inflammatory cytokines, expression of inducible nitric oxide synthase (NOS), and inappropriate vasodilation were deemed culpable and inhibition of NO production was explored as a therapeutic strategy. Early single center clinical studies indicated a dramatic benefit from inhibition of nitric oxide synthase [73,74]. The phase 2, dose-ranging trial SHOCK -2 (Should We Inhibit Nitric Oxide Synthase in cardiogenic Shock 2) demonstrated modest early changes in hemodynamic parameters, but no effect on survival [75]. The large multicenter Tilarginine Acetate Injection in a Randomized International Study in Unstable MI Patients with Cardiogenic Shock (TRIUMPH) trial was recently halted after no benefit was seen during an interim analysis [76].

There is intense clinical and basic science activity exploring delivery of stem cells to the infracted myocardium to improve LV recovery. While the early studies remain inconclusive, it is likely that cardiogenic shock patients will be enrolled in the pivotal trials once an effective strategy to salvage or revive the infarcted myocardium is discovered.

Summary

Cardiogenic shock remains the leading cause of death for patients hospitalized with MI. Rapid diagnosis should be pursued using clinical, electrocardiographic, and echocardiographic information. Institution of supportive therapy including vasopressor and inotropic agents, mechanical ventilatory support, and IABP counterpulsation are important interventions. Critical to improving the grave prognosis, however, is rapid reperfusion of the occluded infarct artery. Revascularization by either PCI or CABG is the only intervention been shown to reduce mortality rates, which can be as high as 70% to 80%. Fibrinolytic therapy with IABP counterpulsation should be considered if revascularization therapy is not rapidly available. Survivors, however, should be transferred to hospitals with revascularization capability as soon as feasible. When IABP counterpulsation fails to improve hemodynamic stability, percutaneous or surgically placed VADs may be useful in select patients. Novel therapies are needed to further decrease mortality rates, which remain high despite reperfusion therapy.

References

[1] Goldberg RJ, Samad NA, Yarzebski J, et al. Temporal trends in cardiogenic shock complicating acute myocardial infarction. N Engl J Med 1999;340:1162–8.

[2] Babaev A, Frederick PD, Pasta DJ, et al. Trends in management and outcomes of patients with acute myocardial infarction complicated by cardiogenic shock. JAMA 2005;294: 448–54.

[3] Bates ER, Moscucci M. Postmyocardial infarction cardiogenic shock. In: Brown DL, editor. Cardiac intensive care. Philadelphia: WB Saunders Co; 1998. p. 215–27.

[4] Reynolds HR, Hochman JS. Cardiogenic shock complicating acute myocardial infarction: current concept and improving outcomes. Circulation, in press.

[5] Hochman JS, Sleeper LA, Webb JG, et al. Early revascularization in acute myocardial infarction complicated by cardiogenic shock. SHOCK Investigators. SHould we

emergently revascularize Occluded Coronaries for cardiogenic shocK. N Engl J Med 1999; 341:625–34.

[6] Hochman JS, Sleeper LA, White HD, et al. One-year survival following early revascularization for cardiogenic shock. JAMA 2001;285:190–2.

[7] Hochman JS, Sleeper LA, Webb JG, et al. Early revascularization and long-term survival in cardiogenic shock complicating acute myocardial infarction. JAMA 2006;295:2511–5.

[8] Menon V, White H, LeJemtel T, et al. The clinical profile of patients with suspected cardiogenic shock due to predominant left ventricular failure: a report from the SHOCK Trial Registry. SHould we emergently revascularize Occluded Coronaries in cardiogenic shocK? J Am Coll Cardiol 2000;36:1071–6.

[9] Jacobs AK, Leopold JA, Bates E, et al. Cardiogenic shock caused by right ventricular infarction: a report from the SHOCK registry. J Am Coll Cardiol 2003;41:1273–9.

[10] Thompson CR, Buller CE, Sleeper LA, et al. Cardiogenic shock due to acute severe mitral regurgitation complicating acute myocardial infarction: a report from the SHOCK Trial Registry. SHould we use emergently revascularize Occluded Coronaries in cardiogenic shocK? J Am Coll Cardiol 2000;36:1104–9.

[11] Menon V, Webb JG, Hillis LD, et al. Outcome and profile of ventricular septal rupture with cardiogenic shock after myocardial infarction: a report from the SHOCK trial registry. J Am Coll Cardiol 2000;36:1110–6.

[12] Slater J, Brown RJ, Antonelli TA, et al. Cardiogenic shock due to cardiac free-wall rupture or tamponade after acute myocardial infarction: a report from the SHOCK trial registry. J Am Coll Cardiol 2000;36:1117–22.

[13] Holmes DR Jr, Berger PB, Hochman JS, et al. Cardiogenic shock in patients with acute ischemic syndromes with and without ST-segment elevation. Circulation 1999;100:2067–73.

[14] Jacobs AK, French JK, Col J, et al. Cardiogenic shock with non-ST-segment elevation myocardial infarction: a report from the SHOCK Trial Registry. SHould we emergently revascularize Occluded Coronaries for cardiogenic shocK? J Am Coll Cardiol 2000;36: 1091–6.

[15] Webb JG, Sleeper LA, Buller CE, et al. Implications of the timing of onset of cardiogenic shock after acute myocardial infarction: a report from the SHOCK Trial Registry. SHould we emergently revascularize Occluded Coronaries for cardiogenic shocK? J Am Coll Cardiol 2000;36:1084–90.

[16] Menon V, Slater JN, White HD, et al. Acute myocardial infarction complicated by systemic hypoperfusion without hypotension: report of the SHOCK trial registry. Am J Med 2000; 108:374–80.

[17] Sanborn TA, Sleeper LA, Webb JG, et al. Correlates of one-year survival in patients with cardiogenic shock complicating acute myocardial infarction. Angiographic findings from the SHOCK trial. J Am Coll Cardiol 2003;42:1373–9.

[18] Hollenberg SM. Clinical assessment and initial management of cardiogenic shock. In: Hollenberg SM, Bates ER, editors. Cardiogenic shock. Armonk (NY): Futura; 2002. p. 45–59.

[19] Nishimura RA, Tajik AJ, Shub C, et al. Role of two-dimensional echocardiography in the prediction of in-hospital complications after acute myocardial infarction. J Am Coll Cardiol 1984;4:1080–7.

[20] Picard MH, Davidoff R, Sleeper LA, et al. Echocardiographic predictors of survival and response to early revascularization in cardiogenic shock. Circulation 2003;107:279–84.

[21] Fincke R, Hochman JS, Lowe A, et al. Cardiac power is the strongest hemodynamic correlate of mortality in cardiogenic shock: a report from the SHOCK trial registry. J Am Coll Cardiol 2004;44:340–8.

[22] Topol EJ, Goldschlager N, Ports TA, et al. Hemodynamic benefit of atrial pacing in right ventricular myocardial infarction. Ann Intern Med 1982;96:594–7.

[23] Hudson MP, Ohman EM. Intra-aortic balloon counterpulsation for cardiogenic shock complicating acute myocardial infarction. In: Hollenberg SM, Bates ER, editors. Cardiogenic shock. Armonk (NY): Futura; 2002. p. 81–102.

[24] Kern MJ, Aguirre F, Bach R, et al. Augmentation of coronary blood flow by intra-aortic balloon pumping in patients after coronary angioplasty. Circulation 1993;87:500–11.

[25] Scheidt S, Wilner G, Mueller H, et al. Intra-aortic balloon counterpulsation in cardiogenic shock. Report of a cooperative clinical trial. N Engl J Med 1973;288:979–84.

[26] O'Rourke MF, Norris RM, Campbell TJ, et al. Randomized controlled trial of intra-aortic balloon counterpulsation in early myocardial infarction with acute heart failure. Am J Cardiol 1981;47:815–20.

[27] Anderson RD, Ohman EM, Holmes DR Jr, et al. Use of intra-aortic balloon counterpulsation in patients presenting with cardiogenic shock: observations from the GUSTO-I study. J Am Coll Cardiol 1997;30:708–15.

[28] Kovach PJ, Rasak MA, Bates ER, et al. Thrombolysis plus aortic counterpulsation: improved survival in patients who present to community hospitals with cardiogenic shock. J Am Coll Cardiol 1997;29:1454–8.

[29] Barron HV, Every NR, Parsons LS, et al. The use of intra-aortic balloon counterpulsation in patients with cardiogenic shock complicating acute myocardial infarction: data from the National Registry of Myocardial Infarction 2. Am Heart J 2001;141:933–9.

[30] Sanborn TA, Sleeper LA, Bates ER, et al. Impact of thrombolysis, intra-aortic balloon pump counterpulsation, and their combination in cardiogenic shock complicating acute myocardial infarction: a report from the SHOCK trial registry. J Am Coll Cardiol 2000;36:1123–9.

[31] Ohman EM, Nanas J, Stomel RJ, et al. Thrombolysis and counterpulsation to improve survival in myocardial infarction complicated by hypotension and suspected cardiogenic shock or heart failure: results of the TACTICS Trial. J Thromb Thrombolysis 2005;19: 33–9.

[32] Ohman EM, George BS, White CJ, et al. Use of aortic counterpulsation to improve sustained coronary artery patency during acute myocardial infarction. Results of a randomized trial. The Randomized IABP Study Group. Circulation 1994;90:792–9.

[33] Ishihara M, Sato H, Tateishi H, et al. Intra-aortic balloon pumping as adjunctive therapy to rescue coronary angioplasty after failed thrombolysis in anterior wall acute myocardial infarction. Am J Cardiol 1995;76:73–5.

[34] Stone GW, Marsalese D, Brodie BR, et al. A prospective, randomized evaluation of prophylactic intra-aortic balloon counterpulsation in high-risk patients with acute myocardial infarction treated with primary angioplasty. J Am Coll Cardiol 1997;29:1459–67.

[35] Antman EM, Anbe DT, Armstrong PW, et al. ACC/AHA guidelines for the management of patients with ST-elevation myocardial infarction: a report of the American College of Cardiology/American Heart Association Task Force on Practice Guidelines (Committee to Revise the 1999 Guidelines for the Management of Patients with Acute Myocardial Infarction). Circulation 2004;110:e82–292.

[36] Fibrinolytic Therapy Trialists' (FTT) Collaborative Group. Indications for fibrinolytic therapy in suspected acute myocardial infarction: collaborative overview of early mortality and major morbidity results from all randomised trials of more than 1000 patients. Lancet 1994; 343:311–22.

[37] Meinertz T, Kasper W, Schumacher M, et al. The German multicenter trial of anisoylated plasminogen streptokinase activator complex versus heparin for acute myocardial infarction. Am J Cardiol 1988;62:347–51.

[38] Wilcox RG, von der Lippe G, Olsson CG, et al. Trial of tissue plasminogen activator for mortality reduction in acute myocardial infarction; Anglo-Scandinavian Study of Early Thrombolysis (ASSET). Lancet 1988;2:525–30.

[39] AIMS Trial Study Group. Long-term effects of intravenous anistreplase in acute myocardial infarction: final report of the AIMS study. Lancet 1990;335:427–31.

[40] The International Study Group. In-hospital mortality and clinical course of 20,891 patients with suspected acute myocardial infarction randomised between alteplase and streptokinase with or without heparin. Lancet 1990;336:71–5.

[41] ISIS-3 (Third International Study of Infarct Survival) Collaborative Group. ISIS-3: a randomised comparison of streptokinase vs tissue plasminogen activator vs anistreplase and of aspirin plus heparin vs aspirin alone among 41,299 cases of suspected acute myocardial infarction. Lancet 1992;339:753–70.

[42] The Global Use of Strategies to Open Occluded Coronary Arteries (GUSTO III) Investigators. A comparison of reteplase with alteplase for acute myocardial infarction. N Engl J Med 1997;337:1118–23.

[43] Neuhaus KL, von Essen R, Tebbe U, et al. Improved thrombolysis in acute myocardial infarction with front-loaded administration of alteplase: results of the rt-PA-APSAC patency study (TAPS). J Am Coll Cardiol 1992;19:885–91.

[44] The GUSTO investigators. An international randomized trial comparing four thrombolytic strategies for acute myocardial infarction. N Engl J Med 1993;329:673–82.

[45] International Joint Efficacy Comparison of Thrombolytics. Randomised, double-blind comparison of reteplase double-bolus administration with streptokinase in acute myocardial infarction (INJECT): trial to investigate equivalence. Lancet 1995;346:329–36.

[46] Bates ER, Topol EJ. Limitations of thrombolytic therapy for acute myocardial infarction complicated by congestive heart failure and cardiogenic shock. J Am Coll Cardiol 1991; 18:1077–84.

[47] Becker RC. Hemodynamic, mechanical, and metabolic determinants of thrombolytic efficacy: a theoretic framework for assessing the limitations of thrombolysis in patients with cardiogenic shock. Am Heart J 1993;125:919–29.

[48] Prewitt RM, Gu S, Garber PJ, et al. Marked systemic hypotension depresses coronary thrombolysis induced by intracoronary administration of recombinant tissue-type plasminogen activator. J Am Coll Cardiol 1992;20:1626–33.

[49] Urban P, Stauffer JC, Bleed D, et al. A randomized evaluation of early revascularization to treat shock complicating acute myocardial infarction. The (Swiss) Multicenter Trial of Angioplasty for Shock—(S)MASH. Eur Heart J 1999;20:1030–8.

[50] Hochman JS, Buller CE, Sleeper LA, et al. Cardiogenic shock complicating acute myocardial infarction—etiologies, management and outcome: a report from the SHOCK Trial Registry. SHould we emergently revascularize Occluded Coronaries for cardiogenic shocK? J Am Coll Cardiol 2000;36:1063–70.

[51] Dzavik V, Sleeper LA, Cocke TP, et al. Early revascularization is associated with improved survival in elderly patients with acute myocardial infarction complicated by cardiogenic shock: a report from the SHOCK trial registry. Eur Heart J 2003;24:828–37.

[52] Antoniucci D, Valenti R, Migliorini A, et al. Comparison of impact of emergency percutaneous revascularization on outcome of patients > or = 75 to those < 75 years of age with acute myocardial infarction complicated by cardiogenic shock. Am J Cardiol 2003;91: 1458–61.

[53] Dauerman HL, Ryan TJ Jr, Piper WD, et al. Outcomes of percutaneous coronary intervention among elderly patients in cardiogenic shock: a multicenter, decade-long experience. J Invasive Cardiol 2003;15:380–4.

[54] Prasad A, Lennon RJ, Rihal CS, et al. Outcomes of elderly patients with cardiogenic shock treated with early percutaneous revascularization. Am Heart J 2004;147:1066–70.

[55] Antoniucci D, Valenti R, Santoro GM, et al. Systematic direct angioplasty and stent-supported direct angioplasty therapy for cardiogenic shock complicating acute myocardial infarction: in-hospital and long-term survival. J Am Coll Cardiol 1998;31: 294–300.

[56] Chan AW, Chew DP, Bhatt DL, et al. Long-term mortality benefit with the combination of stents and abciximab for cardiogenic shock complicating acute myocardial infarction. Am J Cardiol 2002;89:132–6.

[57] Huang R, Sacks J, Thai H, et al. Impact of stents and abciximab on survival from cardiogenic shock treated with percutaneous coronary intervention. Catheter Cardiovasc Interv 2005;65: 25–33.

[58] Yip HK, Wu CJ, Chang HW, et al. Comparison of impact of primary percutaneous transluminal coronary angioplasty and primary stenting on short-term mortality in patients with cardiogenic shock and evaluation of prognostic determinants. Am J Cardiol 2001;87:1184–8.

[59] Giri S, Mitchel J, Azar RR, et al. Results of primary percutaneous transluminal coronary angioplasty plus abciximab with or without stenting for acute myocardial infarction complicated by cardiogenic shock. Am J Cardiol 2002;89:126–31.

[60] De Luca G, Suryapranata H, Stone GW, et al. Abciximab as adjunctive therapy to reperfusion in acute ST-segment elevation myocardial infarction: a meta-analysis of randomized trials. JAMA 2005;293:1759–65.

[61] Antoniucci D, Valenti R, Migliorini A, et al. Abciximab therapy improves survival in patients with acute myocardial infarction complicated by early cardiogenic shock undergoing coronary artery stent implantation. Am J Cardiol 2002;90:353–7.

[62] Zeymer U, Vogt A, Zahn R, et al. Predictors of in-hospital mortality in 1333 patients with acute myocardial infarction complicated by cardiogenic shock treated with primary percutaneous coronary intervention (PCI). Results of the primary PCI registry of the Arbeitsgemeinschaft Leitende Kardiologische Krankenhausarzte (ALKK). Eur Heart J 2004;25: 322–8.

[63] White HD, Assmann SF, Sanborn TA, et al. Comparison of percutaneous coronary intervention and coronary artery bypass grafting after acute myocardial infarction complicated by cardiogenic shock: results from the SHould we emergently revascularize Occluded Coronaries for cardiogenic shocK (SHOCK) trial. Circulation 2005;112:1992–2001.

[64] Vogel RA, Shawl F, Tommaso C, et al. Initial report of the National Registry of Elective Cardiopulmonary Bypass Supported Coronary Angioplasty. J Am Coll Cardiol 1990;15:23–9.

[65] Nichol G, Karmy-Jones R, Salerno C, et al. Systematic review of percutaneous cardiopulmonary bypass for cardiac arrest or cardiogenic shock states. Resuscitation 2006;70:381–94.

[66] Bartlett RH, Roloff DW, Custer JR, et al. Extracorporeal life support: the University of Michigan experience. JAMA 2000;283:904–8.

[67] Thiele H, Lauer B, Hambrecht R, et al. Reversal of cardiogenic shock by percutaneous left atrial-to-femoral arterial bypass assistance. Circulation 2001;104:2917–22.

[68] Vranckx P, Foley DP, de Feijter PJ, et al. Clinical introduction of the Tandemheart, a percutaneous left ventricular assist device, for circulatory support during high-risk percutaneous coronary intervention. Int J Cardiovasc Intervent 2003;5:35–9.

[69] Atiemo AD, Conte JV, Heldman AW. Resuscitation and recovery from acute right ventricular failure using a percutaneous right ventricular assist device. Catheter Cardiovasc Interv 2006;68:78–82.

[70] Thiele H, Sick P, Boudriot E, et al. Randomized comparison of intra-aortic balloon support with a percutaneous left ventricular assist device in patients with revascularized acute myocardial infarction complicated by cardiogenic shock. Eur Heart J 2005;26:1276–83.

[71] Magliato KE, Kleisli T, Soukiasian HJ, et al. Biventricular support in patients with profound cardiogenic shock: a single-center experience. ASAIO J 2003;49:475–9.

[72] Hochman JS. Cardiogenic shock complicating acute myocardial infarction: expanding the paradigm. Circulation 2003;107:2998–3002.

[73] Cotter G, Kaluski E, Blatt A, et al. L-NMMA (a nitric oxide synthase inhibitor) is effective in the treatment of cardiogenic shock. Circulation 2000;101:1358–61.

[74] Cotter G, Kaluski E, Milovanov O, et al. LINCS: L-NAME (a NO synthase inhibitor) in the treatment of refractory cardiogenic shock: a prospective randomized study. Eur Heart J 2003;24:1287–95.

[75] Dzavik V, Cotter G, Reynolds HR, et al. Effect of nitric oxide synthase inhibition on hemodynamics and outcome of patients with persistent cardiogenic shock complicating acute myocardial infarction: a phase II dose-ranging study. Eur Heart J 2007;28:1009–16.

[76] The TRIUMPH Investigators. Effect of tilarginine acetate in patients with acute myocardial infarction and cardiogenic shock. The TRIUMPH randomized controlled trial. JAMA 2007; 297:1657–66.

ELSEVIER
SAUNDERS

CRITICAL
CARE
CLINICS

Crit Care Clin 23 (2007) 779–800

Acute Aortic Dissection

Desikan Kamalakannan, MBBS, MRCP[a],*,
Howard S. Rosman, MD, FACC[a],
Kim A. Eagle, MD, FACC[b]

[a]St. John Hospital and Medical Center, 22151, Moross Road, Suite 126,
Detroit, MI 48236, USA
[b]University of Michigan Cardiovascular Center, 300, N. Ingalls, Ann Arbor, MI 48109, USA

Acute aortic dissection (AAD) is an uncommon but potentially cata-strophic illness with high mortality. Significant advances in the understand-ing, diagnosis, and management have been made since the first reported case of aortic dissection 3 centuries ago. This comprehensive review discusses the pathophysiology, classification, clinical manifestations, early diagnosis, and management of this important cardiovascular emergency.

Pathophysiology

A classic aortic dissection begins with a tear in the aortic intima and inner layer of the aortic media allowing blood to enter and split the aortic media [1]. This process is responsible for the formation of true and false lumen separated by the intimal flap. Cystic medial necrosis or degeneration of aortic media is thought to be a prerequisite for dissection [2]. Spontaneous hypertension-related rupture of the vasa vasorum of the aorta may cause intramural hematoma (IMH) and subsequently to intimal tear due to weak-ening of the media by intramural hemorrhage [1]. Mechanical forces con-tributing to aortic dissection include flexion forces of the vessel at fixed sites, the radial impact of the pressure pulse, and the shear stress of the blood [3]. Hypertension adds to a mechanical strain on the aortic wall to the shearing forces exerting a longitudinal stress along the aortic wall [3]. A combination of these factors results in an intimal tear and the propaga-tion of dissection in to the aortic media, especially in patients who have medial degeneration and weakening.

* Corresponding author.
E-mail address: desikan.kamalakannan@stjohn.org (D. Kamalakannan).

Incidence

The incidence of aortic dissection is related to the prevalence of risk factors for aortic dissection in the population that is studied. The estimated incidence is about 5 to 30 cases per million per year [4–7]. About 65% of dissections originate in the ascending aorta, 20% in the descending thoracic aorta, 10% in the aortic arch, and the remainder in the abdominal aorta. There is male predominance with a male-to-female ratio of 2:1 and with peak incidence in the sixth and seventh decades of life [4].

Predisposing factors

Mechanisms that lead to weakening of the aortic media may lead to higher wall stress that then leads to aortic dilatation, aneurysm formation, intramural hemorrhage and eventually to dissection or rupture. A variety of inherited and acquired conditions predispose a person to aortic dissection (Box 1). Systemic hypertension is thought to be the most important predisposing factor; a history of systemic hypertension was reported in 72% of patients in the International Registry of Aortic Dissection (IRAD) [4]. Other acquired predisposing conditions include direct trauma, iatrogenic retrograde dissection from catheter-related aortic intimal injury, and previous valvular or coronary bypass or aortic surgery. Cocaine use also predisposes to aortic dissection by the sudden increase in aortic wall stress caused by catecholamine surge. An unexplained relationship may exist between aortic dissection and pregnancy, with about half of all dissections in young women occurring during pregnancy, typically in the third trimester [8]. In younger patients, inherited conditions such as Marfan's syndrome, Ehlers-Danlos syndrome, biscuspid aortic valve, aortic coarctation, and Turner's syndrome predispose to AAD.

Classification

Aortic dissections can be classified according to the anatomic location and the duration from the onset of symptoms to medical evaluation. A dissection presenting less than 2 weeks from symptom onset is defined as acute; those that have been present 2 weeks or more are defined as chronic. Most dissections are acute at diagnosis, and about one third are chronic [5]. The De Bakey and Stanford (or Daily) systems commonly are used for anatomic classification of aortic dissections. In the Stanford classification (Fig. 1), type A (proximal) dissection involves the ascending aorta, and type B (distal) dissection does not involve the ascending aorta [10]. In the De Bakey classification, type I dissection involves the entire aorta, type II dissection involves only the ascending aorta, and type III dissection involves only the descending aorta, sparing the ascending aorta and the arch [11]. For simplification, De Bakey types I and II can be grouped as Stanford type A because both involve the ascending aorta. These classifications are helpful

Box 1. Predisposing conditions for aortic dissection [9]

Long-standing arterial hypertension
Smoking
Dyslipidemia
Use of cocaine/crack

Connective tissue disorders
Hereditary fibrillinopathies
    Marfan's syndrome
    Ehlers-Danlos syndrome
Hereditary vascular diseases
    Biscuspid aortic valve
    Coarctation
Vascular inflammation
    Giant cell arteritis
    Takayasu arteritis
    Behcet's disease
    Syphilis
    Ormond's disease

Deceleration trauma
Car accident
Fall from height

Iatrogenic factors
Catheter/Instrument intervention
Valvular/aortic surgery
    Side- or cross-clamping/aortotomy
    Graft anastomosis
    Patch aortoplasty
    Cannulation site
    Aortic wall fragility

Other
Pregnancy
Turner's syndrome

Adapted from Nienaber CA, Eagle KA. Aortic dissection: new frontiers in diagnosis and management: part I: from etiology to diagnostic strategies. Circulation 2003;108(5):629; with permission.

for distinguishing dissections with and without ascending aortic involvement for therapeutic and prognostic reasons. A newer subclassification of these types has been proposed to include IMH and aortic ulcers that are considered precursors of typical aortic dissection [12].

Type A (proximal)   Type B (Distal)

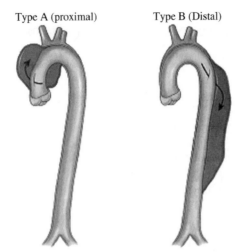

Fig. 1. Stanford classification of aortic dissection. Type A (proximal) dissection involves the ascending aorta. Type B (distal) dissection does not involve the ascending aorta. (*Adapted from* Isselbacher EM. Diseases of the aorta. In: Zipes DP, Libby P, Bonow RO, et al, editors. Braunwald's heart disease: a textbook of cardiovascular medicine, vol. 2. 7th edition. Philadelphia: Elsevier Saunders; 2005. p. 1416; with permission.)

Intramural hematomas

IMH originates from ruptured vasa vasorum in the aortic medial wall layers and is characterized by blood in the aortic wall in the absence of an intimal tear. IMH may be a precursor for classic aortic dissection [13,14]. IMH has a prevalence of 10% to 30% in patients suspected of having aortic dissection [9]. It is estimated that IMH can lead to AAD in 28% to 47% of affected patients and is associated with aortic rupture in 21% to 47% of cases [9]. The management is similar to that of classic aortic dissection, depending on anatomic location. Fig. 2 shows a representative IMH.

Clinical manifestations

Symptoms

The most common initial symptom of AAD is pain, which is present in 96% of cases [4]. The pain of aortic dissection is usually in midline and is felt in the front and back of the trunk, depending on the location of the dissection. The pain typically is of sudden/abrupt onset and is severe at onset, in contrast to that of myocardial infarction, which builds up over a period of time. Sudden onset of pain was reported in 85% of the 464 patients reviewed in the IRAD [4]. The classical quality of pain is described as

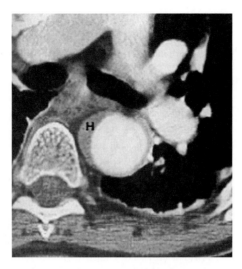

Fig. 2. Intramural hematoma. An axial contrast-enhanced CT scan demonstrating crescentic thickening of the aortic wall (H) that does not enhance, confirming the presence of an intramural hematoma. Note that neither the size nor the shape of the aortic lumen is distorted, as it typically would be in the presence of a classic aortic dissection. (*Adapted from* Isselbacher EM. Diseases of the aorta. In: Zipes DP, Libby P, Bonow RO, et al, editors. Braunwald's heart disease: a textbook of cardiovascular medicine, vol. 2. 7th edition. Philadelphia: Elsevier Saunders; 2005. p. 1429; with permission.)

tearing or ripping (51%), although sharp pain (64%) was reported even more often [4]. Radiating or migratory pain has also been reported. The pain of aortic dissection may radiate to jaw, neck, shoulder, or arms, which also is found in acute coronary syndromes. Anterior chest pain is typical for type A dissection, whereas pain in the posterior chest (interscapular), back, or abdomen is typical for type B dissection, although there can be substantial overlap [4]. To diagnose or even to suspect AAD, all patients presenting with severe chest pain should be asked about three features of pain: (1) the quality of the pain, rather than simply its presence, (2) radiation, and (3) pain intensity at onset. In one study, when all three questions were asked, 30 of 33 patients (91%) were suspected of having dissection before imaging or death, compared with only 22 of 45 patients (49%) when none or only one or two of the questions were posed [15]. Painless aortic dissection is relatively uncommon and is seen predominantly in patients who have coma, stroke, or syncope. Initial pain followed by a pain-free interval lasting from hours to days followed by return of pain is common and may be falsely reassuring. The return of pain after a pain-free interval is an ominous sign of extension of dissection or impending rupture [16].

Syncope with or without pain occurs in about 13% of patients who have AAD [17]. It is more common in patients who have type A dissections than in those who have type B dissection. There are several pathophysiologic mechanisms for syncope in AAD. Cardiac tamponade from rupture of type A dissection in to the pericardium can result in hypotension and syncope [18]. Stroke from carotid artery involvement in type A dissection can lead to decreased cerebral blood flow resulting in syncope [19]. Other mechanisms include vasovagal phenomenon associated with intense pain of dissection [18] or direct stretching of the aortic baroreceptors [20]. Patients who have syncope have been found to have higher mortality than patients without syncope in AAD and also are more likely to have cardiac tamponade or stroke [17].

Dyspnea and symptoms of heart failure usually are secondary to severe aortic regurgitation in this setting and are reported in 7% of patients who have AAD [4]. Other symptoms often are related to malperfusion syndromes from dissection-related side branch occlusion or ischemia. Cerebrovascular accident manifestations with neurologic symptoms, paraplegia, and symptoms of limb ischemia can occur because of involvement of the aortic branch vessels by dissection at the origin or obliteration of the vessel by expanding false lumen. Anuria can result from renal artery involvement, and abdominal symptoms may result from involvement of arteries supplying the gastrointestinal system.

Systemic manifestations such as high fever are uncommon but can occur from release of pyrogenic substances from the aortic wall [21].

Physical findings

The physical examination can provide important clues as to the presence and origin of aortic dissection. Hypertension is common and occurs in 70% of patients who have type B dissection but in only 36% of those who have type A dissection in the IRAD [4]. Hypotension can occur at presentation or later in the course of the disease and usually is the result of cardiac tamponade, aortic rupture, or severe aortic regurgitation. Hypotension is more common in type A (25%) than type B dissection (4%) [4]. Pseudohypotension—inaccurate measurement of blood pressure—can result from compromise of the brachial arteries in dissection involving the brachiocephalic trunk.

Pulse deficits represent a significant difference in the pulse volume and/or blood pressure between two upper extremities or sudden loss of a peripheral pulse. Pulse deficits are a manifestation of impaired blood flow to peripheral vessels, and their presence in a patient who has chest pain should raise the suspicion for AAD. A pulse deficit is more common in type A dissection (19%–30%) than in type B dissection (9%–21%) [4,22,23]. Pulse deficits are reported to be associated with higher inhospital complications and mortality [22].

A diastolic murmur of aortic regurgitation is present in about one third to one half of patients who have type A dissection [4,24]. The murmur can be quite soft, and the typical peripheral signs of severe aortic regurgitation such as wide pulse pressure may be absent in the acute setting. Acute aortic regurgitation in AAD can result from aortic root dilatation resulting in malcoaptation of the aortic leaflets, by detachment of one or more aortic leaflets by extension of the dissection into the aortic root, or by intussusception of the intimal flap in to the left ventricular outflow tract [8].

Neurologic manifestations occur more commonly in type A dissection and may represent involvement of cerebral or spinal circulation. This involvement may manifest as focal neurologic deficits. Obstruction of the aortic branch vessel may present as signs of limb or organ (eg, renal/mesenteric) ischemia. In 1% to 2% of cases retrograde extension of dissection into the aortic root and sinus of Valsalva affects the coronary artery ostia, (the right more often than the left) and can result in myocardial ischemia/infarction [8].

Signs of pericardial involvement such as pericardial friction rub, jugular venous distension, and pulsus paradoxus should suggest the possibility of pericardial effusion/tamponade. Pleural effusions may result from contained rupture of aorta into the pleural space, usually in the left side. Inflammatory reaction from the aortic wall also can produce pleural effusion. Other rare clinical manifestations include compression of the left recurrent laryngeal nerve causing vocal cord paralysis, dysphagia caused by compression of esophagus, hemoptysis or hematemesis caused by rupture into tracheobronchial tree or esophagus, superior vena caval syndrome, pulsating neck masses, and Horner's syndrome [21]. Table 1 gives the frequencies of the common presenting symptoms and physical examination findings of AAD from the IRAD.

Differential diagnosis

A variety of conditions, including myocardial ischemia/infarction with or without ST elevation, pulmonary embolism, pericarditis, aortic aneurysm without dissection, acute aortic regurgitation without dissection, mediastinal tumors, perforating peptic ulcer, acute pancreatitis, cholecystitis, cholesterol or atherosclerotic embolism, and musculoskeletal pain should be considered in the differential diagnosis of AAD [21]. Up to 30% of patients later found to have aortic dissection initially are suspected of having a different condition [21]. A missed diagnosis of AAD typically is catastrophic. Treatment of other suspected conditions such as myocardial infarction or pulmonary embolism with antithrombotics/anticoagulants delays the diagnosis and exacerbates bleeding. Thus, when there is clinical suspicion of aortic dissection, diagnostic imaging and (in nearly certain cases) initiation of intravenous beta-blocker therapy should be performed emergently before presumptive treatment for other conditions.

Biomarkers

Currently no biomarkers are available or recommended for clinical use for a rapid, noninvasive diagnosis of AAD. Of the several markers that have been evaluated, D-dimer [25–28], soluble elastin fragments [29],

Table 1

Presenting symptoms and physical examination of patients who had acute aortic dissection form the International Registry of Aortic Dissection: (N = 464)

Category	Present/No. Reported (%)	No. Type A (%)	No. Type B (%)
Presenting symptoms			
Any pain reported	443/464 (95.5)	271 (93.8)	172 (98.3)
Abrupt onset	379/447 (84.8)	234 (85.4)	145 (83.8)
Chest pain	331/455 (72.7)	221 (78.9)	110 (62.9)
Anterior chest pain	262/430 (60.9)	191 (71)	71 (44.1)
Posterior chest pain	149/415 (35.9)	85 (32.8)	64 (41)
Back pain	240/451 (53.2)	129 (46.6)	111 (63.8)
Abdominal pain	133/449 (29.6)	60 (21.6)	73 (42.7)
Severity of pain: severe or worst ever	346/382 (90.6)	211 (90.1)	135 (90)
Quality of pain: sharp	174/270 (64.4)	103 (62)	71 (68.3)
Quality of pain: tearing or ripping	135/267 (50.6)	78 (49.4)	57 (52.3)
Radiating	127/449 (28.3)	75 (27.2)	52 (30.1)
Migrating	74/446 (16.6)	41 (14.9)	33 (19.3)
Syncope	42/447 (9.4)	35 (12.7)	7 (4.1)
Physical examination			
Hemodynamics (n = 451)			
Hypertensive (SBP ≥ 150 mm Hg)	221 (49)	99 (35.7)	122 (70.1)
Normotensive (SBP 100–149 mm Hg)	156 (34.6)	110 (39.7)	46 (26.4)
Hypotensive (SBP < 100 mm Hg)	36 (8)	32 (11.6)	4 (2.3)
Shock or Tamponade (SBP ≤ 80 mm Hg)	38 (8.4)	36 (13)	2 (1.5)
Murmur of aortic insufficiency	69/457 (15.1)	117 (44)	20 (12)
Pulse deficit	69/457 (15.1)	53 (18.7)	16 (9.2)
Cerebrovascular accident	21/447 (4.7)	17 (6.1)	4 (2.3)
Congestive heart failure	29/440 (6.6)	24 (8.8)	5 (3)

Abbreviation: SBP, systolic blood pressure.

Adapted from Hagan PG, Nienaber CA, Isselbacher EM, et al. The International Registry of Acute Aortic Dissection (IRAD): new insights into an old disease. JAMA 2000;283(7):900; with permission.

smooth muscle heavy chain protein [30], and metalloproteinase-9 [31] show some promise for future clinical use.

Imaging

Chest radiography

Conventional chest radiography is neither specific nor sensitive for the diagnosis of AAD. The radiologic signs of AAD include mediastinal widening and abnormalities of aortic contour [3,32,33]. Other findings include displaced calcification, aortic kinking, opacification of the aorticopulmonary window, and pleural effusion. In a study of 216 patients suspected of having acute aortic syndromes over a 6-year period, Von Kodolitsch and colleagues [34] report a sensitivity of 67% for overt aortic dissection and of 63% for intramural hemorrhage or penetrating ulcer. The sensitivity for proximal aorta was 47% and for distal aortic dissection was 77% [34]. These observations indicate that chest radiography is of limited value in the diagnosis of AAD. If the aorta or mediastinum appears to be wide on chest radiography, it raises suspicion for AAD. If it does not, AAD within a normal or only modestly widened aorta is still possible.

Aortography

Contrast aortography was the reference standard before cross-sectional imaging was available but now largely has been abandoned because of a high false-negative rate of 10% [20,35]. Cineangiography and intra-arterial and intravenous digital subtraction angiography have been used for imaging the aorta. Intra-arterial digital subtraction angiography has the advantage of a large field of view and is used most frequently. Diagnosis of AAD requires the visualization of two lumens and the intimal flap. Other findings may include compression of the true lumen, thickening of the aortic wall, abnormalities of branch vessels, and aortic regurgitation [36,37]. Aortography has high specificity (94%) and lower sensitivity (88%) [38]. False-negative results are caused by difficulties in identifying intramural hematoma, thrombosed false lumen, and simultaneous opacification of the true and false lumens when the imaging plane renders the intimal flap invisible [38]. The invasive nature, limited accuracy, procedural time, and rate of complications have decreased the use of aortography for diagnosis of AAD. With the growth of percutaneous approaches to treat distal AAD, aortography may become more commonplace in the future.

Echocardiography

Transthoracic echocardiography (TTE) has limited value in the evaluation for AAD, primarily because of its inadequacy in visualizing the distal ascending, transverse, and descending aorta. Furthermore, image quality is affected adversely by obesity, chronic obstructive pulmonary disease, mechanical ventilation, and chest wall deformities [35]. When imaging planes are excellent, diagnostic findings include a mobile intimal flap that is visualized in more than one view and has a defined motion that is not parallel to motion of any other cardiac or aortic root structure [35]. The sensitivity and specificity of TTE for diagnosing AAD have been reported to be in the range of 59% to 85% and 63% to 96%, respectively [35]. The low sensitivity limits the usefulness of TTE for the diagnosis of AAD, although it is useful in assessing the complications of AAD such as aortic regurgitation, pericardial effusion, and left ventricular function.

Transesophageal echocardiography (TEE) overcomes many of the limitations of TTE because of the proximity of the esophagus to the aorta. It also is widely available, relatively safe, and easy to perform at the bedside even in unstable patients. In addition to the visualization of intimal flap within the aortic lumen with high spatial resolution, the true and false lumen usually can be identified, and the flow within and between them can be characterized using color Doppler. Thrombosis within the false lumen, aortic regurgitation, pericardial effusion, and the proximal coronary arteries also can be visualized. When the false lumen is thrombosed, a central displacement of the intimal calcification and a thickening of aortic wall may suggest the presence of AAD [39]. Intramural hematoma typically appears as smooth, homogenous, crescentic thickening of the aortic wall, usually more than 7 mm, does not have active flow within the lumen, and has no identifiable tear in the intima [40]. The sensitivity of TEE for AAD has been reported to be as high as 98%, and specificity ranges from 63% to 96% [41–48]. False positives are caused mainly by reverberation artifacts. The area of the ascending aorta, where the trachea interposes between esophagus and aorta, is a blind spot in monoplane TEE, but these blind spots can be reduced with currently available biplane and multiplane TEE [43,49]. False-negative or nondiagnostic TEE studies can occur when a dissection flap is not observed in patients who have dilated aorta and/or pericardial effusion or when a proximal dissection involving the aortic valve is mistaken for endocarditis with vegetation and flail aortic valve leaflets [50]. The important disadvantage of TEE is its limited ability to visualize the distal thoracic and abdominal aorta and its strong operator dependence. Representative TEE images are shown in Fig. 3.

CT

CT is a noninvasive, fast, and accurate method that is readily available in most hospitals. Continuing technical improvements and the availability of CT angiography and helical and multislice CT scanners have increased the resolution and permit three-dimensional reconstruction of the aorta and its branches. These advances have improved the accuracy of CT in diagnosing AAD. Multislice CT is useful in identifying the intimal flap, the extent of the dissection, branch vessel involvement, the size of the aorta, the patency of false lumen, and pericardial effusion and can visualize proximal coronary arteries [51]. Diagnosis of AAD is made by the identification of intimal flap separating the true and false lumens. Intramural hematoma appears as a crescent-shaped, high-attenuation signal within the wall of aorta on noncontrast CT. It also may appear as a localized thickening of the aortic wall with internal displacement of intimal calcifications [51,52]. The sensitivity and specificity of CT for the diagnosis of AAD range from 83% to 100% and from 87% to 100%, respectively [51,52]. The limitations include visualization of intimal flap in less than 75% of cases and inability to

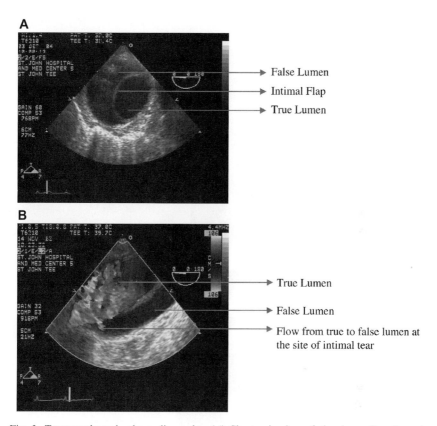

Fig. 3. Transesophageal echocardiography. (*A*) Short-axis view of the descending thoracic aorta showing true and false lumens separated by the intimal flap. (*B*) Long-axis view of the descending thoracic aorta showing true and false lumens separated by the intimal flap. Color Doppler shows flow from true to false lumen at the site of intimal tear.

identify readily the site of intimal tear [53]. Other disadvantages include use of iodinated contrast and inability to assess aortic regurgitation. Representative CT images are shown in Fig. 4.

MRI

MRI can detect AAD accurately, can delineate the extent of dissection, and can reveal extent of branch vessel involvement [54]. The double lumen and intimal flap are identified readily. Contrast-enhanced MRI is superior to black-blood MRI in detecting intimal flaps and branch vessel involvement. Cine-MRI and gradient echo techniques can provide dynamic information about flow within the true and false lumens and also can assess aortic regurgitation [55,56]. The sensitivity and specificity of MRI for diagnosing AAD are in the range of 95% to 100% [57]. The advantages include noninvasiveness, high resolution, 3D reconstruction, the use of less-toxic

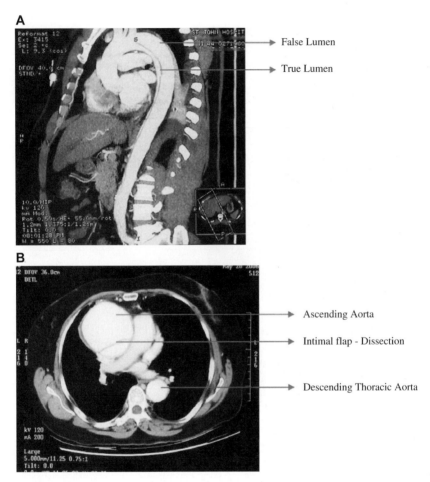

Fig. 4. Contrast-enhanced CT scans. (*A*) Reconstruction showing type B aortic dissection extending from the arch to the abdominal aorta. The intimal flap separates the true and false lumen. (*B*) Transverse section at the level just above the aortic valve showing aneurysmally dilated ascending aorta with dissection.

gadolinium as contrast agent, and the absence of ionizing radiation. The disadvantages are inconvenience, lack of availability on emergency basis, limited applicability in patients who have metallic implants, and concerns about patient monitoring and prolonged scanning time, especially in unstable patients. Representative images are shown in Fig. 5.

Medical treatment

The aims of medical therapy in AAD are to reduce the force of left ventricular contraction, to decrease the steepness of the rise in aortic pulse wave (ie, dp/dt), and to reduce the systemic arterial pressure as low as

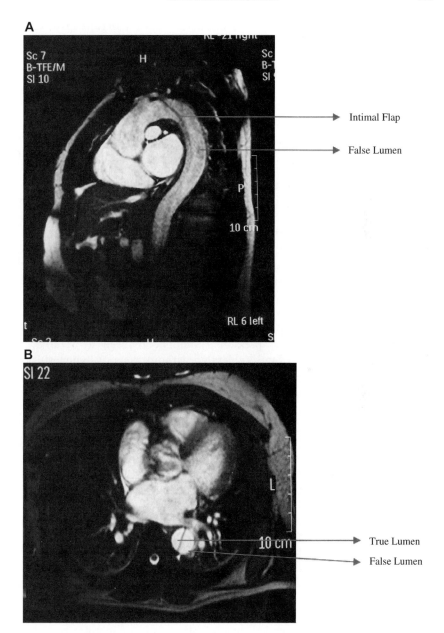

Fig. 5. Gadolinium-enhanced MRI. (*A*) Reconstruction showing type B aortic dissection. (*B*) Transverse section demonstrating true and false lumens separated by an intimal flap in the descending aorta.

possible without compromising perfusion to the vital organs [57]. These measures will decrease the aortic shear stress and minimize further dissection.

Every patient suspected of having AAD should be admitted to the ICU while appropriate testing is being arranged. Intravenous access should be obtained for fluid and drug administration. In unstable patients who require hemodynamic monitoring, central venous lines may be necessary to guide fluid replacement. In unstable patients, a radial arterial line should be placed for blood pressure monitoring. Blood pressure should be obtained in both arms because pseudohypotension in one arm may occur because of aortic branch vessel occlusion. The arm with the higher blood pressure should be used for titrating antihypertensives. Intubation and mechanical ventilation are essential to stabilize the unstable patients. ECGs should be obtained, because 20% of patients who have AAD have evidence of acute cardiac ischemia [58]. Patients who have ST-segment elevation on ECG and are suspected of having AAD should undergo diagnostic imaging before administration of thrombolytic therapy, because this therapy may be detrimental for patients who have AAD.

Adequate pain control with intravenous morphine is necessary to allay anxiety and to reduce sympathetic stimulation, which may raise the blood pressure. The systolic blood pressure should be reduced to a target of 110 mm Hg or the lowest that is tolerated without signs of hypoperfusion [59]. Intravenous beta-blockers are the first-line drugs for reduction of blood pressure in AAD because they have the desirable effect of reducing the aortic shear stress [21]. Esmolol (administered at a loading dose of 0.5 mg/kg over 2–5 min followed by an infusion of 0.1–0.2 mg/kg/min), propranolol (0.05–0.15 mg/kg every 4–6 hours), or labetalol (20-mg bolus followed by 20–80 mg every 10 minutes to a total dose of 300 mg or an infusion at 0.5 to 2 mg/min) should be used as initial therapy. If blood pressure remains high after adequate beta-blockade (at maximum dose or at heart rate < 60 beats/min) additional vasodilator therapy should be initiated. Direct vasodilators should not be used alone, because they can cause an increase in sympathetic drive that will increase the force of left ventricular ejection and risk further dissection [21]. Sodium nitroprusside (initial dose of 0.25 μg/kg/min and then titrated to target blood pressure) is the preferred vasodilator in combination with a beta-blocker. Angiotensin-converting enzyme inhibitors are an alternative to nitroprusside [59]. Other direct vasodilators (eg, hydralazine) are less desirable because they increase aortic shear stress and have less predictable control of blood pressure. In patients for whom beta-blockers are contraindicated, such as those who have severe bronchial asthma, calcium-channel blockers such as diltiazem or verapamil can be used, although there are no data supporting or refuting their benefit in this condition [21]. In normotensive or hypotensive patients, evaluation for blood loss, heart failure, or pericardial effusion with tamponade is mandatory before volume administration [59]. Inotropic agents should be avoided, because they may worsen dissection by increasing the shear stress. In patients who have cardiac tamponade, percutaneous pericardiocentesis should not be attempted, because it can accelerate bleeding and shock [60].

While initial treatment and stabilization are in progress, emergency diagnostic imaging should be performed to confirm the diagnosis and plan definitive treatment without delay. Bedside TEE is the test of choice in unstable patients [59]. An algorithm for management of patients suspected of having AAD is provided in Fig. 6. The European Society of

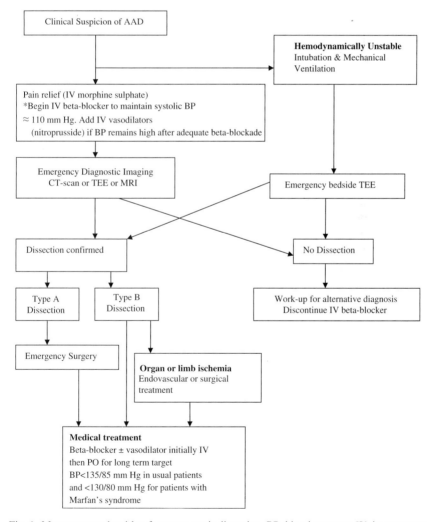

Fig. 6. Management algorithm for acute aortic dissection. BP, blood pressure; IV, intravenous; PO, by mouth; TEE, transesophageal echocardiogram; *, cautious use of beta-blocker if patient is normotensive at presentation.

Cardiology recommendations for initial management of patients suspected of having AAD are shown in Table 2.

Surgical treatment

Type A AAD is a true surgical emergency, because these patients have a high risk of life-threatening complications including cardiac tamponade, acute aortic regurgitation, coronary flow obstruction, and occlusion of aortic branch vessels. The mortality rate is 1% to 2% per hour early after symptom onset [9]. No randomized comparing medical and surgical treatments for type A AAD are available. In an IRAD review of 547 patients

Table 2
European Society of Cardiology guidelines for the initial management of patients suspected of having aortic dissection

Recommendation	Class[a]	Level of Evidence[b]
Detailed medical history and complete physical examination (whenever possible)	I	C
Intravenous line, blood sample (creatine kinase, troponin T or I, myoglobin, white blood cell count, D-dimer, hematocrit, lactase dehydrogenase)	I	C
ECG: documentation of ischemia	I	C
Heart rate and blood pressure monitoring	I	C
Pain relief (morphine sulfate)	I	C
Reduction of systolic blood pressure using beta-blockers (intravenous propranolol, metoprolol, esmolol, or labetalol)	I	C
Transfer to ICU	I	C
In patients who have severe hypertension additional vasodilator (intravenous sodium nitroprusside to titrate blood pressure to 100–120 mm Hg)	I	C
In patients who have obstructive pulmonary disease, blood pressure lowering with calcium-channel blockers	II	C
Imaging in patients who have ECG signs of ischemia before thrombolysis if aortic pathology is suspected	II	C
Chest radiograph	III	C

[a] Class I conditions are conditions for which there is evidence and/or general agreement that a given procedure or treatment is useful and effective. Class II conditions are conditions for which there is conflicting evidence and/or divergence of opinion about the usefulness/efficacy of a procedure or treatment. Class III conditions are conditions for which there is evidence and/or general agreement that the procedure/treatment is not useful and in some cases may be harmful.

[b] Level of evidence C: consensus statement.

Adapted from Erbel R, Alfonso F, Boileau C, et al. Diagnosis and management of aortic dissection. Eur Heart J 2001;22(18):1653; with permission.

who had type A dissection, the inhospital mortality rate of patients treated medically (reasons for nonsurgical treatment were comorbid conditions, old age, and patient refusal) was 56%, compared with 27% for those treated with surgery [61]. This degree of difference may result in part from comorbid conditions in the medically treated patients. Because of high mortality with medical therapy alone, surgical treatment is indicated in all patients who have type A dissections, with the exception of patients who have serious concomitant conditions that, in the opinion of the surgical team, preclude surgery [62]. New ischemic and hemorrhagic stroke often is a relative contraindication to surgery because of the increased risk of intracranial hemorrhage caused by intraoperative heparinization and restoration of blood flow to ischemic brain. The presence of acute myocardial infarction does not preclude surgical intervention. Knowledge of coronary anatomy by angiography, especially in patients who have a known history of significant coronary artery disease, may be desirable in the setting of aortic repair with cardiopulmonary bypass, because additional coronary artery bypass grafts can be performed without significant increases in operative mortality. Retrospective analysis of patients from a large registry, however, suggests that that coronary angiography before emergency aortic surgery does not impact survival and may delay the time to operation [63]. Newer 64-slice CT angiography may provide the details of coronary anatomy without delays caused by going through traditional coronary angiography. Preoperative TEE is helpful to determine the severity and mechanism of aortic regurgitation to decide on aortic valve repair or replacement [24]. The approach to and extent of surgery depends on the presence or absence and mechanism of aortic regurgitation, pericardial involvement, the extent of dissection in to major aortic branches, the localization of entry and re-entry sites, and the presence of thrombosis in the false lumen [64]. The different surgical techniques and selection of patients for them is beyond the scope of this article. The operative mortality ranges from 15% to 30% [65], although some single-center series report mortality as low as 6.3% [66]. In IRAD, the overall surgical mortality was 25.1% in the 526 patients who underwent surgery for type A dissection at a large number of aortic centers [65]. The independent preoperative predictors of operative mortality include a history of aortic valve replacement (odds ratio, 3.12), migrating chest pain (odds ratio, 2.77), hypotension as a sign of AAD (odds ratio, 1.95), shock or tamponade (odds ratio, 2.69), preoperative cardiac tamponade (odds ratio, 2.22), and preoperative limb ischemia (odds ratio, 2.10), [65]. The patients who do the best are those receiving surgery before any hemodynamic instability or complication develops.

Medical therapy is the treatment of choice for uncomplicated type B AAD because there is no proven superiority of surgery or interventional treatment in these patients [59]. Optimal medical therapy is thought to include control of blood pressure and heart rate with beta-blockers and additional antihypertensive drugs as necessary to reduce shear stress and propagation of dissection. Interventional (percutaneous fenestration and stenting) or surgical treatment is reserved for life-threatening complications such as intractable pain, rapidly expanding aortic diameter, occlusion of a major aortic branch, dissection extension, aortic rupture, or evidence of imminent rupture such as mediastinal or periaortic hematoma [59]. In IRAD, of the 384 patients who had type B aortic dissection, 282 (73%) were treated medically, 56 (15%) were treated surgically, and 46 (12%) were treated with percutaneous intervention. The unadjusted inhospital mortality rates were 9.6%, 32.1%, and 6.5%, respectively. Surgical treatment was performed primarily for complicated type B dissections, and interventional therapy usually was reserved for patients who had undergone at least 8 weeks of medical treatment [23]. The high short-term mortality for surgically treated patients is not surprising, because these were the most complicated cases. The reported long-term survival rates for medical therapy for type B dissection is about 60% to 80% at 5 years and 40% to 45% at 10 years [67–69]. With technical advances and experience in percutaneous endovascular treatments, there is growing interest in treating type B dissections with stent-graft placement. Whether stent grafting will evolve as an adjunctive treatment to medical therapy alone needs to be assessed by randomized, controlled trials with long-term follow-up. One such trial, with 2-year follow-up, is underway currently [70].

Long-term management

Optimal long-term management of operated and medically treated AAD involves aggressive medical therapy, regular follow-up visits, patient education, and serial imaging. It has been estimated that one third of patients surviving initial treatment for AAD experience dissection extension or aortic rupture or will require surgery for aortic aneurysm formation within 5 years of initial presentation [59]. Treatment with beta-blockers and additional antihypertensives as necessary to control hypertension is critical. Current guidelines recommend target blood pressure lower than 135/85 mm Hg in usual patients and lower than 130/80 mm Hg in patients who have Marfan's syndrome [59]. The authors prefer even lower blood pressure targets when feasible. Serial imaging is recommended at 1, 3, 6, and 12 months after discharge and annually thereafter [21]. Imaging should not be confined simply to the region of initial involvement, because dissection and aneurysm formation can occur anywhere along the length of aorta. The choice of imaging modality (MRI, TEE, or CT) depends on institutional expertise and availability. Patients must be cautioned to avoid extreme isometric exercises and major contact sports and must be counseled carefully about symptoms to watch for that might indicate aortic instability. They also must understand that any potential recurrence of symptoms should be treated as an emergency until proven otherwise.

Summary

Despite several advances in diagnosis and treatment, the mortality of AAD remains high. The keys to success are immediate clinical suspicion rapidly leading to appropriate imaging tests to confirm the diagnosis and prompt initiation of appropriate medical and, when indicated, surgical therapy. Further research is needed to identify and define the potential role of biomarkers in establishing early diagnosis, optimal medical therapy, and the proper role of percutaneous intervention for this deadly disease.

References

[1] Coady MA, Rizzo JA, Elefteriades JA. Pathologic variants of thoracic aortic dissections: penetrating atherosclerotic ulcers and intramural hematomas. Cardiol Clin 1999;17(4): 637–57.

[2] Larson EW, Edwards WD. Risk factors for aortic dissection: a necropsy study of 161 cases. Am J Cardiol 1984;53(6):849–55.

[3] Macura KJ, Corl FM, Fishman EK, et al. Pathogenesis in acute aortic syndromes: aortic dissection, intramural hematoma, and penetrating atherosclerotic aortic ulcer. AJR Am J Roentgenol 2003;181(2):309–16.

[4] Hagan PG, Nienaber CA, Isselbacher EM, et al. The International Registry of Acute Aortic Dissection (IRAD): new insights into an old disease. JAMA 2000;283(7):897–903.

[5] Spittell PC, Spittell JA Jr, Joyce JW, et al. Clinical features and differential diagnosis of aortic dissection: experience with 236 cases (1980 through 1990). Mayo Clin Proc 1993; 68(7):642–51.

[6] Bickerstaff LK, Pairolero PC, Hollier LH, et al. Thoracic aortic aneurysms: a population-based study. Surgery 1982;92(6):1103–8.

[7] Eisenberg MJ, Rice SA, Paraschos A, et al. The clinical spectrum of patients with aneurysms of the ascending aorta. Am Heart J 1993;125(5):1380–5.

[8] Isselbacher EM, et al. Diseases of the aorta. In: Zipes DP, Libby P, Bonow RO, editors. Braunwald's heart disease: a textbook of cardiovascular medicine, vol. 2. 7th edition. Philadelphia: Elsevier Saunders; 2005. p. 1403–35.

[9] Nienaber CA, Eagle KA. Aortic dissection: new frontiers in diagnosis and management: part I: from etiology to diagnostic strategies. Circulation 2003;108(5):628–35.

[10] Daily PO, Trueblood HW, Stinson EB, et al. Management of acute aortic dissections. Ann Thorac Surg 1970;10(3):237–47.

[11] DeBakey ME, Beall AC Jr, Cooley DA, et al. Dissecting aneurysms of the aorta. Surg Clin North Am 1966;46(4):1045–55.

[12] Svensson LG, Labib SB, Eisenhauer AC, et al. Intimal tear without hematoma: an important variant of aortic dissection that can elude current imaging techniques. Circulation 1999; 99(10):1331–6.

[13] O'Gara PT, DeSanctis RW. Acute aortic dissection and its variants. Toward a common diagnostic and therapeutic approach. Circulation 1995;92(6):1376–8.

[14] Nienaber CA, Sievers HH. Intramural hematoma in acute aortic syndrome: more than one variant of dissection? Circulation 2002;106(3):284–5.

[15] Rosman HS, Patel S, Borzak S, et al. Quality of history taking in patients with aortic dissection. Chest 1998;114:793–5.

[16] Meszaros I, Morocz J, Szlavi J, et al. Epidemiology and clinicopathology of aortic dissection. Chest 2000;117(5):1271–8.

[17] Nallamothu BK, Mehta RH, Saint S, et al. Syncope in acute aortic dissection: diagnostic, prognostic, and clinical implications. Am J Med 2002;113(6):468–71.

[18] Slater EE. Aortic dissection: presentation and diagnosis. In: Doroghazi RM, Slater EE, editors. Aortic dissection. New York: McGraw-Hill; 1983. p. 61–70.

[19] Gore I, Hirst AE. The etiology and pathology of aortic dissection. In: Doroghazi RM, Slater EE, editors. Aortic dissection. New York: McGraw-Hill; 1983. p. 13–53.

[20] Sanders JS, Ferguson DW, Mark AL. Arterial baroreflex control of sympathetic nerve activity during elevation of blood pressure in normal man: dominance of aortic baroreflexes. Circulation 1988;77(2):279–88.

[21] Erbel R, Alfonso F, Boileau C, et al. Diagnosis and management of aortic dissection. Eur Heart J 2001;22(18):1642–81.

[22] Bossone E, Rampoldi V, Nienaber CA, et al. Usefulness of pulse deficit to predict in-hospital complications and mortality in patients with acute type A aortic dissection. Am J Cardiol 2002;89(7):851–5.

[23] Suzuki T, Mehta RH, Ince H, et al. Clinical profiles and outcomes of acute type B aortic dissection in the current era: lessons from the International Registry of Aortic Dissection (IRAD). Circulation 2003;108(Suppl 1):II312–7.

[24] Movsowitz HD, Levine RA, Hilgenberg AD, et al. Transesophageal echocardiographic description of the mechanisms of aortic regurgitation in acute type A aortic dissection: implications for aortic valve repair. J Am Coll Cardiol 2000;36(3):884–90.

[25] Hazui H, Fukumoto H, Negoro N, et al. Simple and useful tests for discriminating between acute aortic dissection of the ascending aorta and acute myocardial infarction in the emergency setting. Circ J 2005;69(6):677–82.

[26] Weber T, Hogler S, Auer J, et al. D-dimer in acute aortic dissection. Chest 2003;123(5): 1375–8.

[27] Ohlmann P, Faure A, Morel O, et al. Diagnostic and prognostic value of circulating D-dimers in patients with acute aortic dissection. Crit Care Med 2006;34(5):1358–64.

[28] Eggebrecht H, Naber CK, Bruch C, et al. Value of plasma fibrin D-dimers for detection of acute aortic dissection. J Am Coll Cardiol 2004;44(4):804–9.

[29] Shinohara T, Suzuki K, Okada M, et al. Soluble elastin fragments in serum are elevated in acute aortic dissection. Arterioscler Thromb Vasc Biol 2003;23(10):1839–44.

[30] Suzuki T, Katoh H, Tsuchio Y, et al. Diagnostic implications of elevated levels of smooth-muscle myosin heavy-chain protein in acute aortic dissection. The smooth muscle myosin heavy chain study. Ann Intern Med 2000;133(7):537–41.

[31] Sangiorgi G, Trimarchi S, Mauriello A, et al. Plasma levels of metalloproteinases-9 and -2 in the acute and subacute phases of type A and type B aortic dissection. J Cardiovasc Med 2006;7(5):307–15.

[32] Jagannath AS, Sos TA, Lockhart SH, et al. Aortic dissection: a statistical analysis of the usefulness of plain chest radiographic findings. AJR Am J Roentgenol 1986;147(6): 1123–6.

[33] Earnest F, Muhm JR, Sheedy PF. Roentgenographic findings in thoracic aortic dissection. Mayo Clin Proc 1979;54(1):43–50.

[34] von Kodolitsch Y, Nienaber CA, Dieckmann C, et al. Chest radiography for the diagnosis of acute aortic syndrome. Am J Med 2004;116(2):73–7.

[35] Cigarroa JE, Isselbacher EM, DeSanctis RW, et al. Diagnostic imaging in the evaluation of suspected aortic dissection. Old standards and new directions. N Engl J Med 1993;328(1): 35–43.

[36] Petasnick JP. Radiologic evaluation of aortic dissection. Radiology 1991;180(2): 297–305.

[37] Dinsmore RE, Rourke JA, DeSanctis RD, et al. Angiographic findings in dissecting aortic aneurysm. N Engl J Med 1966;275(21):1152–7.

[38] Erbel R, Engberding R, Daniel W, et al. Echocardiography in diagnosis of aortic dissection. Lancet 1989;1(8636):457–61.

[39] Erbel R. Role of transesophageal echocardiography in dissection of the aorta and evaluation of degenerative aortic disease. Cardiol Clin 1993;11(3):461–73.

[40] Vilacosta I, San Roman JA, Ferreiros J, et al. Natural history and serial morphology of aortic intramural hematoma: a novel variant of aortic dissection. Am Heart J 1997;134(3): 495–507.

[41] Hashimoto S, Kumada T, Osakada G, et al. Assessment of transesophageal Doppler echography in dissecting aortic aneurysm. J Am Coll Cardiol 1989;14(5):1253–62.

[42] Erbel R, Borner N, Steller D, et al. Detection of aortic dissection by transoesophageal echocardiography. Br Heart J 1987;58(1):45–51.

[43] Keren A, Kim CB, Hu BS, et al. Accuracy of biplane and multiplane transesophageal echocardiography in diagnosis of typical acute aortic dissection and intramural hematoma. J Am Coll Cardiol 1996;28(3):627–36.

[44] Vignon P, Gueret P, Vedrinne JM, et al. Role of transesophageal echocardiography in the diagnosis and management of traumatic aortic disruption. Circulation 1995;92(10):2959–68.

[45] Adachi H, Omoto R, Kyo S, et al. Emergency surgical intervention of acute aortic dissection with the rapid diagnosis by transesophageal echocardiography. Circulation 1991; 84(5 Suppl):III14–9.

[46] Ballal RS, Nanda NC, Gatewood R, et al. Usefulness of transesophageal echocardiography in assessment of aortic dissection. Circulation 1991;84(5):1903–14.

[47] Farah MG, Suneja R. Diagnosis of circumferential dissection of the ascending aorta by transesophageal echocardiography. Chest 1993;103(1):291–2.

[48] Goldman AP, Kotler MN, Scanlon MH, et al. The complementary role of magnetic resonance imaging, Doppler echocardiography, and computed tomography in the diagnosis of dissecting thoracic aneurysms. Am Heart J 1986;111(5):970–81.

[49] Tardif JC, Schwartz SL, Vannan MA, et al. Clinical usefulness of multiplane transesophageal echocardiography: comparison to biplanar imaging. Am Heart J 1994;128(1):156–66.

[50] Patel S, Alam M, Rosman H. Pitfalls in the echocardiographic diagnosis of aortic dissection. Angiology 1997;48:939–46.

[51] Gotway MB, Dawn SK. Thoracic aorta imaging with multislice CT. Radiol Clin North Am 2003;41(3):521–43.

[52] Ledbetter S, Stuk JL, Kaufman JA. Helical (spiral) CT in the evaluation of emergent thoracic aortic syndromes. Traumatic aortic rupture, aortic aneurysm, aortic dissection, intramural hematoma, and penetrating atherosclerotic ulcer. Radiol Clin North Am 1999; 37(3):575–89.

[53] Sommer T, Fehske W, Holzknecht N, et al. Aortic dissection: a comparative study of diagnosis with spiral CT, multiplanar transesophageal echocardiography, and MR imaging. Radiology 1996;199(2):347–52.

[54] Amparo EG, Higgins CB, Hricak H, et al. Aortic dissection: magnetic resonance imaging. Radiology 1985;155(2):399–406.

[55] Nienaber CA, von Kodolitsch Y, Nicolas V, et al. The diagnosis of thoracic aortic dissection by noninvasive imaging procedures. N Engl J Med 1993;328(1):1–9.

[56] Sechtem U, Pflugfelder PW, Cassidy MM, et al. Mitral or aortic regurgitation: quantification of regurgitant volumes with cine MR imaging. Radiology 1988;167(2):425–30.

[57] Khan IA, Nair CK. Clinical, diagnostic, and management perspectives of aortic dissection. Chest 2002;122(1):311–28.

[58] Kamp TJ, Goldschmidt-Clermont PJ, Brinker JA, et al. Myocardial infarction, aortic dissection, and thrombolytic therapy. Am Heart J 1994;128:1234–7.

[59] Nienaber CA, Eagle KA. Aortic dissection: new frontiers in diagnosis and management: Part II: therapeutic management and follow-up. Circulation 2003;108(6):772–8.

[60] Isselbacher EM, Cigarroa JE, Eagle KA. Cardiac tamponade complicating proximal aortic dissection. Is pericardiocentesis harmful? Circulation 1994;90(5):2375–8.

[61] Mehta RH, Suzuki T, Hagan PG, et al. Predicting death in patients with acute type a aortic dissection. Circulation 2002;105(2):200–6.

[62] Borst HG, Laas J. Surgical treatment of thoracic aortic aneurysms. Adv Card Surg 1993;4: 47–87.

[63] Penn MS, Smedira N, Lytle B, et al. Does coronary angiography before emergency aortic surgery affect in-hospital mortality? J Am Coll Cardiol 2000;35(4):889–94.

[64] Jamieson WR, Munro AI, Miyagishima RT, et al. Aortic dissection: early diagnosis and surgical management are the keys to survival. Can J Surg 1982;25(2):145–9.

[65] Trimarchi S, Nienaber CA, Rampoldi V, et al. Contemporary results of surgery in acute type A aortic dissection: the International Registry of Acute Aortic Dissection experience. J Thorac Cardiovasc Surg 2005;129(1):112–22.

[66] Westaby S, Saito S, Katsumata T. Acute type A dissection: conservative methods provide consistently low mortality. Ann Thorac Surg 2002;73(3):707–13.

[67] Doroghazi RM, Slater EE, DeSanctis RW, et al. Long-term survival of patients with treated aortic dissection. J Am Coll Cardiol 1984;3(4):1026–34.

[68] Umana JP, Lai DT, Mitchell RS, et al. Is medical therapy still the optimal treatment strategy for patients with acute type B aortic dissections? J Thorac Cardiovasc Surg 2002;124(5): 896–910.

[69] Bernard Y, Zimmermann H, Chocron S, et al. False lumen patency as a predictor of late outcome in aortic dissection. Am J Cardiol 2001;87(12):1378–82.

[70] Nienaber CA, Zannetti S, Barbieri B, et al. Investigation of stent grafts in patients with type B aortic dissection: design of the INSTEAD trial–a prospective, multicenter, European randomized trial. Am Heart J 2005;149(4):592–9.

ELSEVIER
SAUNDERS

CRITICAL
CARE
CLINICS

Crit Care Clin 23 (2007) 801–834

Pulmonary Hypertension in the Critical Care Setting: Classification, Pathophysiology, Diagnosis, and Management

Melvyn Rubenfire, MD*, Melike Bayram, MD,
Zachary Hector-Word, MD

*Division of Cardiovascular Medicine and Department of Internal Medicine,
University of Michigan, Ann Arbor, MI, USA*

Pulmonary hypertension (PH) is common in the critical care setting, and may be a target for specific therapy. Moderate degrees of PH are most often the consequence of acute or chronic heart failure, hypoxemia, or acute pulmonary embolism (PE), and may be relatively rapidly reversible. The consequences of more severe forms of PH, both acute and chronic, can include hypotension; low cardiac output; right heart failure with congestion of the liver, gut, and kidneys; and varying degrees of hypoxemia, each of which can lead to death or severe disability. We will review the physiology, definitions, classification, pathogenesis, diagnostic tools and algorithms for the diagnosis and specific treatments for the various causes of PH as seen in the critical care setting.

Physiology, definition, and classification

Normally the pulmonary artery pressure is about one fifth of systemic pressure. The pulmonary vasculature in adults and children has excellent vasodilator reserve and accommodates increases in flow. However, the pulmonary vasculature, like the systemic vasculature, can respond in varying degrees and pathologically to several triggers including pressure, flow, hypoxemia, toxins, and emboli, which can induce endothelial dysfunction, loss of elastance, smooth muscle vasoconstriction, and cellular hypertrophy resulting in decreased luminal diameter of the resistance vessels, the pulmonary arterioles.

* Corresponding author. University of Michigan Preventive Cardiology, 24 Frank Lloyd Wright Drive, Ann Arbor, MI 48106-0363.
  E-mail address: mrubenfi@umich.edu (M. Rubenfire).

0749-0704/07/$ - see front matter © 2007 Elsevier Inc. All rights reserved.
doi:10.1016/j.ccc.2007.07.006   *criticalcare.theclinics.com*

Significant PH is most commonly defined as an sPA or right ventricular systolic pressure (RVSP) >40 mm Hg or mean PA (mPA) >25 mm Hg at rest or > 30 mm Hg during exercise. Additional criteria for PAH are a PCW ≤ 15 mm Hg, and pulmonary vascular resistance (PVR) ≥ 3 Wood units (also known as RU or resistance units) [2]. This definition has been used to characterize PAH for epidemiologic studies and new drug evaluation. Lesser degrees of PH with lower pulmonary vascular resistance can be found in mildly symptomatic persons with early PAH. With an increase in stroke volume from obesity, anemia, or sepsis, the sPA or right ventricular systolic pressure (RVSP) estimated from the echo-Doppler may exceed 40 mm Hg.

In the intensive care unit (ICU) patient, PH may be suspected due to characteristic signs and symptoms, discovered incidentally on an echo-Doppler, or its presence may be known at the time of ICU admission. Of course, multifactorial pulmonary hypertension is common and more often the rule in the ICU. The Venn diagram in Fig. 1 depicts the potential relationship between the various etiologies of PH. For example, pulmonary emboli, both acute and chronic, could result in PH from hypoxemia, pulmonary vasoconstriction, decrease in the pulmonary vascular volume, and often occurs in the setting of congestive heart failure (CHF). Chronic left heart failure or mitral valve disease can result in pulmonary congestion and interstitial lung disease, hypoxemia, hypertrophy of the pulmonary arterioles, and noncompliance of the major pulmonary arteries.

The determinants of the systolic pulmonary artery pressure (sPA) include the right ventricular stroke volume and compliance of the main pulmonary artery and its branches. The diastolic pulmonary artery pressure (dPA) determinants include the tone of the pulmonary arterioles, the size of the pulmonary vascular bed (> 100,000 pulmonary arterioles), the pulmonary capillary wedge

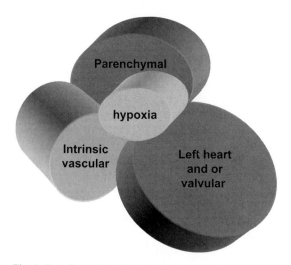

Fig. 1. Paradigm of multifactorial pulmonary hypertension.

Box 1. Classification of pulmonary hypertension (modified from Venice Classification 1)

Class I. Pulmonary arterial hypertension
Idiopathic (familial or sporadic)
Related to or associated with:
  Collagen vascular diseases (especially scleroderma and lupus)
  Portal hypertension
  HIV infection
  Congenital heart disease with right to left shunting (repaired, nonrepaired, small, large),
  Drugs and toxins such as anorexigens (fenfluramine derivatives), cocaine
  Other including Gaucher disease, hereditary hemorrhagic telangiectasia, hemoglobinopathies, hemolytic anemia, splenectomy, myeloproliferative disorders
Persistent pulmonary hypertension of the newborn associated with significant venous or capillary involvement
  Pulmonary veno-occlusive disease (idiopathic or associated with scleroderma/lupus)
  Pulmonary capillary hemangiomatosis

Class II. Pulmonary venous hypertension
Left-sided atrial, ventricular, or valvular diseases or disorders
Secondary to veno-occlusive diseases due to fibrosing mediastinitis, compression by adenopathy/tumors, fibrosis by drugs, ie, bleomycin, mitomycin C, cyclophosphamide, etoposide)

Class III. Pulmonary hypertension secondary to disorders of respiratory system and/or hypoxemia
Chronic obstructive pulmonary disease
Interstitial lung disease
Sleep-disordered breathing, obstructive sleep apnea
Alveolar hypoventilation disorders
Chronic exposure to high altitude,
Alveolar capillary dysplasia, neonatal lung disease

Class IV. Pulmonary hypertension due to chronic thrombotic and/or embolic disease
Thromboembolic obstruction of proximal and/or distal arteries
In situ thrombotic disease, sickle cell disease
Nonthrombotic pulmonary embolism (parasites [schistosomiasis], foreign body, tumors)

Class V. Miscellaneous
Sarcoidosis, histiocytosis X, lymphangiomatosis,
Other

pressure (PCW) or pulmonary artery occlusive pressure (PAOP), which is a reflection of the pulmonary venous pressure, left atrial pressure, mitral valve function, and left ventricular diastolic pressure.

The World Health Organization (WHO) classification of PH (Box 1) [1], most recently updated in 2003 at the Third World Symposium of Pulmonary Hypertension in Venice, Italy, provides a comprehensive scheme that groups disorders according to similarities in pathophysiology and treatment. The terms "primary pulmonary hypertension" and "secondary pulmonary hypertension" have been abandoned due to marked heterogeneity in the conditions to which the later term applied. Idiopathic pulmonary arterial hypertension (IPAH), formerly called primary pulmonary hypertension, is the prototype of pulmonary arterial hypertension (PAH). It is useful to first consider the mechanism/etiology of PH from an anatomic perspective as precapillary, postcapillary, or both.

Pathogenesis

The pathogenesis of diseases associated with acute and chronic PH as listed in Box 1 share much in common. PH associated with chronic thromboembolism (CTEPH) is unique in that it results from an occluding thrombus of major and secondary branches that become a fibrotic mass with occlusion or significant stenosis following varying degrees of lysis. Additionally, in a significant percentage there is further development of down-stream resistance vessel disease that is similar to that found in other causes of precapillary PH, including PAH and hypoxemia.

There are 3 major components in the pathogenesis of chronic PAH: endothelial dysfunction and vasoconstriction, vascular remodeling, and in situ thrombosis, each of which is a target for treatment (Fig. 2) [3,4]. The fourth, which occurs in severe forms or late PAH (including IPAH, scleroderma, Eisenmenger's), is the development of plexiform lesions that irreversibly obliterate the pulmonary arterioles.

Impaired endothelial function is the earliest abnormality and results in vasoconstriction due to decreased endothelial-derived nitric oxide, decreased prostacyclin, and an increase in the vasoconstrictor endothelin (ET). Abnormal endothelial function also results in in situ thrombi within the pulmonary arterioles and secondary branches due to increased thrombosis and diminished thrombolysis. Aggravating factors in both acute and chronic settings include hypoxia, acidosis (ie, in the setting of infection), and increased cardiac output (stroke volume), as occurs with pregnancy, anemia, and hyperthyroidism.

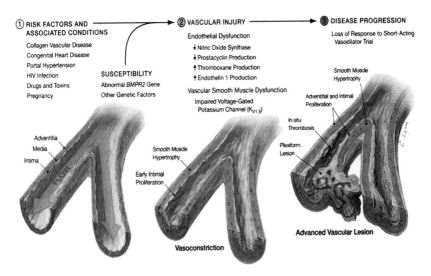

Fig. 2. Pathogenesis of pulmonary arterial hypertension. (*From* Gaine S. Pulmonary hypertension. JAMA 2000;284(24):3160–8; with permission.)

PH from any cause can result in increasing right ventricular afterload and contributes to right ventricular failure [4]. The clinical significance of PH is highly dependent on the rate of progression of the inciting disease, which influences the ability of the RV to compensate. For example, Eisenmenger's reaction in congenital heart disease has a relatively good long-term prognosis because of longstanding RV hypertrophy, while IPAH and PAH associated with scleroderma can progress to death within months to a few years.

Diagnosis, clinical characteristics, and clinical assessment

The diagnosis of PH involves detection of elevated pulmonary pressures and characterization of severity, associated findings, and hemodynamic parameters [2]. It is essential that PH is adequately characterized at the time of diagnosis, whether it is chronic or acute, since appropriate and specific treatment depends on the results. This requires measurement of pressures, mixed venous oxygen saturations, cardiac output, and assessment of right ventricular function. A stepwise approach to the diagnosis of PH has been outlined by the American College of Chest Physicians (ACCP) [5] and may be modified in the ICU as in Figs. 3 and 4.

The major determinant of symptoms in PAH is right ventricular function at rest and during exercise. Patients present with fatigue and shortness of breath due to impaired oxygen transport and reduced cardiac output, syncope from systemic hypotension resulting from systemic vasodilation and underfilling of the RV and LV, angina associated with right ventricular ischemia, and right sided failure symptoms such as lower extremity edema, hepatic congestion, and ascites. When the jugular venous pressure (JVP) exceeds 10 to

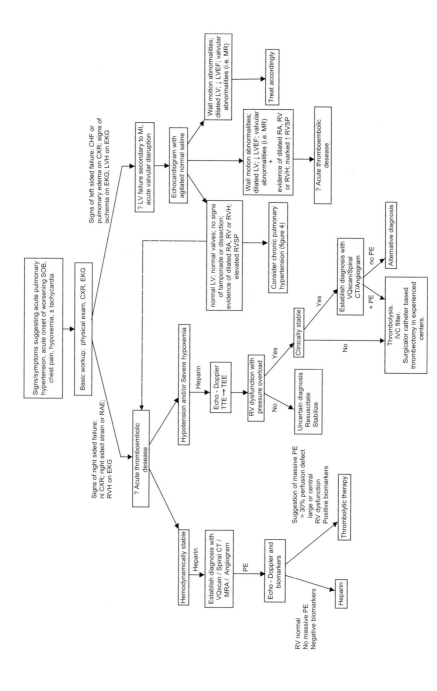

Fig. 3. Diagnostic algorithm for acute onset pulmonary hypertension. (*Adapted from* Wood KE. Major pulmonary embolism: review of a pathophysiologic approach to the golden hour of the hemodynamically significant pulmonary embolism. Chest 2002;121:877–905; with permission.)

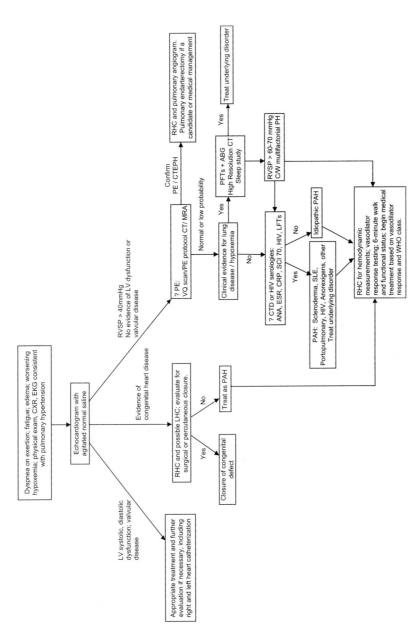

Fig. 4. Diagnostic algorithm for chronic pulmonary hypertension.

15 mm Hg, patients may have early satiety, anorexia, and gut edema, which can be associated with constipation, abdominal pain, and malabsorption. The combination of low cardiac output and high venous pressure can lead to mesenteric ischemia, pancreatitis, and ischemic nephropathy.

The severity of clinical symptoms is classified using the WHO terminology, classes I to IV, which is similar to the New York Heart Association (NYHA) classification for heart failure (Box 2).

In the ICU, patients with PH often present with severe hypoxemia, hypotension, and right-sided heart failure. The differential diagnosis in acutely decompensated PAH is described in Boxes 3 and 4.

Sudden severe precapillary PH is most commonly a result of a massive or submassive PE defined as occlusion of at least 30% of the pulmonary vascular bed in previously healthy persons, but can be less in persons with previous cardiopulmonary disease and particularly the elderly. Mild to moderate degrees of PH may be seen with acute hypoxemia, chronic obstructive pulmonary disease (COPD), pneumonia, pneumothorax, acute thromboemboli, or a left-sided event such as an acute myocardial infarction (MI) or valvular dysfunction causing pulmonary edema. Sudden severe PH can be seen when an acute insult (hypoxemia, pulmonary embolism) occurs in the setting of moderate degrees of PH associated with CHF. History and physical exam together with simple studies such as routine labs, chest x-ray (CXR), EKG, and arterial blood gases (ABG) help to clarify many of the possible etiologies.

Electrocardiogram

The ECG findings in PH lack both the sensitivity and specificity to distinguish among the various causes of PH, but the ECG should be obtained in

---

Box 2. WHO pulmonary hypertension functional assessment classification

Class I: Ordinary physical activity does not cause undue dyspnea or fatigue, chest pain, or near syncope.

Class II: Slight limitation of physical activity; ordinary physical activity causes undue dyspnea or fatigue, chest pain, or near syncope.

Class III: Marked limitation of physical activity; comfortable at rest, but less-than-ordinary activity causes undue dyspnea or fatigue, chest pain, or near syncope; signs of right-sided heart failure may be present.

Class IV: Inability to carry out any physical activity without symptoms; dyspnea and/or fatigue may even be present at rest; discomfort is increased by any physical activity; signs of right-sided heart failure are usually present.

Box 3. Causes of rapid deterioration in PAH

1. Natural history of the disease
2. Catheter occlusion or pump malfunction (prostacyclin)
3. Pneumonia
4. Indwelling catheter infection
5. RV ischemia, stunning, infarction
6. Pulmonary embolism
7. In situ pulmonary thrombus
8. Gastrointestinal (GI) bleeding
9. Anemia
10. Ischemic bowel
11. Pancreatitis
12. Acute renal failure
13. Hypothyroidism
14. Hyperthyroidism
15. Arrhythmias (atrial fibrillation/flutter)
16. Subdural hematoma (confusion/central nervous system (CNS) symptoms)
17. Hyponatremia
18. Hypokalemia
19. Dehydration (rare)

patients with dyspnea to assess for right ventricular hypertrophy (RVH) and its effects and ischemic disease, which can overlap. Care must be taken in interpretation of certain ECG findings. The $S_1Q_3T_3$ pattern (S wave in lead I, Q wave and inverted T wave in lead III), for example, reflects RVH and

Box 4. Causes of acute worsening of hypoxemia in PAH

1. RV failure and decrease cardiac output
2. Pump or catheter malfunction in patients who are on continuous therapy (ie, prostacyclin analogues)
3. In situ thrombosis
4. Pulmonary embolism (unlikely for patients who are therapeutic on warfarin and/or who are on prostacyclin analogues)
5. Pneumonia/atelectasis
6. Sepsis
7. Right to left shunt via a patent patent foramen ovale (PFO) or atrial septal defect (ASD)
8. Large pleural effusion
9. Pneumothorax

RV strain and is of no value in distinguishing PE from other causes of PH unless it appears suddenly. Left atrial abnormality or enlargement (LAE) may suggest pulmonary venous pressure elevation such as would occur in LVH, but an LAE pattern is not specific and may reflect right atrial (RA) enlargement. The typical ST-T findings in the right-sided precordial leads and inferior leads in RVH with RV strain mimic those seen in inferior MI and "anterior ischemia," and must be interpreted in the context of other available information. Automatic computerized interpretations are frequently misleading in PH [6]. An example is shown in Fig. 5.

Gas exchange and pulmonary function testing

Hypoxemia is common in PH, and usually occurs in the setting of increased minute ventilation and normal or low pCO_2. It is multifactorial in etiology, resulting from ventilation-perfusion inequality, loss of vascular bed volume, decreased cardiac output, and, in some cases, intracardiac shunting or associated interstitial lung disease. Neither the overall oxygen content nor the alveolar-arterial (A-a) oxygen gradient are useful in the diagnosis of PE [7], nor are they useful in distinguishing various causes of PH. An exception occurs when 100% oxygen does not change the arterial oxygen tension, which suggests an intracardiac shunt. In IPAH and CTEPH, pulmonary function

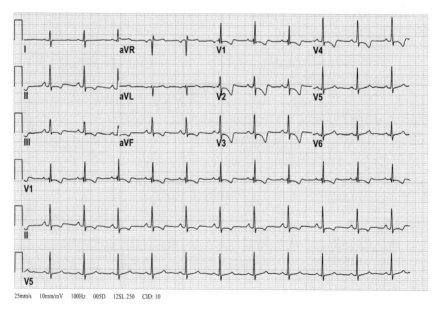

25mm/s   10mm/mV   100Hz   005D   12SL 250   CID: 10

Fig. 5. Sample ECG from a patient with IPAH. This was interpreted as "ST and T wave abnormality, consider anterior ischemia, ST and T wave abnormality, consider inferior ischemia" by the computer and a cardiologist unaware of the clinical history. With the clinical history known, a more accurate interpretation would be right ventricular hypertrophy with RV strain pattern in the inferior and anterior leads (V1–V4), borderline right atrial enlargement.

tests show a restrictive pattern and a reduction in diffusion capacity (DLCO), both of which are usually mild unless the cardiac output is very low. Obstructive disease and more severe restrictive disease suggest comorbid parenchymal lung disease and should prompt a high-resolution CT scan. Severe reduction in DLCO suggests associated interstitial lung disease, a very low cardiac output, or both.

Echocardiographic evaluation of pulmonary hypertension

The transthoracic echocardiogram (TTE) can be done at the bedside in unstable patients and provides an estimate of chamber pressures and volumes and valve competence, and can be used to distinguish pulmonary venous hypertension from PAH (see diagnostic algorithm Figs. 3 and 4). RVSP is calculated based on the peak Doppler derived systolic tricuspid regurgitation (TR) velocity, and equals the sPA in the absence of RV outflow obstruction. RVSP higher than 40 mm Hg represents PH, but this measurement must be interpreted in the context of other information. RVSP higher than 80 to 90 mm Hg suggests chronic disease, since the acutely stressed right ventricle cannot generate very high pressures. Other echocardiographic features of PH include RV hypokinesis, dilation of RA and RV, tricuspid annular dilatation with TR, and abnormal systolic bowing of the intraventricular septum toward the LV causing a D-shaped LV (Fig. 6) [8].

Echo-Doppler is useful in the unstable patient with evidence of RV dysfunction. One should keep in mind, however, that elevated right-sided pressures alone without RA/RV dilation, RV failure, or abnormal systolic bowing of the interventricular septum (IVS) may not be sufficient to explain

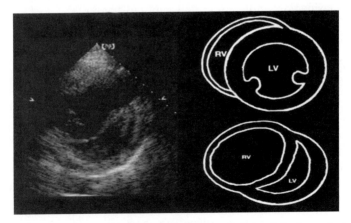

Fig. 6. Taken from a patient with hypotensive response to nifedipine. Left, short axis view shows diminished LV size and left-to-right septal bowing. Right above, normal; right below, diagram of echocardiogram on left. (*From* Ricciardi MJ, Bossone E, Bach DS, et al. Echocardiographic predictors of an adverse response to nifedipine trial in primary pulmonary hypertension: diminished left ventricular size and leftward ventricular septal bowing. Chest 1999;116(5):1221; with permission.)

hemodynamic instability. In the acutely unstable patient, TTE and/or trans-esophageal echocardiography (TEE) is useful for assessing LV and mitral and aortic valvular function, and to eliminate pericardial tamponade, aortic dissection, and myocardial infarction. Agitated saline should be routinely used and supplemented by cough and Valsalva's maneuver to detect intra-cardiac shunts such as atrial septal defect (ASD) and patent foramen ovale. The TTE may be useful in suspected PE with PH including visualization of clots in transit and by assessment of RV function, determination of progno-sis, and to decide the treatment paradigm. McConnell's sign can be used to differentiate RV hypokinesis secondary to PE from other causes. It refers to the sparing of contractility in the RV apex with hypokinesis of the right ven-tricular base. McConnell's sign is 77% sensitive and 94% specific for PE [9].

Evaluation for pulmonary thromboembolic disease

The combination of elevated jugular venous pressure, clear lungs, hypox-emia, and cool extremities with a narrow pulse pressure is highly suggestive of acute right heart failure and the differential diagnosis in this setting includes massive PE, cardiac tamponade, right ventricular infarction, pericardial con-striction, and decompensated PAH. In patients not known to have PH who present with severe hypoxemia and/or evidence of isolated right heart failure, PE should be the working diagnosis. Echo-Doppler is appropriate in some pa-tients (see Fig. 3) while others will require computer tomographic angiography (CTA), ventilation perfusion scanning, or conventional angiography to con-firm or exclude the diagnosis. In extremely unstable patients with RV failure and no underlying cardiopulmonary disease, empiric thrombolytic therapy may be considered without confirmation of the diagnosis.

Multiple strategies exist for the exclusion of PE as a potential diagnosis. Findings that are considered to exclude the diagnosis include a normal invasive pulmonary angiography, normal ventilation/perfusion scanning (V/Q), a negative D-Dimer combined with a low clinical probability of venous thromboembolic disease (VTE), and negative serial compression ultrasonogra-phy [10]. Multidetector-row CT angiography has rapidly penetrated clinical practice to become the most frequently employed modality for diagnosis of VTE in many centers, although fewer prospective data on its predictive value are available. In patients with nonacute presentation who are suspected of hav-ing PAH, central and or peripheral CTEPH must first be excluded by a V/Q scan and if necessary confirmed with a PE protocol CT or pulmonary angiogram.

Pulmonary embolism protocol computed tomography

Prospective studies evaluating the accuracy of spiral CTA in the diagno-sis of PE [11,12] suggest anticoagulation can safely be withheld in clinically stable patients with low to moderate clinical probability and a negative CTA. A major advantage of CT is its ability to evaluate pulmonary parenchyma and mediastinal structures, whereby diagnoses other than PE are made in a large proportion of patients scanned [11]. In the event of PE, as with the echo-Doppler, the finding of an enlarged right ventricle and septal bowing on CT imply an increased risk of morbidity and mortality and potential value of therapies beyond anticoagulation.

In the recently completed Prospective Investigation of Pulmonary Embolism Diagnosis (PIOPED II) study, multidetector row CT angiography had a sensitivity of 90% and a specificity of 95% for the diagnosis of PE, when combined with accompanying CT venography. Results that were discordant with clinical probability (ie, negative CT scan in a patient with high clinical probability or positive CT scan in a patient with low clinical probability) had significantly lower predictive values [12]. Critically ill patients were excluded from PIOPED II, however, and data regarding the use of CTA in this population are limited. A study of multidetector row CT in ICU patients revealed that 25% of CTA examinations were considered nondiagnostic on technical grounds, most commonly due to poor contrast bolus or artifact from motion or hardware [13].

Findings on CTA in CTEPH include increased size of the main pulmonary artery and branches, sharp vessel cutoffs, intraluminal thrombi or fibrotic material in the main PA and major and secondary branches, subpleural densities, bronchial artery collateral flow (arteriovenous malformations), and mosaic attenuation of pulmonary parenchyma. Negative results on CTA do not exclude CTEPH as reliably as V/Q and the latter is therefore recommended as the initial study in stable patients being evaluated for PH. CT angiography may be used for anatomic characterization in patients with intermediate or high probability V/Q scans.

Ventilation/perfusion scanning

Ventilation/perfusion scintigraphy (V/Q scan) has long been the initial diagnostic study of choice for suspected PE, but is being eclipsed by CTA, despite lack of data on reproducibility in the clinical setting as opposed to expert academic centers. In the PIOPED study [14], high probability V/Q scans with concordant clinical probability had a positive predictive value of 96% and normal scans had a negative predictive value of 96%. The principal drawback of V/Q scanning is the frequent low and intermediate probability results, which occurred in 73% of patients in the PIOPED study, and must be considered nondiagnostic. Critically ill patients, many of whom have underlying cardiopulmonary disease, are even less likely than the population at large to have a normal V/Q scan, making its utility in eliminating PE as a diagnostic possibility low. High probability results have positive predictive value in critically ill patients similar to that in other populations, and strongly suggest the diagnosis of PE, especially if clinical suspicion is also high [15]. High probability V/Q scans can be seen with tumors, vasculitis, pulmonary veno-occlusive disease, and pulmonary capillary hemangiomatosis [15].

Pulmonary angiography

Right heart catheterization and pulmonary angiography (PA) has largely been replaced in clinical practice by CTA because of its difficulty, expense, and the added risks associated with use of an invasive diagnostic procedure. Invasive angiography allows for localization of the embolism and measurement of hemodynamic parameters, but its primary advantage is that it allows for simultaneous therapeutic intervention. Inferior vena cava (IVC) filters can be placed and thrombi can be fragmented or extracted via catheter-based techniques. Since most patients with PE are hemodynamically stable and are not candidates for therapy beyond anticoagulation, noninvasive diagnosis is adequate. In the critically ill, the ability to make a definitive diagnosis quickly, and provide potential for therapeutic intervention, makes pulmonary angiography an attractive first-line modality. It is also useful when noninvasive testing is not definitive and empiric treatment is not justified.

PA and right heart catheterization are necessary in CTEPH patients who are unstable or at least WHO class II. Clinical, hemodynamic, and anatomic data are used to determine candidacy for surgical intervention with a pulmonary thromboendarterectomy. It may be preferable to defer angiography and hemodynamic assessment to experienced centers.

Biomarkers in pulmonary hypertension

The D-dimer assay can be helpful in excluding VTE in hemodynamically stable patients, especially if the pretest probability of VTE is low, but its role in the acutely ill or unstable patient is limited by the need to make a definitive diagnosis rapidly [10] and the high prevalence of comorbidities that can cause false-positive results.

Elevations in cardiac troponin I and troponin T occur in PE and can be useful in risk stratification. The degree of troponin elevation correlates with right ventricular dysfunction, mortality, and complicated hospital course [16]. Patients with a normal troponin have a low risk of in-hospital death, and can be safely treated with anticoagulation alone [17]. The presence of detectable troponin T is also associated with a poorer prognosis in PAH [18]. Detectable levels do not necessarily imply an acute event in PAH and CTEPH patients who may have chronic elevations.

Brain natriuretic peptide (BNP) and N-terminal brain natriuretic peptide (NT-BNP) are released in response to myocardial wall stress, and have been useful for differentiating pulmonary and cardiac causes of dyspnea. However, both are elevated in left or right ventricular pressure overload, including PE, CTEPH, and the various forms of PAH. Levels of BNP expected in WHO class IV or hypotension associated with PH range from 500 to 3000 pg/mL. BNP may be falsely low in obesity and elevated in acute or chronic renal failure of even mild to moderate degree. A normal BNP indicates a favorable prognosis in PE [19] and IPAH [20].

Hemodynamics in pulmonary hypertension

The normal range of directly measured and derived parameters obtained on a right heart catheterization is summarized in Box 5. In healthy adults,

---

Box 5. Normal hemodynamic parameters

Hemodynamic Parameter	Normal Value
Right atrial pressure (RA)	≤ 6 mm Hg
Right ventricular pressure	Systolic 15–25 mm Hg
	Diastolic 0–8 mm Hg
Pulmonary artery pressure	sPA 15–30 mm Hg
(PA, electrical mean	dPA 8–15 mm Hg
PA = sPA + 2dPA/3)	mPA 6–19 mm Hg
Pulmonary artery occlusive pressure (mean PAOP) or PCW	≤12 mm Hg
Mean arterial pressure = (SBP + 2DBP)/3	70–100 mm Hg
Cardiac output (CO)	4–8 L/min
Fick = Oxygen consumption/ [Hgb(g/dL) × 13.6 × (SaO$_2$ – SvO$_2$)]	
Mixed venous O$_2$ (SvO$_2$) – as measured in RA, RV, or PA if no shunt; In presence of shunt, SvO$_2$ = [3 × (O$_2$ sat in SVC) + (O$_2$ sat in IVC)]/4	65%–75% (without anemia)
Cardiac index (CI) = CO/BSA	2.6–4.2 L/min/m^2
Systemic vascular resistance (SVR) = [(mean arterial pressure – mean RA)/CO]	800–1200 dynes × sec/cm^5
Pulmonary vascular resistance (PVR) = [(mPA – mean PAOP)/ CO] × 80. RU or Wood units are the absolute value not multiplied by 80.	40–120 dynes × sec/cm^5 0.5–1.2 RU or Wood units
Pulmonary vascular resistance index (PVRI) = PVR/CI	≤ 2.8 (ages 6 to 10) ≤ 3.2 (ages 32 to 45) ≤ 4.6 (ages 60 to 83)

the normal mean pulmonary artery pressure (mPA) range is 9 to 19 mm Hg. An mPA of 20 to 24 is characterized as mild PH; 25 to 35 mm Hg mild to moderate; mPA 35 to 45 mm Hg moderate; and mPA greater than 45 mm Hg is severe PH [21,22]. In PAH the PAOP or PCW is equal to or less than 15 mm Hg, whereas in pulmonary venous hypertension PAOP is greater than 15 mm Hg. Obtaining an accurate PAOP can be difficult in PH patients due to high-velocity TR jets, and enlarged and thickened vessels and elevated pressures that prevent the balloon from occluding the vessel. Special flotation catheters are available through which a stiffening wire can be carefully advanced to stabilize the catheter in place. These catheters must be used with caution to avoid perforation of the RA, RV, or pulmonary artery. When the PAOP or PCW is elevated in the setting of PH, a left heart catheterization is necessary to determine the accuracy of the PCW and contribution of left ventricular filling pressure to the mPA, dPA, and PVR. As per the Venn diagram in Fig. 1, multifactorial PH should always be a consideration when interpreting the hemodynamic data and deciding treatment strategies. For example, in scleroderma, each of the following can occur together: systemic hypertension and LV diastolic dysfunction; scleroderma heart disease; interstitial lung disease; and intrinsic pulmonary arterial disease. The presence of an elevated LV diastolic pressure and PAOP does not exclude a contribution of pulmonary arteriole vasculopathy, which could be a therapeutic target. The latter can be suspected when the mean PA to PAOP gradient is greater than 10 mm Hg, and the dPA to PAOP gradient is greater than 5 to 10 mm Hg.

Cardiac output (CO) can and should be determined by both the thermodilution and Fick methods. In the presence of significant tricuspid regurgitation (TR), the thermodilution technique may underestimate CO, whereas in the presence of a left to right intracardiac shunt it overestimates the systemic CO. In the absence of left to right or bidirectional intracardiac shunts, both techniques are useful together. Particularly since the oxygen consumption is estimated, patients are usually on supplemental oxygen, and may be anemic. A single measure or continuous monitoring of the mixed venous oxygen saturation (mVO_2) is useful for estimating cardiac output and prognosis. An mVO_2 less than 60% is associated with a poor prognosis in PAH. The implications of the mVO_2 need to be considered in light of the hemoglobin, since it will decrease proportionately.

A mean right atrial pressure (mRA) $\geq$ 8 and RV end diastolic pressure $\geq$ 12 are consistent with RV failure. The mRA correlates with the RV filling pressure unless there is more than mild tricuspid insufficiency characterized by RA v-wave > a-wave. Severe degrees of RV failure (RA usually > 10 to 12 mm Hg and as high as 25 mm Hg with giant "V" waves) results in a marked increase in RV diastolic pressure (mid-diastolic 10 to 15 mm Hg, end-diastolic 15 to 20 mm Hg), which can compress the LV causing an increased LV filling pressure and reduced LV filling volume. The dynamic interaction between the RV and LV can be associated with an increase in PCW in precapillary PH. The underfilling of the left ventricle can result in a marked reduction in LV stroke volume and cardiac output, which will be demonstrated in the section on echo-Doppler. Markedly increased right ventricular pressures together with decreased left ventricular stroke volume and systemic pressure can compromise the right coronary artery flow resulting in right ventricular ischemia and further contributing to the right-sided failure.

Vasodilator response during hemodynamic measurements

PH specialists use the hemodynamic response to vasodilators to help decide treatment and prognosis. Vasodilator reserve infers a better prognosis [23] and treatment response to calcium channel blocker (CCB) therapy. Vasodilators that can be used include inhaled nitric oxide (iNO), intravenous (IV) epoprostenol, and IV adenosine. There is no utility to IV nitroglycerin. We prefer iNO because of its rapid onset of action and short half-life, ease of administration, and no effect on systemic pressures. Testing should be done by physicians experienced with the agents and the pitfalls with the interpretation. A positive response includes a reduction in mean PA $\geq$ 10 mm Hg to achieve a mean PA $\leq$ 40 mm Hg with an increased or unchanged cardiac output [23]. About 10% to 20% of PAH patients have a positive response, which could warrant consideration of CCB therapy. CCB therapy is never given in unstable patients, or those with right heart failure.

Treatment of acute and chronic thromboembolic disease

Acute pulmonary embolism

Fig. 3 is an algorithm for the evaluation and management of patients with symptoms and signs consistent with acute PE. In the absence of a contraindication, anticoagulation with unfractionated heparin (UFH) should be started in patients with suspected major PE. Recent meta-analyses comparing low molecular weight heparin (LMWH) to UFH in patients with nonmassive PE have demonstrated trends toward decreased recurrence and decreased bleeding with LMWH [24,25], but there are no data in massive PE (defined as hemodynamic instability and severe hypoxemia). Once the diagnosis has been confirmed, oral anticoagulation with warfarin should be continued for at least 6 months if the event was related to a reversible risk factor, and up to 5 years or longer if not [26,27].

Additional therapies may be warranted in certain patient populations. Mortality in PE increases with right ventricular dysfunction on echo-Doppler [28] or CT [29], systemic hypotension, shock, and cardiac arrest [30]. Surgical embolectomy and catheter-based interventions are options in acute PE with systemic hypotension, shock, or cardiac arrest, although the use of such modalities is not well supported by large randomized clinical trials in any population. In experienced hands, aggressive protocols for intervention in patients with severe RV dysfunction due to PE have resulted in mortality rates below what would be expected based on historical data [31]. There are no trials comparing the effectiveness of thrombolytic therapy with surgical or catheter-based approaches. In patients with significant hypoxemia, hypotension, and other high-risk indices, thrombolytic therapy is used unless contraindicated. Surgical embolectomy and catheter-based thrombus extraction are appropriate in experienced centers in patients with hypotension who require cardiac surgery for an alternate indication and those with contraindication to thrombolytics, although the contraindications for the two approaches overlap.

Appropriate treatment of patients with RV dysfunction and preserved systemic blood pressure is controversial. Such patients face mortality rates approximately twice as high as those with uncomplicated PE [28], and some authorities advocate aggressive intervention, but improved outcomes with this approach have yet to be clearly demonstrated. In the Management Strategies and Prognosis of Pulmonary Embolism-3 (MAPPET-3) study, normotensive patients with RV dysfunction who were given IV thrombolytic therapy had decreased need for escalation of therapy, including endotracheal intubation, pressor support, and use of open-label thrombolytics, but there was no difference in mortality [32]. A recent meta-analysis of thrombolytics in PE showed no benefit overall, but there was a decrease in death or recurrent PE, which was confined to studies that enrolled patients with hemodynamic instability [33]. Larger trials are needed to definitively elucidate the role of thrombolysis and embolectomy (surgical or catheter-based) in PE. Until such studies are done, practice patterns will continue to differ by experience and intuitive bias.

IVC filters are warranted in patients who cannot be anticoagulated, have failed anticoagulation, or are thought to have insufficient cardiopulmonary reserve to tolerate further thromboemboli including those with chronic thromboembolic PH. In patients who can tolerate oral anticoagulation there is little advantage to a filter. The short-term reduction in pulmonary emboli that can be achieved via IVC filter placement is no longer evident 2 years after placement, presumably because of propagation of thrombus through the filter and formation of collateral vessels, and is balanced by a long-term increase in deep vein thrombosis [34].

Hypotension in acute PE is usually a reflection of RV failure and its treatment is similar to that in RV failure due to PAH. The use of fluids and catecholamines in RV failure is discussed later in this article.

Chronic thromboembolic pulmonary hypertension (CTEPH)

CTEPH is thought to follow incomplete resolution of one or more acute massive or submassive PE. The concept that recurrent small pulmonary emboli result in severe PH is not supported by clinical or pathologic findings.

Following occlusion of primary and secondary pulmonary artery branches, both loss of volume in the pulmonary vasculature and a progressive secondary vasculopathy [35] that is histologically indistinguishable from other forms of PH contribute to elevated pulmonary vascular resistance. Hemodynamic parameters found in significant CTEPH are similar to those found in PAH, but symptoms can occur with lower degrees of PH, particularly when associated with anemia, COPD, or CHF.

Patients with CTEPH require lifelong anticoagulation with warfarin, regardless of the presence or absence of acute PE by history. Anticoagulation does not affect the chronic emboli/thrombi that are replaced with fibrous tissue, nor prevent the progression of the pulmonary vasculopathy, but may reduce in situ thrombi and recurrent thromboembolus. Because these patients cannot tolerate further acute emboli, an inferior vena cava filter is indicated.

A pulmonary thromboendarterectomy (PEA) is indicated in CTEPH in patients who are WHO class III or greater and have a PVR of at least 3 Wood units [36]. While the risk of PEA can be as high as 25% and depends on the experience of the surgical team and patient risk factors, more than 90% of survivors benefit from surgery. At the University of California in San Diego, where the procedure was developed and refined, the mortality in the recent past is 4.4% [36]. Experience, however, is that a percentage of survivors may have persistent PH or gradual worsening of PH that requires treatments similar to PAH. There are, as yet, no clear guidelines on selection of patients for surgery. The location of the emboli influences the technical feasibility of the operation with more distal thrombus being less accessible. The degree of distal vessel vascular remodeling has important prognostic implications for patients undergoing surgery with later stage disease being associated with increased perioperative mortality and decreased postoperative hemodynamic improvement. Patients found to have CTEPH should be referred to an experienced center for determination of candidacy.

Medical therapy with IV epoprostenol has been used as a bridge to PEA in patients with CTEPH and severe peripheral pulmonary vasculopathy [37]. Improving hemodynamics by treatment of the pulmonary vasculopathy in non-occluded vessels may improve surgical outcomes, given that higher preoperative PVR confers a worse prognosis. Treatment of CTEPH patients who are not surgical candidates or who have failed PEA includes inhaled iloprost [38], sildenafil [39], and bosentan [40]. Improvements in clinical outcomes and 6-minute walk distance, and hemodynamic outcomes including PVR have been noted with each of these agents. Continuous infusion of sub-Q treprostinil was associated with an improved survival in CTEPH compared to historic controls [41]. Intravenous prostacyclins, treprostinil, and epoprostenol can be effective in WHO class III and IV CTEPH.

Treatment of pulmonary arterial hypertension

Drug treatment options for PAH or pre-capillary pulmonary hypertension are complex, vary considerably, and each has a particular role. It is important to understand the indications and complications of each. For patients with known PAH who deteriorate or with newly diagnosed WHO class III or IV PAH requiring hospitalization, referral to an experienced PAH center should be made as early as possible.

Rapid deterioration in PAH is associated with marked fatigue and dyspnea, increasing edema and ascites (anasarca), renal failure, malnutrition and malabsorption, hypoxemia, hypotension, and CNS symptoms including confusion. Box 4 summarizes the most common causes. Management of acute deterioration must be urgently targeted toward the underlying mechanisms.

Hypotension

Hypotension in WHO class IV PAH is rarely related to low intravascular volume with the exception of acute GI bleeding, overdiuresis, vomiting, and diarrhea. The risk of both upper and lower GI bleeding is increased in PH with RV failure and hypotension due to decreased gastric emptying; hypoperfused ischemic and congested bowel; warfarin; and prostacyclin, a potent platelet antagonist that causes thrombocytopenia (not immune mediated and usually 40-75 K platelet count) in 10% of cases.

More commonly, hypotension is due to worsening RV failure. If a drug delivery pump failure or Hickman catheter occlusion is found, the drug should be restarted through alternative access (including peripheral) as soon as possible. Considerations for hypotension include systemic vasodilation from CCBs (which should be avoided), sildenafil, ACEi or ARBs, and the negative inotropic effect of beta blockers and diltiazem. An excessive dose of IV prostacyclin (epoprostenol, treprostinil) may cause hypotension, which would often be accompanied by a headache, macular rash, or diarrhea. If suspected, the infusion rate can be reduced by 25% after a 1-minute interruption to test for overdose. If there is no change, that may be repeated in 5 minutes. If blood pressure is adversely affected, the previous dose should be resumed.

A quick infectious workup should be completed and broad-spectrum antibiotics should be started if infection is suspected. Central line infection occurs in 2% to 3% of patients each year in those receiving chronic IV prostacyclin therapy and is often subclinical.

It is difficult to determine volume status in PH given the RV dysfunction, low stroke volume and decreased arterial pulse pressure. An elevated jugular venous pressure (JVP) (> 12–15 cm) is inconsistent with significant volume depletion, but intravascular volume can be low in patients with edema and ascites. Rapid fluid administration should be limited to those patients who are clearly volume depleted until invasive or echo-Doppler assessment of volume can be made. Fluid administration in the setting of right ventricular pressure overload, as evidenced by septal bowing and a compressed left ventricle on echo (Fig. 7), will result in further dilatation and decrease in RV function and decreasing LV stroke volume. When volume status is not clear, it is reasonable to rapidly infuse 200 mL of saline over 10 minutes to assess the effect on systemic pressure.

Hypotension in patients with severe PAH *must be rapidly reversed* to avoid spiraling decrease in RV function and cardiac output. Super-systemic RV and PA pressures combined with systemic hypotension can result in critically low oxygen transport; severe hypoxemia (due to low flow and right to left shunt via a patent foramen ovale [PFO] or ASD); decrease in coronary blood flow, and RV ischemia, stunning, and infarction followed by electrical-mechanical dissociation or ventricular fibrillation. In patients not able to maintain a mean arterial pressure of at least 60 to 70 mm Hg, agents with α1 receptor activity (phenylephrine, norepinephrine, high dose dopamine [Table 1]) are preferred. The α1 receptor activity increases systemic arterial pressure and coronary perfusion pressure, systemic resistance and LV afterload, and reduces RV compression of the LV and LV outflow tract, which improves LV stroke volume and cardiac output. When systemic pressure is adequate, inotropic drugs such as dobutamine and milrinone can be added to improve cardiac output. Once systemic pressure is reasonable, IV epoprostenol can be used to increase cardiac output and reduce pulmonary pressures. On occasion, in de novo patients with PAH presenting with hypotension, iNO (not approved by the Food and Drug Administration [FDA] for this indication), a selective pulmonary vasodilator, will reduce the pulmonary artery pressure, improve cardiac output, and reverse hypotension, which gives time for long-term treatment options. Survival is rare in patients

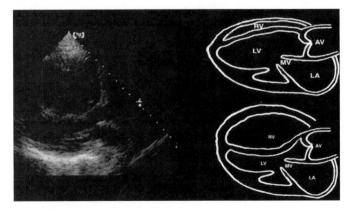

Fig. 7. Left is a parasternal long axis view taken from a patient with nifedipine hypotension. Demonstrates the decreased LV size and septal bowing occluding the LV outflow tract. Right above is normal; right below is a diagram of the echocardiogram on the left. (*From* Ricciardi MJ, Bossone E, Bach DS, et al. Echocardiographic predictors of an adverse response to nifedipine trial in primary pulmonary hypertension: diminished left ventricular size and leftward ventricular septal bowing. Chest 1999;116(5):1221; with permission.)

Table 1
Vasopressor and inotropic agents used in hypotension/shock

Agent	Receptor activity and dose (IV)	Effect	Onset and duration of action	Pitfalls
Dopamine	$D1 = D2 \gg \beta \gg \alpha$ Dopamine receptors: 0.5–2 μg/kg/min Beta receptors: 5–10 μg/kg/min Mixed alpha and beta: 10–20 μg/kg/min Predominantly alpha: >20 μg/kg/min	Effects on dopaminergic receptors produce renal and mesenteric vasodilation. β1 receptor activity has inotropic and chronotropic effects; β2 vasodilatory effects. Overall effect on α1 and α2 receptors causes peripheral vasoconstriction.	Onset within 5 min. Duration < 10 min after discontinuation	Initial titration may result in further hypotension. Increases ventricular ectopy and arrhythmias especially at high doses; hypertension at high doses; peripheral ischemia in presence of peripheral vascular disease.
Phenylephrine Neosynephrin	$\alpha1 > \alpha2 \ggg \beta$ Start 100–180 μg/min, once BP is stable decrease dose to 40–60 μg/min for maintenance.	Potent vasoconstrictor secondary to α1 receptor activity	Immediate onset of action. Duration 15–20 min after discontinuation.	Hypertension; headaches restlessness; reflex bradycardia; peripheral ischemia in presence of peripheral vascular disease.
Norepinephrine Levophed	$\alpha1 = \alpha2; \beta1 \gg \beta2$ Start with 0.05–0.1 μg/kg/min, adjust dose to blood pressure response to a maximum of 1.5 μg/kg/min.	Main action is on the β1 and α receptors, thus has inotropic, and chronotropic effects and causes peripheral vasoconstriction.	Onset is in 1–2 min; duration is 1–2 min after discontinuation.	Dose-related hypertension; reflex bradycardia; arrhythmias.
Dobutamine	$\beta1 > \beta2 \ggg \alpha$ Start with 2.5 μg/kg/min, increasing gradually in 2.5-μg/kg/min increments to 20 μg/kg/min, adjusting dosage to response	Major action is inotropic effect via dopaminergic receptors and β1. The clinical effect is a potent β1 agonist with mild vasodilatory properties. Effective in combination with vasoconstrictor phenylephrine	Onset very rapid (< 2 min), peak within 10 min; duration <10 min	Arrhythmias, ventricular and atrial. May worsen hypotension given without vasoconstrictors.

with long-standing PAH on treatment who develop cardiogenic shock without a clear alternative explanation.

Hypoxemia

A similar search for a superimposed insult should be undertaken when a PAH patient becomes acutely hypoxemic, with the differential diagnosis in Box 5. When each has been excluded, the cause is deteriorating RV function and morbidly low cardiac output. Very often it is a combination of factors. Pulmonary emboli are rare in patients on warfarin and epoprostenol. Supplemental oxygen should be provided to maintain arterial saturation above 92% if possible. To maintain adequate oxygen transport (the product of arterial oxygen content [Hgb × 1.34 × sAO$_2$%] × cardiac output), blood transfusions should be considered. Blood products may be life saving, but could increase the antigen burden so as to preclude lung or heart-lung transplant.

Continuous positive pressure ventilation may improve oxygenation temporarily. Intubation and ventilator support may be needed for adequate oxygenation, particularly in the setting of pneumonia.

Arrhythmias

Sinus tachycardia in chronic PH is unusual and generally a manifestation of infection, hypovolemia, hypoxemia, or low output. Atrial fibrillation and flutter are the most common types of dysrhythmia and can result in rapid clinical worsening. The loss of atrial contraction and increasing rate result in decreasing LV filling pressure and volume, and decreasing RV and LV stroke volume, CO, and hypotension. Treatment of tachyarrhythmia follows the advanced cardiac life support (ACLS) algorithm with DC cardioversion of unstable patients (hypotension, hypoxemia). IV diltiazem and adenosine should be avoided in PH with markedly impaired RV function and hypotension. Rate slowing can be achieved with IV digoxin, carefully administered short-acting IV beta blockers, and IV amiodarone. For maintenance of sinus rhythm, amiodarone and type 1C agents including propafenone and flecainide can be used with caution. Disopyramide should be avoided.

Ventricular arrhythmias occur primarily in end-stage disease and their treatment, according to ACLS algorithms, is minimally effective in improving outcomes. Cardiopulmonary resuscitation (CPR) status should be discussed with PH patients and families, preferably before they become critically ill, so they can make an informed end-of-life decision. CPR is uniformly ineffective in PAH when associated with end-stage disease and severe right heart failure [42].

Adjunctive therapy in PAH

Nonspecific adjunctive therapy in PAH includes warfarin, supplemental oxygen, diuretics, digoxin, nutrition to ideal weight, salt restriction, and regular exercise. Warfarin has been shown to improve survival in IPAH (prior to the prostacyclin era), possibly by preventing in-situ thrombi [43]. While there are no supporting data, it is also considered appropriate for PAH from associated conditions (eg, scleroderma, Eisenmenger's) [2]. Target international normalized ratio (INR) is usually 2 to 3, but is reduced to 1.5 to 2.5 when used with prostacyclins. Unlike in thromboembolic PH, there is no need to transition to warfarin with heparin or LMWH.

Patients should be assessed for the need of supplemental O_2 to maintain arterial oxygen saturation higher than 90% at rest, during sleep, and during activity. Diuretics are used to prevent RV volume overload, and the discomfort and complications of edema, ascites, and malabsorption associated with bowel edema. Electrolytes and renal function should be observed closely. Spironolactone can be used as an adjunctive and potassium-sparing diuretic and thiazides can be used sparingly to augment loop diuretics. Digoxin increases baroreceptor sensitivity, and may increase cardiac output, but there are no controlled studies. Predose blood levels should not exceed 1 ng/mL.

Because of their complexity and the need for frequent, intensive, and skilled physician and nurse monitoring, initiation of PAH-specific therapies should generally be deferred to experienced physicians and centers with dedicated programs and appropriate nursing support. Fig. 8 shows the portion of the treatment algorithm developed at the third World Symposium on Pulmonary Arterial Hypertension [44], applicable to acutely ill patients. The algorithm is based on drug safety, efficacy, ease of use, and need for rapid effectiveness. The degree and duration of benefit from each available treatment option is not predictable, and is dependent upon many factors including the duration of the disease/symptoms, WHO class, RV function, severity of PH, and etiology (eg, scleroderma worst prognosis). Combination therapies are required in most WHO class III and IV patients. The goal is to improve the patient to at least WHO class II without evidence for right heart failure. Patients are generally begun on a single agent and reevaluated every 3 months with clinical and functional assessment that includes presence of RH failure, BNP level, distance achieved on a 6-minute hall walk, oxygen requirements, and periodic repeat right heart catheterization. If patients have not improved to WHO class II with improvement in the other parameters, a second agent and/or third agent is added. If they deteriorate from WHO class III to IV, a prostacyclin analogue is added, which is usually parenteral.

CCB treatment is rarely effective and generally should be avoided, in particular empiric unmonitored use. A retrospective analysis of survival on long-term CCB therapy showed that only 54% of patients with response to acute vasodilator therapy continued to have long-term response (> 1 year) [23]. The use of CCBs can result in systemic hypotension and rapid progression to death in minutes to hours.

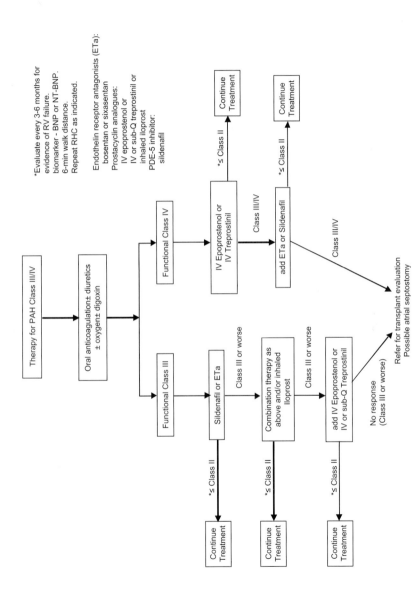

Fig. 8. Treatment algorithm for pulmonary arterial hypertension WHO classes III and IV.

Specific treatment for pulmonary hypertension

Table 2 summarizes each of the drug therapies for PAH. The material has been extracted from FDA-approved drug information inserts, references, and is supplemented by experience.

Endothelin antagonists

Endothelin antagonists (ETa) are the first oral drug class found specifically effective in PAH. Endothelin-1 is a potent vasoconstrictor and smooth muscle mitogen capable of inducing smooth muscle cell hypertrophy and is increased in patients with IPAH. There are two types of endothelin receptors—ET-A (involved in vasoconstriction and smooth muscle proliferation) and ET-B (vasodilation and involved in clearance of endothelin). Bosentan, a nonspecific ETa, and sitaxsentan (6000 times more specific for ET-A) are the two endothelin receptor antagonists that have been studied extensively. Bosentan (Tracleer) is FDA approved for PAH WHO classes III and IV. Following approval by third-party insurance, it is distributed via special pharmacies. In IPAH and scleroderma-related disorders, it improves symptoms, hemodynamics, and exercise capacity [45]. The major risk is hepatic toxicity, and liver function tests (LFTs) must be monitored monthly (see Table 2). About 10% of patients require discontinuation because of ALT/AST rise by more than threefold upper lab limits, and a small percentage for unexplained anemia. Double birth-control precautions are recommended. Other considerations include the interaction with drugs using the P-450 system, and the effects on spermatogenesis and teratogenesis. Sitaxsentan (Thelin) has been evaluated in WHO functional class II-IV patients with IPAH, PAH secondary to connective tissue diseases and congenital heart disease. It improves exercise capacity and functional class [46] and is associated with less hepatotoxicity than bosentan (3% versus 11%) [46], but still requires regular monitoring for hepatoxicity. Sitaxsentan can reduce the required dose of warfarin and increase bleeding risk if the INR is not monitored appropriately (see Table 2). A third endothelin antagonist, ambrisentan, which is intermediate regarding selectivity, is in phase III clinical trials.

Phosphodiesterase-5 inhibitor

Sildenafil (Revatio), a potent inhibitor of phosphodiesterase-5 (PDE-5), used for erectile dysfunction, is an effective treatment option for PAH. Nitric oxide (NO), the endothelial-derived relaxing factor, has vasodilatory effects that are by mediated by activation of guanylate cyclase and increased cGMP production. PDE-5 inhibition increases intracellular cGMP and prolongs its vasodilatory effects. When sildenafil is used in combination with iNO, it has been shown to augment and prolong the hemodynamic effects

Table 2
Pulmonary arterial hypertension specific drug therapy

Drug class	Dosing	Pharmacology	Effect	Adverse effect	Other benefits/pitfalls
Prostacyclin Analogue: Epoprostenol (intravenous) Flolan	Start 2 ng/kg/min; titrate 1–2 ng/kg/min daily for 3–4 days. Wait at least 15 min between dose changes. Dose adjust q 1–2 weeks as tolerated until improved. Long-term dosing averages 45 ng/kg/min; range 10–>100 ng/kg/min. Adjust dose with weight loss and symptoms.	Half life <4–6 min. Reaches steady state in 15 min. Clinical improvement may be seen within hours.	Potent vasodilator of the systemic and pulmonary vasculature; antiplatelet; Major effect is long-term effect is improved RV function and cardiac output and vascular remodeling. Benefit in days, but major effects at 3–6 mos.	Headache; flushing; jaw pain; diarrhea; nausea; body aches; hypotension; dizziness rash; anemia; thrombocytopenia; hypersplenism, hyper- and hypothyroid, goiter	Unstable at room temperature, needs to be kept at 2–8°C at all times; mixed by the patients in sterile fashion; requires central venous access for long term; interruption may cause rebound worsening of PH and death; infusion line infections not uncommon. May be infused via peripheral IV. Can use standard high-precision infusion pump in the hospital setting. Monitor regularly for thrombocytopenia (40–80K) that occurs in 10% of long-term users and is an indication to stop warfarin

(continued on next page)

Table 2 (*continued*)

Drug class	Dosing	Pharmacology	Effect	Adverse effect	Other benefits/pitfalls
Treprostinil (intravenous; subcutaneous). Remodulin	Sub Q and IV: start 1.25 ng/kg/min and increase by 1.25 ng/kg/min/wk × 4 wks then by 2.5 ng/kg/min/wk as tolerated. Dose range 15–100 ng/kg/min. Experienced centers will titrate faster.	Half life 3 h. Almost 100% bioavailable. Reaches steady state in 10 h.	Similar to epoprostenol.	Sub-Q: pain, induration or erythema at infusion site; otherwise as with epoprostenol for IV with possibly less side effects.	Stable at room temperature; comes premixed; catheter can be replaced or pump switched without serious complications given the long half-life; used sub Q need to change the infusion site every 2–30 days to prevent infusion site reaction. Dosing IV and sub Q are the same. Dosing experience less than epoprostenol, In unstable patients would prefer epoprostenol.
Iloprost (inhaled) Ventavis	Start 2.5 μg/inh × 6–8/ day. Increase to 5 μg/ inh in 1–2 wks as tolerated. Daily doses >45 μg has not been studied in randomized control studies.	Half-life 20–30 min. Acts within 30 min. Not detectable in plasma 30 min–1 h after inhalation	Similar to others but less potent	Jaw pain; headache; mild cough; flushing; dizziness; hypotension.	Inconvenient given frequency and duration of inhalations. Can be used safely with sildenafil and endothelin antagonists. When combined with sildenafil may need less frequent dosing. No clinical trial data with ventilators or during anesthesia

Drug	Dosing	Pharmacokinetics	Effect	Side Effects	Metabolism/Contraindications
Endothelin Antagonists: Bosentan (oral) Tracleer	Initiate at 62.5 mg twice a day × 4 wks then increase to 125 mg twice a day.	Half-life is 5 h. Max plasma concentration is attained in 3–5 h.	Causes vasodilation in the systemic and pulmonary vasculature. First effect at 2–4 wks maximal effect 3–6 mo.	Liver toxicity (10%); headache; flushing; hypotension; edema; anemia; decreases efficacy of oral contraceptives	Teratogenic. Liver toxicity is enhanced when used with glyburide. Metabolized by and inducer of CYP2C9 and CYP3A4 and caution with drugs affecting this system (ketaconazole). Contraindicated with cyclosporine and glyburide.
Sitaxsentan (oral) Thelin	100 mg daily	Half-life is 10 h and steady state reached in about 6 d.	Causes vasodilation in the systemic and pulmonary vasculature with remodeling. Initial effect seen at 2–4 wks and continues to improve 3–6 mos.	Liver toxicity 3%; peripheral edema; nausea; nasal congestion; headache; dizziness	Primarily metabolized by and inhibitor of CYP2C9, which interferes with warfarin metabolism and elevates INR. Teratogenic.
PDE-5 inhibitors: Sildenafil (oral) Revatio	20 mg, 3 times a day, with 4–6 h between doses.	Half-life is 4 h. Peak levels in 60 min after ingestion.	Systemic and pulmonary vasodilation and remodeling likely. Onset may be in hours to days with maximal effects in 3–6 mos.	Visual changes; dyspepsia; flushing; headache; hypotension.	Metabolized by CYP 450 system. Contraindicated with nitrates.

and prevent rebound vasoconstriction when iNO is discontinued [47]. Silde-nafil has been evaluated extensively in a large randomized placebo-controlled trial in PAH WHO classes II to IV. At both 12-week and 1-year follow-up there was an improvement in functional class and exercise toler-ance, and a very good safety profile [48]. Hemodynamic benefits are similar to those found with the endothelin antagonists. Clinical experience suggests it is safe and effective in combination with prostacyclin and ETa, each of which is being evaluated in clinical trials. Sildenafil is approved for PAH regardless of WHO class.

Prostacyclin analogues

IV epoprostenol (Flolan) is the first available drug specific for PAH and remains the most appropriate first-line agent in the critically ill. Epoproste-nol improves symptoms, hemodynamics, and long-term survival in PAH classes III and IV [48,49], and is FDA approved for use in WHO classes III to IV. It has a sustained benefit on survival; 62.8% at 3 years compared to expected 35.4% survival based on historical controls [49].

Because it is a complicated drug with a very short half-life requiring con-tinuous IV delivery via an indwelling catheter (see Table 2), patients initi-ated on epoprostenol and their significant others require a great deal of education and support to manage the drug and its delivery system. Compli-cations of therapy include failure of the infusion pump; dislodgement, occlu-sion, or fracture of the indwelling catheter; and catheter infections ranging from local abscess and cellulitis to bacteremia and sepsis, which can be mono- and poly-microbial. Any bacterial pathogen including diptheroids can seed the catheter and result in bacteremia.

Treprostinil (Remodulin), a newer prostacyclin analogue with a half-life of 3 to 4 hours, can be given by continuous subcutaneous or IV infusion. IV epoprostenol, IV treprostinil, and subcutaneous treprostinil have similar he-modynamic effects [50]. Because of less long-term experience, IV treprostinil is best used in patients who are stable. The largest treprostinil trial included WHO class II to IV patients (IPAH, scleroderma, and congenital heart dis-ease) and showed improved exercise capacity with 6-minute walk distance [51]. There is a long-term survival benefit in PAH and CTEPH, when com-pared to historic controls [41]. Both sub-Q and IV treprostinil are easier to administer than epoprostenol because of its longer half-life and stability at room temperature (see Table 2). Sub-Q administration is safe and effective, and avoids the risks of the indwelling catheter. However, it is associated with injection site pain, which is tolerated by most patients. With appropri-ate correction of dosing, transitions between epoprostenol and IV and sub-Q treprostinil can be done safely and quickly in the hospital setting.

Iloprost (Ventavis), a prostacyclin analogue, is an effective treatment for PAH that is delivered by inhalation six to eight times a day. Because of the limited dosing delivery that can be achieved by inhalation, it is potentially less effective than parental prostacyclin. It has been shown to improve hemodynamics, exercise capacity, quality of life, and survival (see Table 2) [38,49,52]. It can be used as an alternative to parental prostacyclins in patients who refuse or do not have the ability to tolerate the complexity of those agents. It is generally used in combination with oral agents in patients who remain symptomatic (>WHO class II) or have had inadequate improvement in 6-minute hall walk or invasive hemodynamic parameters, particularly cardiac output.

Inhaled NO

Although not FDA approved for children and adults with PAH, iNO is a treatment option for the hemodynamically unstable patient in the ICU and postoperatively. It has the advantage of increasing pulmonary perfusion only in ventilated areas, which can improve gas exchange and decrease PVR without increasing intrapulmonary shunting, as could occur with epoprostenol (presumably by vasodilating unventilated lung segments). Inhaled NO is rapidly inactivated in the alveolar capillaries preventing effects on the systemic vasculature. Patients stabilized with iNO may be converted to IV epoprostenol therapy for longer-term use. Sildenafil prolongs the effect of NO by preventing breakdown of its second messenger, cGMP, and may mitigate the rebound effect seen with discontinuation of iNO.

Surgical options for PAH

The mortality in PAH remains high despite advances in therapy, particularly for those WHO class III and IV who do not improve within the first 3 to 6 months. The average life expectancy of 2 years in IPAH has been extended to beyond 5 years with epoprostenol [53]. Death is usually a result of progressive right ventricular failure. As discussed, the markedly dilated RV progressively compresses the LV resulting in hypotension and low cardiac output and worsening RV function. Based on better survival in PAH with a PFO or ASD, catheter-based balloon and blade atrial septostomy have been used to create right to left shunting at the atrial level. By reducing the RV systolic and diastolic load and increasing flow to the underfilled left ventricle, the induced shunt can increase systemic pressure and cardiac output. While high risk, atrial septostomy can improve functional capacity at the expense of profound hypoxemia if the hemoglobin is adequate. In the United States it is generally reserved as a bridge to lung or heart lung transplantation. Lung and heart-lung transplantation are options for relatively young PAH patients who remain WHO class III and IV, and do not achieve adequate quality of life and hemodynamic improvement after 3 to 6 months on prostacyclin and combination therapies [53]. The 1-year survival following lung transplantation is about 80% to 90%, but posttransplant survival time averages about 5 years. Patients in extremis are not candidates for transplantation. Patients whose life expectancy is less than 1 to 2 years should be referred to a lung transplant center, preferably one with experience in PH.

References

[1] Simonneau G, Galie N, Rubin LJ, et al. Clinical classification of pulmonary hypertension. J Am Coll Cardiol 2004;43(12 Suppl S):5S–12S.

[2] Barst RJ, McGoon M, Torbicki A, et al. Diagnosis and differential assessment of pulmonary arterial hypertension. J Am Coll Cardiol 2004;43(12 Suppl S):40S–7S.

[3] Gaines S. Pulmonary hypertension. JAMA 2000;284:3160–8.

[4] Humbert M, Morrell NW, Archer SL, et al. Cellular and molecular pathobiology of pulmonary arterial hypertension. J Am Coll Cardiol 2004;43(12 Suppl S):13S–24S.

[5] McGoon M, Gutterman D, Steen V, et al. Screening, early detection, and diagnosis of pulmonary arterial hypertension: ACCP evidence-based clinical practice guidelines. Chest 2004; 126(Suppl 1):14S–34S.

[6] Bossone E, Butera G, Bodini BD, et al. The interpretation of the electrocardiogram in patients with pulmonary hypertension: the need for clinical correlation. Ital Heart J 2003; 4(12):850–4.

[7] Stein PD, Goldhaber SZ, Henry JW, et al. Arterial blood gas analysis in the assessment of suspected pulmonary embolism. Chest 1996;109:78–81.

[8] Bossone E, Duong-Wagner T, Paciocco G, et al. Echocardiographic features of primary pulmonary hypertension. J Am Soc Echocardiogr 1999;12(8):655–62.

[9] McConnell MV, Solomon SD, Rayan ME, et al. Regional right ventricular dysfunction detected by echocardiography in acute pulmonary embolism. Am J Cardiol 1996;78(4):469–73.

[10] Kruip MJ, Leclercq MG, van der Heul C, et al. Diagnostic strategies for excluding pulmonary embolism in clinical outcome studies. A systematic review. Ann Intern Med 2003; 138(12):941–51.

[11] van Strijen MJ, de Monye W, Schiereck J, et al. Single-detector helical computed tomography as the primary diagnostic test in suspected pulmonary embolism: a multicenter clinical management study of 510 patients. Ann Intern Med 2003;138(4):307–14.

[12] Stein PD, Fowler SE, Goodman LR, et al. Multidetector computed tomography for acute pulmonary embolism. N Engl J Med 2006;354(22):2317–27.

[13] Kelly AM, Patel S, Carlos RC, et al. Multidetector row CT pulmonary angiography and indirect venography for the diagnosis of venous thromboembolic disease in intensive care unit patients. Acad Radiol 2006;13(4):486–95.

[14] The PIOPED Investigators. Value of the ventilation/perfusion scan in acute pulmonary embolism: result of the prospective investigators of pulmonary embolism diagnosis (PIOPED). JAMA 1990;263:2753–9.

[15] Henry JW, Stein PD, Gottschalk A, et al. Scintigraphic lung scans and clinical assessment in critically ill patients with suspected acute pulmonary embolism. Chest 1996;109(2):462–6.

[16] Konstantinides S, Geibel A, Olschewski M, et al. Importance of cardiac troponins I and T in risk stratification of patients with acute pulmonary embolism. Circulation 2002;106(10): 1263–8.

[17] Kucher N, Goldhaber SZ. Cardiac biomarkers for risk stratification of patients with acute pulmonary embolism. Circulation 2003;108(18):2191–4.

[18] Torbicki A, Kurzyna M, Kuca P, et al. Detectable serum cardiac troponin T as a marker of poor prognosis among patients with chronic precapillary pulmonary hypertension. Circulation 2003;108:844–8.

[19] Kucher N, Printzen G, Goldhaber SZ. Prognostic role of brain natriuretic peptide in acute pulmonary embolism. Circulation 2003;107(20):2545–7.

[20] Nagaya N, Nishikimi T, Uematsu M, et al. Plasma brain natriuretic peptide as a prognostic indicator in patients with primary pulmonary hypertension. Circulation 2000;102(8):865–70.

[21] Chemla D, Castelain V, Herve P, et al. Hemodynamic evaluation of pulmonary hypertension. Eur Respir J 2002;20:1314–31.

[22] McLaughlin VV, Presberg KW, Doyle RL, et al. Prognosis of pulmonary arterial hypertension: ACCP evidence-based clinical practice guidelines. Chest 2004;126:78–92.

[23] Sitbon O, Humbert M, Jaïs X, et al. Long-term response to calcium channel blockers in idiopathic pulmonary arterial hypertension. Circulation 2005;111:3105–11.

[24] Quinlan DJ, McQuillan A, Eikelboom JW. Low-molecular-weight heparin compared with intravenous unfractionated heparin for treatment of pulmonary embolism: a meta-analysis of randomized, controlled trials. Ann Intern Med 2004;140:175–83.

[25] Mismetti P, Quenet S, Levine M, et al. Enoxaparin in the treatment of deep vein thrombosis with or without pulmonary embolism: an individual patient data meta-analysis. Chest 2005; 128(4):2203–10.

[26] Ridker PM, Goldhaber SZ, Danielson E, et al. Long-term, low-intensity warfarin therapy for the prevention of recurrent venous thromboembolism. N Engl J Med 2003;348(15): 1425–34.

[27] Kearon C, Ginsberg JS, Kovacs MJ, et al. Comparison of low-intensity warfarin therapy with conventional-intensity warfarin therapy for long-term prevention of recurrent venous thromboembolism. N Engl J Med 2003;349(7):631–9.

[28] Kucher N, Rossi E, De Rosa M, et al. Prognostic role of echocardiography among patients with acute pulmonary embolism and a systolic arterial pressure of 90 mm Hg or higher. Arch Intern Med 2005;165:1777–81.

[29] Quiroz R, Kucher N, Schoepf UJ, et al. Right ventricular enlargement on chest computed tomography: prognostic role in acute pulmonary embolism. Circulation 2004;109: 2401–4.

[30] Kasper W, Konstantinides S, Geibel A, et al. Management strategies and determinants of outcome in acute major pulmonary embolism: results of a multicenter registry. J Am Coll Cardiol 1997;30:1165–71.

[31] Aklog L, Williams CS, Byrne JG, et al. Acute pulmonary embolectomy: a contemporary approach. Circulation 2002;105:1416–9.

[32] Konstantinides S, Geibel A, Heusel G, et al. Heparin plus alteplase compared with heparin alone in patients with submassive pulmonary embolism. N Engl J Med 2002;347: 1143–50.

[33] Wan S, Quinlan DJ, Agnelli G, et al. Thrombolysis compared with heparin for the initial treatment of pulmonary embolism: a meta-analysis of the randomized controlled trials. Circulation 2004;110:744–9.

[34] Decousus H, Leizorovicz A, Parent F, et al. A clinical trial of vena caval filters in the prevention of pulmonary embolism in patients with proximal deep-vein thrombosis. N Engl J Med 1998;338:409–15.

[35] Moser KM, Bloor CM. Pulmonary vascular lesions occurring in patients with chronic major vessel thromboembolic pulmonary hypertension. Chest 1993;103:685–92.

[36] Jamieson SW, Kapelanski DP, Sakakibara N, et al. Pulmonary endarterectomy: experience and lessons learned in 1,500 cases. Ann Thorac Surg 2003;76:1457–62.

[37] Bresser P, Fedullo PF, Auger WR, et al. Continuous intravenous epoprostenol for chronic thromboembolic pulmonary hypertension. Eur Respir J 2004;23:595–600.

[38] Olschewski H, Simonneau G, Galie N, et al. Aerosolized Iloprost Randomized Study Group. Inhaled iloprost for severe pulmonary hypertension. N Engl J Med 2002;347(5):322–9.

[39] Ghofrani HA, Schermuly RT, Rose F, et al. Sildenafil for long-term treatment of nonoperable chronic thromboembolic pulmonary hypertension. Am J Respir Crit Care Med 2003; 167:1139–41.

[40] Hughes RJ, Jais X, Bonderman D, et al. The efficacy of bosentan in inoperable chronic thromboembolic pulmonary hypertension: a 1-year follow-up study. Eur Respir J 2006;28: 138–43.

[41] Lang I, Gomez-Sanchez M, Kneussl M, et al. Efficacy of long-term subcutaneous treprostinil sodium therapy in pulmonary hypertension. Chest 2006;129:1636–43.

[42] Sandroni C, Maggiore SM, Proietti R, et al. Cardiopulmonary resuscitation in patients with pulmonary arterial hypertension. Am J Respir Crit Care Med 2003;167:664–5.

[43] Fuster V, Steele PM, Edwards WD, et al. Primary pulmonary hypertension: natural history and importance of thrombosis. Circulation 1984;70:580–7.

[44] Badesch DB, Abman SH, Ahearn GS, et al. Medical therapy for pulmonary arterial hypertension: ACCP evidence-based clinical practice guidelines. Chest 2004;126:35–62.

[45] Rubin LJ, Badesch DB, Barst RJ, et al. Bosentan therapy for pulmonary arterial hypertension. N Engl J Med 2002;346:896–903.

[46] Barst RJ, Langleben D, Badesch D, et al. STRIDE-2 Study Group. Treatment of pulmonary arterial hypertension with selective endothelin-A receptor antagonist sitaxsentan. J Am Coll Cardiol 2006;47:2049–56.

[47] Galiè N, Ghofrani HA, Torbicki A, et al. Sildenafil citrate therapy for pulmonary arterial hypertension. N Engl J Med 2005;353:2148–57.

[48] Barst RJ, Rubin LJ, Long WA, et al. A comparison of continuous intravenous epoprostenol (prostacyclin) with conventional therapy for primary pulmonary hypertension. N Engl J Med 1996;334:296–302.

[49] McLaughlin VV, Shillington A, Rich S. Survival in primary pulmonary hypertension: the impact of epoprostenol therapy. Circulation 2002;106:1477–82.

[50] McLaughlin VV, Gaine SP, Barst RJ, et al. Efficacy and safety of trepostinil, a prostacyclin analogue for primary pulmonary hypertension. J Cardiovasc Pharmacol 2003;41:293–9.

[51] Simonneau G, Barst RJ, Galie N, et al. Treprostinil Study Group. Continuous subcutaneous infusion of treprostinil, a prostacyclin analogue, in patients with pulmonary arterial hypertension: a double-blind, randomized, placebo-controlled trial. Am J Respir Crit Care Med 2002;165(6):800–4.

[52] Hoeper MM, Schwarze M, Ehlerding S, et al. Long-term treatment of primary pulmonary hypertension with aerolozed iloprost, a prostacyclin analogue. N Engl J Med 2000;342: 1866–70.

[53] Pielsticker E, Martinez F, Rubenfire M. Lung and heart-lung transplant practice patterns in pulmonary hypertension centers. J Heart Lung Transplant 2001;20:1297–304.

ELSEVIER
SAUNDERS

CRITICAL
CARE
CLINICS

Crit Care Clin 23 (2007) 835–853

CT and MRI of Acute Thoracic Cardiovascular Emergencies

Aamer Chughtai, FRCR[a,*],
Ella A. Kazerooni, MD, MS[b]

[a]Department of Radiology, University of Michigan Medical Center, 1500 East Medical Center Drive, Ann Arbor, MI 48109-0326, USA
[b]Department of Radiology, University of Michigan Health System, Cardiovascular Center #5482, 1500 East Medical Center Drive, Ann Arbor, MI 48109-5868, USA

A wide spectrum of acute cardiovascular disorders is seen in patients who are hospitalized in a critical care setting. These consist of several acquired conditions, including aortic dissection, venous thromboembolism, pericardial compromise, myocardial infarction, and acute coronary syndrome. Imaging plays a central role in the diagnosis and management of these conditions. The most frequently used imaging remains chest radiography; however, more advanced modalities, including coronary angiography, echocardiography, and radioisotope scintigraphy, have well established roles in the assessment of patients in the critical care setting. More recently, multidetector row CT (MDCT) and MRI are being used increasingly for evaluation of coronary artery disease (CAD), cardiac structure and function, coronary artery anomalies, cardiac masses, pericardial disease, valvular disease, postoperative cardiovascular abnormalities, venous thromboembolism, and acute aortic syndromes, often with other ancillary findings that can provide important clinical information [1]. Cardiac MRI can evaluate cardiac function accurately by cine gradient echo imaging of the ventricles and flow analysis across cardiac valves and the great vessels and evaluation of cardiac wall motion, ventricular volumes, and ventricular mass [2]. Although MR angiography techniques are well established for evaluating the aorta, CT is preferred in unstable patients. MDCT is readily available in most places around the clock, often with in-house CT technologists, and provides rapid imaging assessment of cardiovascular structures in the thorax.

* Corresponding author.
  E-mail address: aamerc@umich.edu (A. Chughtai).

0749-0704/07/$ - see front matter. Published by Elsevier Inc.
doi:10.1016/j.ccc.2007.08.002

criticalcare.theclinics.com

The three most common life-threatening cardiovascular processes in which advanced imaging plays a role, particularly CT, are discussed, including pulmonary embolism (PE), aortic dissection, and CAD.

Acute pulmonary embolism

Acute PE is associated with high morbidity and mortality, particularly in the acute care setting. It is the third most common cause of cardiovascular death after myocardial infarction and stroke [3]. At postmortem examination, PE is found in 7% to 27% of patients who had been in the ICU and contributes to or is the cause of mortality in up to 12% of patients [4].

The incidence of PE has remained constant, with age- and sex-adjusted rates of 117 cases per 100,000 person-years [5]. The incidence increases sharply after age 60 years in men and women [6]. The mortality associated with PE is highest in the first 3 months following the event and exceeds 15% [7]. The initial clinical manifestation is sudden death in almost one fourth of patients who have acute PE [5].

Although there are a myriad of risk factors associated with acute PE, many of them are common in an acute care or intensive care setting, some predating the ICU admission and others developing over the course of the ICU stay. These include prolonged immobilization, increased age, surgery, trauma, shock, stroke, malignancy, pancreatitis, and coagulation abnormalities, such as polycythemia, platelet abnormalities, and history of venous thrombosis. Pregnancy, oral contraceptive use, and smoking also are associated with a higher risk for PE. Patients in the ICU have more baseline risk factors for PE than do patients who are not in the ICU. These risk factors include age older than 70 years, bed rest for 5 days or longer, and a diagnosis of cancer, chronic obstructive pulmonary disease, or congestive cardiac failure [8,9]. The prevalence of deep vein thrombosis (DVT), at 13% to 33%, also is higher in patients who are admitted to the ICU than in patients who are not, regardless of whether they are receiving DVT prophylaxis [4,10,11]. In one study, a DVT rate of 33% was reported, despite DVT prophylaxis in 61% of the patients [10], whereas in another study of 102 patients in the ICU who specifically were defined as high risk for DVT and all were receiving prophylaxis, the rate of DVT was 12% [12].

Diagnosis of acute pulmonary embolism in the critical care setting

The diagnosis of acute PE in patients in the ICU can be challenging for many reasons and requires an integrated approach using clinical history, physical examination, laboratory data, and imaging. The clinical signs and symptoms are nonspecific and may be absent or masked by other disease processes. The diagnosis is complicated by coexisting diseases. Patients commonly present with dyspnea or tachypnea, often associated with pleuritic pain. Nonproductive cough and hemoptysis can occur if there has been pulmonary infarction; however, this is uncommon. Syncope may occur with massive PE, but also with a lesser extent of PE in patients who have impaired cardiopulmonary reserve. On physical examination, tachypnea is a common finding. If cyanosis is present, it usually indicates massive PE. With smaller emboli, pleural effusions, pleural rub with wheeze, and crackles may be present. Lower extremity edema is found in only a third of patients who have acute PE. The major differential diagnoses to consider in this setting include acute myocardial infarction, heart failure, pneumonia, pneumothorax, and an acute aortic syndrome.

When normal, the D-dimer assay has a high negative predictive value of 95.6% to 96.7% for the absence of venous thromboembolism (VTE) [13]. An elevated D-dimer has a low specificity for VTE, ranging from 35% to 77% [14]. Elevated D-dimer can be seen in many acute systemic conditions that may be present in patients in the ICU, including myocardial infarction, pneumonia, sepsis, cancer, and after surgery [14,15]. Chest radiography—although the most frequently performed imaging examination in patients in the ICU—is of little value in the diagnosis of PE with its low specificity, and it often is confounded by coexisting infection, edema, or acute respiratory distress syndrome (ARDS) [16].

Traditionally, ventilation/perfusion (V/Q) scanning has been the mainstay of evaluation, with catheter pulmonary angiography serving as the gold standard or reference test. The presence of pulmonary disease in most critically ill patients makes V/Q scanning limited in its diagnostic value. In the Prospective Investigation of Pulmonary Embolism Diagnosis (PIOPED) study, most patients (73%) had indeterminate (34%) or low (39%) probability V/Q scans, of which 33% and 12%, respectively, had PE. Only 13% of patients had a high probability scan result, in which the prevalence of PE was 88% [17]. From the abstract of that publication, "Almost all patients with pulmonary embolism had abnormal scans of high, intermediate, or low probability, but so did most without pulmonary embolism (sensitivity, 98%; specificity, 10%)." Most of these patients were not patients in the ICU. Coexisting lung disease increases the likelihood of an indeterminate test by virtue of the interpretation criteria. When a perfusion defect is present in the setting of a radiographic opacity, a low probability test result is converted into an intermediate result. In the ICU setting, only a combination of a low clinical and a low or very low scintigraphic probability renders the diagnosis of PE highly unlikely [18]; the only advantage is that it is possible to perform scintigraphy at the bedside of unstable patients. Catheter angiography has been recognized to be an imperfect gold standard, with considerable interobserver variability at the small artery level [19].

Over the last decade, intravenous contrast-enhanced CT pulmonary angiography (CTPA) has emerged as the single most important imaging modality for the diagnosis of acute PE. CTPA is readily available, and the images are available for review in a matter of minutes. This reduces the time to make the diagnosis and management. The sensitivity and specificity of MDCT pulmonary angiography combined with indirect lower extremity CT venography, as reported recently in the PIOPED 2 study—the largest study of MDCT accuracy for PE—are 90% and 95%, respectively [20]. Several other studies showed a high sensitivity and specificity for CTPA of 90% to 100% and 89% to 94%, respectively, and a high negative predictive value of 98% to 99% [21–23]. Baile and colleagues [24] compared CT and catheter angiography in a porcine model for detecting subsegmental emboli, finding no difference in the sensitivity and specificity of the two modalities for detecting PE.

It is important to consider the specificity of CTPA (95%–97%) [22,23] when PE is found, which allows treatment with a high degree of confidence in the diagnosis, as well as the high negative predictive value and the clinical outcome after a normal CT result. Patel and Kazerooni [25] summarized 18 studies in which 4233 patients with a normal CTPA examination were followed from 3 to 12 months. The weighted average occurrence of venous thromboembolic disease was 1.3%, and the weighted average of fatal PE was 0.4%. By comparison, the rate of PE after a normal catheter pulmonary angiogram is 1.6% to 1.7% [26]. Many thoracic radiologists consider CTPA, not catheter angiography, to be the reference standard for evaluating the pulmonary arteries. This is because catheter angiography is a projectional technique in which a limited number of views are obtained because of the contrast volume required for each injection and radiation concerns, small filling defects are difficult to detect, and even with expert readers, there is considerable interobserver variation when interpreting the subsegmental and smaller arteries [14,19]. In one porcine model study, catheter angiography had a false negative rate of 20%, attributed in many cases to partially occluding thrombi [27].

The use of CTPA in the ICU setting has been questioned [28,29], as has the accuracy of CTPA when there is coexisting lung disease, such as pneumonia, edema, or ARDS. Imaging is complicated further by factors such as tubes and lines, metallic hardware, and impaired cardiopulmonary function, causing streak artifacts and suboptimal contrast delivery. Remy-Jardin and colleagues [30] demonstrated that CTPA performed equally well in patients who did and did not have coexisting lung disease. In a study by Kelly and colleagues [11] specifically of patients in the ICU undergoing CTPA using 4-row MDCT scanners, diagnostic quality images were obtained in most patients (76%); images in the remaining 24% were nondiagnostic, highlighting the challenges in this population. Advances in scanner technology since that time, particularly 16- and 64-row scanners that allow the examination in be acquired in as little as 5 seconds, improve image quality by reducing respiratory motion. Additional strengths of CT are that it can evaluate the lung and pleural disease, which often coexists in patients in the ICU and may be the actual cause of an acute clinical deterioration, as well as the aorta and heart in the same acquisition.

In these high-risk patients, a normal CTPA effectively rules out an acute thromboembolic event. Bourriot and colleagues [31] evaluated the clinical outcomes following a normal CTPA in 117 patients: 70% had a known cardiopulmonary disease and 36% had impaired cardiopulmonary reserve. The rate of recurrent PE in these patients was 1.8% to 4.9%, depending on the defining criteria used. This low recurrence confirms the usefulness of CTPA in excluding PE in patients who are being managed in the critical care setting.

CT pulmonary angiography: technique, image reconstruction, and interpretation

CT angiography of the pulmonary arteries is performed with 80 to 130 mL of iodinated contrast material injected through an antecubital vein at a rate of 4 mL per second. Using a 16-detector row CT scanner, this takes 10 to 12 seconds; with a 64-detector row scanner, it takes less than 5 seconds to complete a high-resolution examination of the entire thorax with collimation of approximately 1 mm. This means that the examination can be performed in a single breath hold, minimizing respiratory motion artifact. For an intubated patient, this minimizes the time that the ventilator is suspended for the image acquisition. With optimal enhancement of the pulmonary arteries, emboli in the main trunk down to subsegmental arteries can be visualized easily (Fig. 1). In situations in which the visualization of pulmonary artery filling defects is doubtful or difficult because of breathing or streak artifacts, multiplanar reformats can be generated on the workstation to review the artery in any desired plane, which may enhance diagnostic confidence (Fig. 2).

After the thoracic part of the examination, the veins of the pelvis and thighs are scanned after an additional 2 to 3 minutes as an indirect CT venogram (CTV) to identify DVT (Fig. 3). Scans are obtained from the iliac crests to the tibial plateaus as a contiguous acquisition using 5- or 7.5-mm

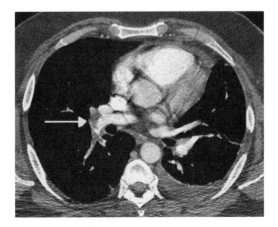

Fig. 1. A 55-year-old man who had sudden-onset chest pain. CTPA demonstrates emboli in right upper lobe lobar, segmental, and subsegmental arteries (*arrow*).

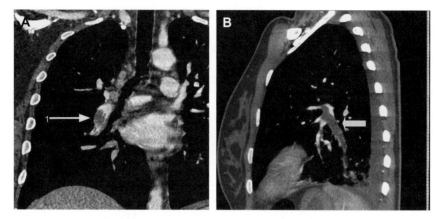

Fig. 2. Multiplanar reformatted images in the coronal (*A*) and sagittal (*B*) planes demonstrate a large embolus in the left lower lobar pulmonary artery and distal branches (*arrow*).

collimation. This one-stop CTPA combined with CTV essentially eliminates the need for a separate ultrasound of lower extremities, reducing the cost and time for the diagnostic workup. Furthermore, it increases the diagnostic yield of the CT examination for disease. In the PIOPED II study, the sensitivity for VTE increased from 83% to 90% when CTV was considered with CTPA [20]. Several other studies showed an excellent correlation between indirect CTV and ultrasound in studies in which patients prospectively underwent both tests, with sensitivity and specificity ranging from 89% to 100% and 94% to 100%, respectively, and a negative predictive value of 97% to 100% [32–38]. The reported interobserver agreement also is good to excellent, with kappa values of 0.59 to 0.88 [35,37,39]. Therefore, combining CTV with CTPA increases confidence in the diagnosis of venous thromboembolic disease. This is particularly useful in patients in the ICU

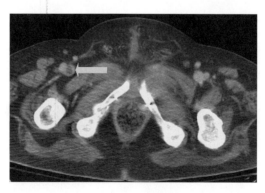

Fig. 3. Indirect CT venography in a patient who recently underwent abdominal surgery and developed lower extremity swelling demonstrates a thrombus in the right superficial femoral vein (*arrow*).

who may not need anticoagulation treatment when results for the pulmonary arteries and leg veins are normal.

Aortic dissection

Aortic dissection occurs most commonly in adults between the ages of 40 and 70 years, with an incidence of 1 to 6 cases per 100,000 per year. It is two to five times more common in men. Risk factors for aortic dissection include hypertension, pregnancy, coarctation of the aorta, bicuspid aortic valve, Marfan syndrome, Ehlers-Danlos syndrome, Bechet's disease, and prior cardiac/aortic surgery [40]. Given the 1% to 2% per hour mortality after symptom onset for the first 24 hours for type A dissection and a 30-day mortality of 10% for type B dissection, early diagnosis is imperative to avoid significant morbidity and mortality.

An aortic dissection is produced when there is penetration of circulating blood into the wall of aorta, through a tear of the intima, for a varying degree. Any mechanism that weakens the media of the aorta may result in aortic dilatation and aneurysm formation and, eventually, intramural hemorrhage, aortic dissection, or rupture [40]. The vessel walls can be affected by congenital connective tissue disorders, such as Marfan's syndrome and Ehlers-Danlos syndrome. Acquired conditions, such as chronic hypertension, may cause aortic aneurysm and dissection [41,42]. Inflammatory processes of the aortic wall or autoimmune processes involving the vasa vasorum supplying the aortic wall, such as Takayasu arteritis, giant cell arteritis, syphilis, and Behcet's disease, lead to weakening, expansion, and dissection, [40]. Iatrogenic aortic dissection can be caused by valve surgery, graft anastomosis, and the cannulation sites, as well as catheter placements [43]. Deceleration trauma, like car accidents and fall from height, can cause aortic dissection, pseudoaneurysm, and rupture, usually at the distal aortic arch just beyond the origin of left subclavian artery. Intramural hematomas of the aorta can lead to a secondary tear on the intima and communicate with the aortic lumen [44].

Aortic dissections generally are classified with respect to what part of the aorta is involved. In the DeBakey classification, type I involves the ascending and descending aorta, type II involves the ascending aorta only, and type III involves the descending aorta only, distal to left subclavian artery [45]. In the more commonly used Stanford classification, a type A dissection is defined as involving the ascending aorta, and type B dissection spares the ascending aorta.

Clinical presentation

Acute-onset chest pain in the midline, radiating to the back, is the most common presenting complaint. The onset usually is sudden and reaches maximal intensity immediately. This abruptness is the most specific characteristic of the pain. The pain is characteristically described as ripping, tearing, chok-ing, or stabbing; it does not commonly radiate to the neck, shoulder, or arm and may be absent in 5% to 10% of cases. Many patients are hypertensive because of preexisting hypertensive disease or increased sympathetic drive.

Clinical findings vary depending on branch artery involvement of differ-ent organ systems, due to ischemia secondary to obstruction of branches of aorta, direct compression of organ by expanding false lumen, or leak or rup-ture of false lumen into surrounding structures. The most common findings are due to cardiovascular and neurologic involvement when coronary ar-teries or aortic arch branches are involved. Cerebral ischemia and stroke is the most common feature. Syncope and myocardial infarction may be seen with coronary artery involvement. Spinal cord lesions are more com-mon with distal dissections and can cause paraplegia. There may be pulse and blood pressure differential between the two arms when the dissection ex-tends into or obliterates the arch vessels [46]. Similarly, acute renal failure can occur with renal artery involvement, and mesenteric ischemia can occur with celiac axis and mesenteric arterial involvement.

Differential diagnosis mainly includes acute myocardial infarction and PE. These can be evaluated easily with a single MDCT scan. Other condi-tions to consider in the differential include mesenteric arterial or venous thrombosis, peptic ulcer, acute appendicitis, intestinal obstruction, pancre-atic/peritoneal cyst, and acute cholecystitis. Conditions associated with aor-tic dissection, such as hypertension and connective tissue disorders, can be helpful in narrowing down the diagnosis.

Diagnosis and advanced imaging

Aortic dissection should be considered in any patient presenting with sudden-onset severe chest pain. A chest radiograph may show a widened mediastinum, irregular aortic contour, deviation of the trachea or the naso-gastric tube in the esophagus, and displacement of calcified intima; however, chest radiograph alone does not confirm the diagnosis and is nonspecific [47]. Historically, invasive catheter aortography was the definitive diagnostic modality. With advances in CT imaging, CT has replaced catheter angiog-raphy in the diagnostic evaluation of the aorta; it is best performed as an ECG-gated CT on a 16- or more detector row scanner, which eliminates aortic pulsation artifact. CT can quickly and noninvasively evaluate the true and false lumens and the intimal flap, including entry and reentry tears, as well complications, such as pericardial and pleural effusions and branch artery involvement. MDCT also is helpful in identifying causes of mediasti-nal widening as seen on chest radiograph other than dissection, such as mediastinal hematomas secondary to central line placement, mediastinal masses, and aortic aneurysms.

Several studies demonstrated that CT is a highly accurate and reliable imaging modality for aortic dissection. In a study by Yoshida and colleagues

[48], the accuracy of CT for the detection of aortic dissection or intramural hematoma of the thoracic aorta was 100%. The sensitivity, specificity, and accuracy, respectively, were 82%, 100%, and 84% for locating the entry tear; 95%, 100%, and 98% for arch branch vessel involvement; and 83%, 100%, and 91% for pericardial effusion. All of these values were 100% for aortic arch anomalies. In a more recent study, Hayter and colleagues [49] evaluated 373 patients who had suspected aortic dissection with MDCT. There were no false positives, 1 false negative, 76 true positives, and 304 true negatives, yielding a sensitivity, specificity, positive predictive value (PPV), negative predictive value (NPV), and accuracy of 99% (67 of 68), 100% (304 of 304), 100% (67 of 67), 99.7% (304 of 305), and 99.5% (371 of 373), respectively. Other studies have reported 100% sensitivity and specificity of MDCT to detect aortic dissections [50,51].

On CT, the primary finding in aortic dissection is the presence of two distinct lumens with a visible intimal flap, which is seen in most cases (Fig. 4); in other cases, the two lumens are identified only by their differing rates of opacification with contrast material or the low attenuation of the false lumen if it is completely thrombosed. An intramural hematoma is a variant of a classic dissection in which only a thickened wall is present, and there are no entry or reentry tears (Fig. 5). One explanation for this is rupture of the vaso vasora that supply the aortic wall. CT examinations done for acute aortic syndromes routinely include noncontrast images first, because acute blood in the aorta appears higher in attenuation than does the blood in the aortic lumen, whereas long-standing hematoma will not (Fig. 6). Indirect signs of dissection include compression of the true lumen by the false lumen, spiraling of a thrombosed false lumen, displaced intimal calcification, widening of the aortic lumen, and ulcerlike projections of contrast material [52]. Three-dimensional reconstructions of the CT data are routine in evaluating the morphology of the dissection and relation to branch vessels

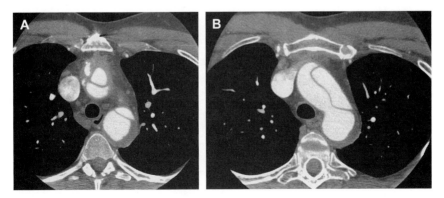

Fig. 4. Type A aortic dissection with intimal separating the true and false lumens at the ascending aorta (A) and at the aortic arch (B).

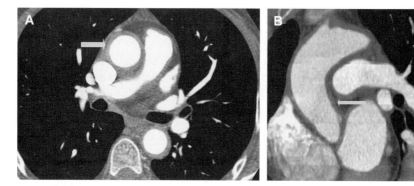

Fig. 5. Acute intramural hematoma manifests as thickening of the ascending and descending thoracic aortic wall (*arrow*), as shown on axial (*A*) and oblique coronal reformatted (*B*) images.

(Fig. 7), which are critical in clinical decision making, particularly when open or endovascular repair is necessary.

Patients who are unable to receive intravenous iodinated contrast for CT can be evaluated with MRI. It also is an accurate noninvasive technique for examining patients who are suspected of having aortic dissection, aortic intramural hematoma, or penetrating aortic ulcer; however, it generally is reserved for stable patients or follow-up imaging, because of the longer examination time and the logistics of doing an MRI examination in a patient who is unstable and requires close monitoring by the health care team. Although MRI has high sensitivity (95%–100%) and specificity (94%–98%) for the detection of aortic dissection, a sensitivity of 100% for detection of aortic intramural hematoma, and a sensitivity of 86% for detection of penetrating aortic ulcer, it has serious limitations [53–55]. Most importantly,

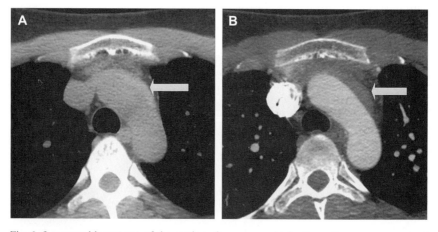

Fig. 6. Intramural hematoma of the aortic arch appears as high attenuation on a noncontrast enhanced image (*A, arrow*) relative to blood in the aortic lumen, indicating that it is acute, and as low attenuation thickening on a contrast-enhanced image (*B, arrow*).

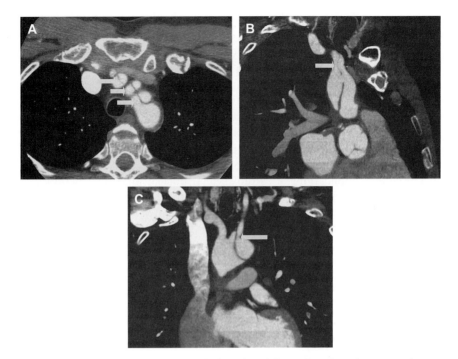

Fig. 7. Acute aortic dissection involving the branches of the aortic arch, as demonstrated on an axial image with flap extending into all three great vessels (*A, arrows*), flap extending into the innominate artery (*B*), and on left common carotid artery on oblique sagittal reconstructions (*C*).

the MRI examination requires approximately 30 minutes or more, compared with the 10 to 30 seconds to acquire the CT data on an MDCT scanner, for which more time is spent moving the patient in and out of the room than on the scan itself. CT scan data are reconstructed so quickly on modern consoles that a physician can review the images and make an assessment before a patient from the ICU and medical team are ready to leave the CT suite. The time it takes for an MRI scan (30 minutes) is a serious limitation, particularly in patients from the ICU who may be unstable, ventilated, or need constant monitoring and who may have MRI incompatible hardware. Also, MRI is less readily available and commonly is at a site at great distance from the ICU or in a remote area of a medical complex, which further limits its role in the diagnosis of an aortic syndrome in the acute setting [49].

Coronary disease and advanced imaging in the critical care setting

A wide variety of cardiac disorders can be found in patients in the ICU; however, CAD with myocardial infarction is among the most common acute conditions and contributes to a significant proportion of the mortality in these patients. The clinical signs and symptoms of an acute cardiac event can be nonspecific (eg, atypical chest pain, nausea, shortness of breath, fatigue, cough, and diaphoresis) and masked by other disease processes. In patients in the ICU who frequently have a complicated clinical presentation, accurate and rapid diagnosis of an acute cardiac event can be challenging. Historically, the diagnosis of an acute coronary syndrome has been based on the ECG and cardiac enzymes, often with a noninvasive stress modality (eg, echocardiography or radionuclide single photon emission computed tomography [SPECT] imaging), with catheter coronary angiography as the final arbiter when the noninvasive test results are not conclusive or discordant with the pretest clinical probability of disease.

The clinical applications of cardiovascular nuclear imaging techniques in the intensive care setting have been well established. These include thallium[201] and Tc[99m]-sestamibi SPECT and Multigated (MUGA) studies to provide quantitative information concerning myocardial perfusion, acute myocardial ischemia, and left ventricular function. These techniques provide objective guidelines for therapy and prognosis [56]. The reported sensitivity and specificity of Tc[99m]-sestamibi SPECT to predict acute coronary ischemia are 94% and 84%, respectively [57,58]; however, the lack of on-site, around-the-clock availability and long examination times are real concerns for its use in patients from the ICU [59].

Rapid advances in MDCT technology over the last few years have greatly facilitated the accurate and rapid evaluation of the coronary arteries using 64-detector MDCT scanners to perform CT coronary angiography. Several studies reported high sensitivity and specificity of MDCT for detecting coronary artery stenoses of 50% or greater, ranging from 90% to 95% and 82% to 98%, respectively [60–65]. Perhaps the most important characteristic of CT coronary angiography is its consistently high NPV of 97% to 99% [22,23,61,62,66]. Mollet and colleagues [66], using vessel-based analysis with 64-slice computerized tomographic angiography (CTA) to detect stenoses of 50% or greater, reported sensitivity, specificity, PPV, and NPV ranging from 97% to 100%, 92% to 99%, 78% to 80%, and 99% to 100%, respectively, depending on the calcium score. The sensitivity for detecting significant disease in the left anterior descending was 96%, whereas in other main coronary arteries the sensitivity was 100%. There was good correlation between CTA and coronary angiography, with a kappa value of 0.85. Ehara and colleagues [67] evaluated 64-slice MDCT for detecting angiographically significant coronary artery stenosis in an unselected consecutive patient population and compared it with conventional invasive angiography. Fifty-seven percent of the patients already had coronary artery stents. They reported that sensitivity for diagnosing significant stenosis ($\geq$50%) was 90%, specificity was 94%, PPV was 89%, and NPV was 95%. For the stented arteries, the sensitivity, specificity, PPV, and NPV were 93%, 96%, 87%, and 98%, respectively.

Raff and colleagues [23] evaluated the diagnostic accuracy of 64-slice coronary CT angiography in 70 consecutive patients undergoing invasive coronary angiography, including patients with high heart rates (23% > 70 beats per minute [bpm], range up to 96 bpm), obesity (50% with body mass index > 30 kg/m^2), and coronary calcification (26% had Agatston score > 400 with range up to 1804), reflecting a more "real world" group of patients. They demonstrated a high NPV of 98% by segment and 97% by artery. They also observed improved image quality with smaller voxel size provided by the 64-slice scanner, which reduced, but did not eliminate, the calcium blooming and beam hardening artifacts. The sensitivity and specificity were 97% and 95%, respectively, with heart rate of less than 70 bpm and 88% and 71%, respectively, with heart rate of 71 to 85 bpm, reinforcing the need to pharmacologically reduce the heart rate during the CT examination. This is done routinely with β-blocker and sometimes calcium channel blockers if there is a contraindication to the former. A high or irregular heart rate decreases the image quality of coronary CT angiography. Achenbach and colleagues [69] evaluated a new dual-source MDCT with the advantage of higher temporal resolution than other 64-detector MDCT scanners, which has made it possible to obtain good quality images at higher heart rates and has reduced, but not eliminated, the need to premedicate patients completely. They reported visualization of 98% of coronary artery segments free of cardiac motion artifacts.

There has been preliminary work on the use of coronary CT angiography in patients who have chest pain presenting to emergency rooms, who are stable clinically, low risk for CAD, and have a normal ECG and cardiac enzymes for at least 4 hours. Patients with a normal scan can be discharged early, leading to a reduction in length of stay and cost of care; unfortunately, the sample sizes have been too small to determine the impact of this strategy on coronary event rates, such as myocardial infarction and intervention [57,68,69]. In a recent study, Rubinshtein and colleagues [70] demonstrated emergency department (ED) MDCT sensitivity of 100%, specificity of 92%, PPV of 87%, and NPV of 100% in a cohort of 58 patients. They concluded that 64-slice cardiac MDCT represents a valuable diagnostic tool in patients in the ED who have chest pain of uncertain origin, providing early direct noninvasive visualization of coronary anatomy.

Technique

Cardiac imaging using CT is a technically demanding procedure, requiring high temporal and spatial resolution to visualize small coronary arteries while the heart is beating continuously. This is achieved using retrospective ECG gating, segmentation, and tailored reconstruction algorithms. Respiratory motion also must be eliminated for cardiac imaging, so scanning is optimally performed in a single breath hold, easily achievable with the 5- to 10-second acquisition times for the examination using 64-slice MDCT scanners.

A stable heart rate of 65 bpm or less is important to obtain diagnostic image quality and to decrease radiation dose and shorten the time for image processing and evaluation. For example, a study of 94 patients reported an inverse correlation between the number of analyzable vessel segments and heart rate [71]. Vessel visibility was highest when the heart rate was less than 65 bpm [71]. If the heart rate is more than 65 bpm or is irregular, β-blocker medication can be administered orally or intravenously before the scan. A single puff (0.4 mg) of sublingual nitroglycerin also is given a few minutes before the scan to dilate the coronary arteries and exaggerate the difference between normal and abnormal segments, as is done before catheter coronary angiography.

A noncontrast enhanced scan using prospective ECG gating is performed through the heart, from which the calcium score is generated and the location of the coronary arteries confirmed. The coronary calcium score is a sensitive marker of CAD; the higher the score, the greater the likelihood of significant coronary event. A large coronary calcium load can potentially degrade the image quality of CTA, however. A timing bolus of 15 to 20 mL of intravenous contrast agent is used to determine the optimum time of arterial peak enhancement for the specific patient, by placing a region of interest in the aortic root. Following this, the contrast-enhanced CTA of the coronary arteries is performed with 70 to 80 mL of low osmolar iodinated contrast material injected intravenously at a rate of 5 mL/s through an

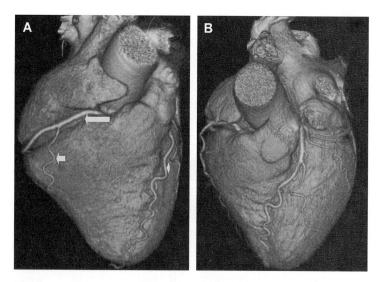

Fig. 8. Volume-rendered images demonstrate excellent visualization of normal coronary anatomy, including the right coronary artery (*arrow*), acute marginal artery (*short arrow*), and left anterior descending coronary artery (*arrowhead*) (*A*) as well as the left main, left anterior descending, and left circumflex coronary arteries and their branches (*B*).

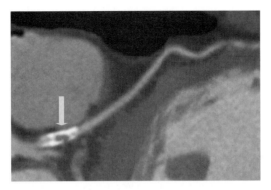

Fig. 9. CT coronary angiography with a high-grade narrowing of the proximal left anterior descending coronary artery due to plaque that has calcified and noncalcified components (*arrow*), as demonstrated on a multiplanar reformatted image.

antecubital vein. During the later part of the contrast injection, the contrast is mixed with saline using a dual-headed power injector, so that the contrast in the right cardiac chambers is not so bright as to cause artifacts in the deep atrioventricular groove where the right coronary artery resides. With 64-slice scanners, the collimation used ranges from 0.5 to 0.625 mm; gantry rotation time is less than 500 milliseconds. The typical scan time is 5 to 10 seconds, short enough to complete the study in a single breath hold.

Following the scan acquisition, processing is performed using retrospective reconstruction of the images at end diastole (70%, 75%, and 80% of the R-R interval), a time of little cardiac motion and the greatest coronary blood flow. The images are reviewed on advanced processing workstations using specialized software for evaluation of the coronary arteries. In a study that compared axial, virtual angioscopic, volume-rendered, and multiplanar reformatted images, the most stenoses were detected on axial images followed by virtual angioscopic, volume-rendered (Fig. 8), and multiplanar reformatted images (Figs. 9 and 10) [72]. Use of all four techniques gave the highest sensitivity.

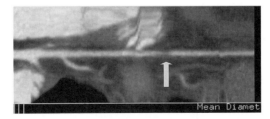

Fig. 10. CT coronary angiography with high-grade stenosis in the mid to distal left anterior descending coronary artery due to circumferential noncalcified plaque (*arrow*).

Summary

ED MDCT is a rapid and accurate test for evaluation of patients who have chest pain in the ED setting. Our understanding about the usefulness and limitations of ED MDCT will improve as more data are made available from ongoing studies.

References

[1] Coche EE, Muller NL, Kim KI, et al. Acute pulmonary embolism: ancillary findings at spiral CT. Radiology 1998;207:753–8.
[2] Greenberg SB. Assessment of cardiac function: magnetic resonance and computed tomography. J Thorac Imaging 2000;15:243–51.
[3] White RH. The epidemiology of venous thromboembolism. Circulation 2003;107:I4–8.
[4] Geerts W, Selby R. Prevention of venous thromboembolism in the ICU. Chest 2003;124:357S–63S.
[5] Heit JA. The epidemiology of venous thromboembolism in the community: implications for prevention and management. J Thromb Thrombolysis 2006;21:23–9.
[6] Silverstein MD, Heit JA, Mohr DN, et al. Trends in the incidence of deep vein thrombosis and pulmonary embolism: a 25-year population-based study. Arch Intern Med 1998;158:585–93.
[7] Piazza G, Goldhaber SZ. Acute pulmonary embolism: Part II: treatment and prophylaxis. Circulation 2006;114:e42–7.
[8] Goldhaber SZ, Visani L, De Rosa M. Acute pulmonary embolism: clinical outcomes in the International Cooperative Pulmonary Embolism Registry (ICOPER). Lancet 1999;353:1386–9.
[9] Flordal PA, Berggvist D, Burmark US, et al. Risk factors for major thromboembolism and bleeding tendency after elective general surgical operations. The Fragmin Multicentre Study group. Eur J Surg 1996;162:783–9.
[10] Hirsch DR, Ingenito EP, Goldhaber SZ. Prevalence of deep venous thrombosis among patients in medical intensive care. JAMA 1995;274:335–7.
[11] Kelly AM, Patel S, Carlos RC, et al. Multidetector row CT pulmonary angiography and indirect venography for the diagnosis of venous thromboembolic disease in intensive care unit patients. Acad Radiol 2006;13:486–95.
[12] Marik PE, Andrews L, Maini B. The incidence of deep venous thrombosis in ICU patients. Chest 1997;111:661–4.
[13] Palareti G, Legnani C, Cosmi B, et al. Risk of venous thromboembolism recurrence: high negative predictive value of D-dimer performed after oral anticoagulation is stopped. Thromb Haemost 2002;87:7–12.
[14] Sadosty AT, Goyal DG, Boie ET, et al. Emergency department D-dimer testing. J Emerg Med 2001;21:423–9.
[15] Goldhaber SZ. The perils of D-dimer in the medical intensive care unit. Crit Care Med 2000;28:583–4.
[16] Worsley DF, Alavi A, Aronchick JM, et al. Chest radiographic findings in patients with acute pulmonary embolism: observations from the PIOPED Study. Radiology 1993;189:133–6.
[17] Value of the ventilation/perfusion scan in acute pulmonary embolism. Results of the prospective investigation of pulmonary embolism diagnosis (PIOPED). The PIOPED investigators. JAMA 1990;263:2753–9.
[18] Jolliet P, Slosman DO, Ricou B, et al. Pulmonary scintigraphy at the bedside in intensive care patients with suspected pulmonary embolism. Intensive Care Med 1995;21:723–8.

[19] Stein PD, Henry JW, Gottschalk A. Reassessment of pulmonary angiography for the diagnosis of pulmonary embolism: relation of interpreter agreement to the order of the involved pulmonary arterial branch. Radiology 1999;210:689–91.

[20] Stein PD, Fowler SE, Goodman LR, et al. Multidetector computed tomography for acute pulmonary embolism. N Engl J Med 2006;354:2317–27.

[21] Qanadli SD, Hajjam ME, Mesurolle B, et al. Pulmonary embolism detection: prospective evaluation of dual-section helical CT versus selective pulmonary arteriography in 157 patients. Radiology 2000;217:447–55.

[22] Leschka S, Alkadhi H, Plass A, et al. Accuracy of MSCT coronary angiography with 64-slice technology: first experience. Eur Heart J 2005;26:1482–7.

[23] Raff GL, Gallagher MJ, O'Neill WW, et al. Diagnostic accuracy of noninvasive coronary angiography using 64-slice spiral computed tomography. J Am Coll Cardiol 2005;46:552–7.

[24] Baile EM, King GG, Muller NL, et al. Spiral computed tomography is comparable to angiography for the diagnosis of pulmonary embolism. Am J Respir Crit Care Med 2000; 161:1010–5.

[25] Patel S, Kazerooni EA. Helical CT for the evaluation of acute pulmonary embolism. AJR Am J Roentgenol 2005;185:135–49.

[26] Henry JW, Relyea B, Stein PD. Continuing risk of thromboemboli among patients with normal pulmonary angiograms. Chest 1995;107:1375–8.

[27] Moser KM, Harsanyi P, Rius-Garriga G, et al. Assessment of pulmonary photoscanning and angiography in experimental pulmonary embolism. Circulation 1969;39:663–74.

[28] Velmahos GC, Vassiliu P, Wilcox A, et al. Spiral computed tomography for the diagnosis of pulmonary embolism in critically ill surgical patients: a comparison with pulmonary angiography. Arch Surg 2001;136:505–11.

[29] Velmahos GC, Toutouzas KG, Vassiliu P, et al. Can we rely on computed tomographic scanning to diagnose pulmonary embolism in critically ill surgical patients? J Trauma 2004;56:518–25 [discussion: 525–6].

[30] Remy-Jardin M, Tillie-Leblond I, Szapiro D, et al. CT angiography of pulmonary embolism in patients with underlying respiratory disease: impact of multislice CT on image quality and negative predictive value. Eur Radiol 2002;12:1971–8.

[31] Bourriot K, Couffinhal T, Bernard V, et al. Clinical outcome after a negative spiral CT pulmonary angiographic finding in an inpatient population from cardiology and pneumology wards. Chest 2003;123:359–65.

[32] Loud PA, Katz DS, Bruce DA, et al. Deep venous thrombosis with suspected pulmonary embolism: detection with combined CT venography and pulmonary angiography. Radiology 2001;219:498–502.

[33] Loud PA, Katz DS, Klippenstein DL, et al. Combined CT venography and pulmonary angiography in suspected thromboembolic disease: diagnostic accuracy for deep venous evaluation. AJR Am J Roentgenol 2000;174:61–5.

[34] Begemann PG, Bonacker M, Kemper J, et al. Evaluation of the deep venous system in patients with suspected pulmonary embolism with multi-detector CT: a prospective study in comparison to Doppler sonography. J Comput Assist Tomogr 2003;27:399–409.

[35] Garg K, Kemp JL, Wojcik D, et al. Thromboembolic disease: comparison of combined CT pulmonary angiography and venography with bilateral leg sonography in 70 patients. AJR Am J Roentgenol 2000;175:997–1001.

[36] Cham MD, Yankelevitz DF, Shaham D, et al. Deep venous thrombosis: detection by using indirect CT venography. The Pulmonary Angiography-Indirect CT Venography Cooperative Group. Radiology 2000;216:744–51.

[37] Ghaye B, Szapiro D, Willems V, et al. Combined CT venography of the lower limbs and spiral CT angiography of pulmonary arteries in acute pulmonary embolism: preliminary results of a prospective study. JBR-BTR 2000;83:271–8.

[38] Duwe KM, Shiau M, Budorick NE, et al. Evaluation of the lower extremity veins in patients with suspected pulmonary embolism: a retrospective comparison of helical CT venography

and sonography. 2000 ARRS Executive Council Award I. American Roentgen Ray Society. AJR Am J Roentgenol 2000;175:1525–31.

[39] Coche EE, Hamoir XL, Hammer FD, et al. Using dual-detector helical CT angiography to detect deep venous thrombosis in patients with suspicion of pulmonary embolism: diagnostic value and additional findings. AJR Am J Roentgenol 2001;176:1035–9.

[40] Nienaber CA, Eagle KA. Aortic dissection: new frontiers in diagnosis and management: Part I: from etiology to diagnostic strategies. Circulation 2003;108:628–35.

[41] Reed D, Reed C, Stemmermann G, et al. Are aortic aneurysms caused by atherosclerosis? Circulation 1992;85:205–11.

[42] Larson EW, Edwards WD. Risk factors for aortic dissection: a necropsy study of 161 cases. Am J Cardiol 1984;53:849–55.

[43] Januzzi JL, Sabatine MS, Eagle KA, et al. Iatrogenic aortic dissection. Am J Cardiol 2002; 89:623–6.

[44] Nienaber CA, Sievers HH. Intramural hematoma in acute aortic syndrome: more than one variant of dissection? Circulation 2002;106:284–5.

[45] Chen K, Varon J, Wenker OC, et al. Acute thoracic aortic dissection: the basics. J Emerg Med 1997;15:859–67.

[46] Ganaha F, Miller DC, Sugimoto K, et al. Prognosis of aortic intramural hematoma with and without penetrating atherosclerotic ulcer: a clinical and radiological analysis. Circulation 2002;106:342–8.

[47] Jagannath AS, Sos TA, Lockhart SH, et al. Aortic dissection: a statistical analysis of the usefulness of plain chest radiographic findings. AJR Am J Roentgenol 1986;147:1123–6.

[48] Yoshida S, Akiba H, Tamakawa M, et al. Thoracic involvement of type A aortic dissection and intramural hematoma: diagnostic accuracy–comparison of emergency helical CT and surgical findings. Radiology 2003;228:430–5.

[49] Hayter RG, Rhea JT, Small A, et al. Suspected aortic dissection and other aortic disorders: multi-detector row CT in 373 cases in the emergency setting. Radiology 2006;238:841–52.

[50] Sommer T, Fehske W, Holzknecht N, et al. Aortic dissection: a comparative study of diagnosis with spiral CT, multiplanar transesophageal echocardiography, and MR imaging. Radiology 1996;199:347–52.

[51] Sebastia C, Pallisa E, Quiroga S, et al. Aortic dissection: diagnosis and follow-up with helical CT. Radiographics 1999;19:45–60, quiz 149–50.

[52] Tisnado J, Cho SR, Beachley MC, et al. Ulcerlike projections: a precursor angiographic sign to thoracic aortic dissection. AJR Am J Roentgenol 1980;135:719–22.

[53] Nienaber CA, von Kodolitsch Y, Petersen B, et al. Intramural hemorrhage of the thoracic aorta. Diagnostic and therapeutic implications. Circulation 1995;92:1465–72.

[54] Nienaber CA, von Kodolitsch Y, Nicolas V, et al. The diagnosis of thoracic aortic dissection by noninvasive imaging procedures. N Engl J Med 1993;328:1–9.

[55] Nienaber CA, Spielmann RP, von Kodolitsch Y, et al. Diagnosis of thoracic aortic dissection. Magnetic resonance imaging versus transesophageal echocardiography. Circulation 1992;85:434–47.

[56] Ell PJ, Donaldson RM. Cardiovascular nuclear medicine and intensive care. Intensive Care Med 1978;4:119–22.

[57] Hoffmann U, Nagurney JT, Moselewski F, et al. Coronary multidetector computed tomography in the assessment of patients with acute chest pain. Circulation 2006;114:2251–60.

[58] Hilton TC, Thompson RC, Williams HJ, et al. Technetium-99m sestamibi myocardial perfusion imaging in the emergency room evaluation of chest pain. J Am Coll Cardiol 1994;23: 1016–22.

[59] White C, Read K, Kuo D. Assessment of chest pain in the emergency room: what is the role of multidetector CT? Eur J Radiol 2006;57:368–72.

[60] Nieman K, Cademartiri F, Lemos PA, et al. Reliable noninvasive coronary angiography with fast submillimeter multislice spiral computed tomography. Circulation 2002;106: 2051–4.

[61] Ropers D, Baum U, Pohle K, et al. Detection of coronary artery stenoses with thin-slice multi-detector row spiral computed tomography and multiplanar reconstruction. Circulation 2003;107:664–6.

[62] Hoffmann U, Moselewski F, Cury RC, et al. Predictive value of 16-slice multidetector spiral computed tomography to detect significant obstructive coronary artery disease in patients at high risk for coronary artery disease: patient- versus segment-based analysis. Circulation 2004;110:2638–43.

[63] Achenbach S, Ropers D, Hoffmann U, et al. Assessment of coronary remodeling in stenotic and nonstenotic coronary atherosclerotic lesions by multidetector spiral computed tomography. J Am Coll Cardiol 2004;43:842–7.

[64] Kuettner A, Beck T, Drosch T, et al. Diagnostic accuracy of noninvasive coronary imaging using 16-detector slice spiral computed tomography with 188 ms temporal resolution. J Am Coll Cardiol 2005;45:123–7.

[65] Mollet NR, Cademartiri F, Krestin GP, et al. Improved diagnostic accuracy with 16-row multi-slice computed tomography coronary angiography. J Am Coll Cardiol 2005;45: 128–32.

[66] Mollet NR, Cademartiri F, van Mieghem CA, et al. High-resolution spiral computed tomography coronary angiography in patients referred for diagnostic conventional coronary angiography. Circulation 2005;112:2318–23.

[67] Ehara M, Surmely JF, Kawai M, et al. Diagnostic accuracy of 64-slice computed tomography for detecting angiographically significant coronary artery stenosis in an unselected consecutive patient population: comparison with conventional invasive angiography. Circ J 2006;70:564–71.

[68] Raff GL, Gallagher MJ, O'Neill WW, et al. Immediate coronary CTA rapidly and definitively excludes CAD in low-risk acute chest pain. Presented at the American College of Cardiology Annual Scientific Session. Atlanta (GA); 2006. p. 807–8.

[69] Achenbach S, Ropers D, Kuettner A, et al. Contrast-enhanced coronary artery visualization by dual-source computed tomography–initial experience. Eur J Radiol 2006;57:331–5.

[70] Rubinshtein R, Halon DA, Gaspar T, et al. Usefulness of 64-slice cardiac computed tomographic angiography for diagnosing acute coronary syndromes and predicting clinical outcome in emergency department patients with chest pain of uncertain origin. Circulation 2007;115:1762–8.

[71] Schroeder S, Kopp AF, Kuettner A, et al. Influence of heart rate on vessel visibility in noninvasive coronary angiography using new multislice computed tomography: experience in 94 patients. Clin Imaging 2002;26:106–11.

[72] Vogl TJ, Abolmaali ND, Diebold T, et al. Techniques for the detection of coronary atherosclerosis: multi-detector row CT coronary angiography. Radiology 2002;223:212–20.

ELSEVIER
SAUNDERS

CRITICAL
CARE
CLINICS

Crit Care Clin 23 (2007) 855–872

Cardiac Arrhythmias: Management of Atrial Fibrillation in the Critically Ill Patient

Thomas C. Crawford, MD, Hakan Oral, MD*

*Cardiac Electrophysiology, Division of Cardiovascular Medicine,
University of Michigan, CVC 1500 E. Medical Center Drive,
SPC 5853, Ann Arbor, MI 48109-5853, USA*

Atrial fibrillation (AF) is a common arrhythmia in the ICU, second only to ventricular tachycardia. A study of prevalence of arrhythmias showed that AF may occur in up to 31% of patients in medical, cardiac, and surgical ICUs [1]. AF is associated with a significantly longer ICU stay. In-hospital mortality associated with acute myocardial infarction (MI) is higher in patients who have AF (25% versus 16%) [2]. AF is associated with a twofold increase in mortality in the community, and it is influenced by the severity of underlying heart disease [3,4].

It is estimated that 2.2 million people in the United States have AF. The prevalence of this disease increases with age. The burden of AF is expected to rise as population ages, and it will continue to be associated with significant health care costs [5].

Etiology and associated conditions

AF is associated with various cardiac or extracardiac conditions, some of which are chronic, while others are short lived. In the setting of acute illness, AF may present de novo, or it may recur in patients who have a history of AF. Surgery, especially cardiac or thoracic, pulmonary embolism or other pulmonary conditions, myocarditis, electrocution, alcohol consumption, thyroid disorders, and other metabolic conditions may contribute to the development of AF.

AF also often is associated with history of hypertension and coronary artery disease (CAD). Eleven percent of patients presenting with acute MI

* Corresponding author.
E-mail address: oralh@umich.edu (H. Oral).

0749-0704/07/$ - see front matter © 2007 Elsevier Inc. All rights reserved.
doi:10.1016/j.ccc.2007.06.005   *criticalcare.theclinics.com*

develop AF during their hospitalization [6]. Left ventricular (LV) hypertrophy and associated diastolic dysfunction likely play a role in the genesis of AF because of an increase in stretch in the left atrium or the pulmonary veins [7]. Valvular heart disease, especially mitral stenosis and mitral regurgitation resulting in left atrial (LA) dilatation, commonly are associated with atrial arrhythmias. AF also may be related to hypertrophic cardiomyopathy (HCM) or dilated cardiomyopathy, and various forms of congenital heart disease in adults, especially atrial septal defect. Less common causes of AF include restrictive cardiomyopathies (such as amyloidosis, hemochromatosis, and endomyocardial fibrosis), pericarditis, and cardiac tumors. The known causes of AF are listed in Box 1.

Among noncardiac chronic conditions, obesity is an important, recently identified risk factor for developing AF [8,9]. There is a direct relationship between LA size and body mass index (BMI). An association between obstructive sleep apnea (OSA) and AF also has been reported [10].

The term lone AF is used to describe AF in individuals younger than 60 years of age who have no clinical or echocardiographic evidence of cardiac disease. In approximately 45% of patients who have paroxysmal AF and 25% of patients who have chronic AF, no cardiac disease can be identified [11]. Fluctuations in autonomic tone appear to play a role in the initiation of AF, especially in structurally normal hearts. Both vagal and sympathetic tone may surge in the minutes that precede initiation of AF [12,13].

Definitions

Various terms have been used in the literature to describe patterns of AF occurrence. The North American Society of Pacing and Electrophysiology and the European Society of Cardiology recently endorsed a new nomenclature [14]. Episodes are classified as first-detected, recurrent, paroxysmal, persistent, or permanent. When a patient has had two or more episodes of AF, AF is considered recurrent. If it terminates spontaneously, AF is designated as paroxysmal; when it is sustained beyond 7 days, it is called persistent. If cardioversion has failed or had not been attempted, and the patient has been in AF for longer than 1 year, AF is referred to as permanent.

Pathophysiology

The mechanisms responsible for AF are multifactorial [15]. Multiple wavelet reentry [16], anisotropic reentry with high-frequency focal sources and centrifugal fibrillatory conduction [17], and perturbations in the autonomic innervation of the atrium [18] have been proposed as potential mechanisms of AF. Pulmonary veins have arrhythmogenic activity and are implicated in the initiation [19] and perpetuation of paroxysmal AF [20]. In patients who have persistent and permanent AF, fibrosis is thought to

Box 1. Etiologies and factors predisposing patients to atrial fibrillation

Electrophysiological abnormalities
- Enhanced automaticity (focal AF)
- Conduction abnormality (reentry)

Increase in atrial pressure
- Mitral or tricuspid valve disease
- Myocardial disease (primary or secondary, leading to systolic or diastolic dysfunction)
- Valvular abnormalities (causing ventricular hypertrophy)
- Systemic or pulmonary hypertension (pulmonary embolism)
- Intracardiac tumors or thrombi

Atrial ischemia
- Coronary artery disease

Inflammatory or infiltrative atrial disease
- Pericarditis
- Amyloidosis
- Myocarditis
- Age-induced atrial fibrotic changes

Drugs
- Alcohol
- Caffeine

Endocrine disorders
- Hyperthyroidism
- Pheochromocytoma

Changes in autonomic tone
- Increased parasympathetic activity
- Increased sympathetic activity

Primary or metastatic disease in or adjacent to the atrial wall

Postoperative
- Cardiac, pulmonary, or esophageal

Congenital heart disease

Neurogenic
- Subarachnoid hemorrhage
- Nonhemorrhagic, major stroke

Idiopathic (lone AF)

Familial AF

Data from Fuster V, Rydén LE, Cannom DS, et al. ACC/AHA/ESC 2006 guidelines for the management of patients with atrial fibrillation—executive summary: a report of the American College of Cardiology/American Heart Association Task Force and the European Society of Cardiology Committee for Practice Guidelines (Writing Committee to Revise the 2001 Guidelines for the Management of Patients With Atrial Fibrillation). J Am Coll Cardiol 2006;48:854–906.

promote AF by facilitating reentry. Loss of intercellular coupling caused by alterations in the number and distribution of gap junctions and connections may be important in creating a substrate capable of maintaining AF [21].

Adrenergic stimulation and inflammation, common among postoperative and critically ill patients, are involved in the genesis of AF by means of complex and incompletely understood mechanisms. AF is associated with an up-regulation of angiotensin subtype 1 receptor [AT (1)] in the left atrium [22]. Renin-angiotensin-aldosterone system (RAAS) promotes development of atrial fibrosis, which is thought to be a substrate for anisotropic reentry. Levels of C-reactive protein (CRP) are higher in patients who have AF, and they increase with higher AF burden [23,24]. AF increases production of superoxide by the left atrium and LA appendage [25]. Pronounced increases in white blood cell (WBC) count have been described as an independent risk factor in patients after cardiac surgery [26]. Statins, which have anti-inflammatory properties, have been shown to suppress electrical remodeling in an animal model of AF [27], and they may reduce the incidence of postoperative AF. This effect may be caused by their inhibition of metalloproteinases, oxidants, and mediators of inflammation [28]. High levels of these stress mediators may be responsible for increased burden of AF in critically ill patients.

Hemodynamic consequences of atrial fibrillation

AF can lead to a decrease in cardiac output, which can manifest as a fall in blood pressure and pulmonary congestion. AF worsens New York Heart Association (NYHA) heart failure class even in patients with relatively well-controlled ventricular response [29]. Hemodynamic deterioration is particularly problematic in patients who have already impaired systolic or diastolic function, and other underlying heart disease, such as significant mitral stenosis and hypertrophic obstructive cardiomyopathy.

Several mechanisms have been proposed to explain the adverse hemodynamic effects of AF. They include a rapid heart rate, loss of atrial systole, irregularity of ventricular rhythm, and activation of neurohormonal mediators such as norepinephrine and angiotensin II [30–33].

Rapid heart rate limits the amount of time available for ventricular filling. Loss of atrial systole may be associated with a 20% reduction in LV stroke volume in patients who have preserved LV function, and up to 35% reduction in patients with recent MI [30] Patients who have diastolic dysfunction or poorly compliant left ventricle rely heavily on atrial systole for filling. In patients who have hypertrophic cardiomyopathy, mitral stenosis, aortic stenosis, and severe cerebrovascular disease, these effects may be more profound.

Irregular rhythm may affect cardiac output adversely by inefficient ventricular mechanics caused by abrupt changes in ventricular cycle length, variations in preload, and in myocardial contractility. Resumption of ventricular regularity with AV nodal ablation and ventricular pacing improves cardiac output beyond what would be expected in patients who have AF and adequate rate control [31].

The fall in cardiac output in critically ill patients who develop AF with rapid ventricular response may activate neurohormonal vasoconstrictors further, which can lead to an increase in systemic vascular resistance (afterload) and coronary vascular resistance (decrease in coronary perfusion). AF episodes are associated with increases in atrial natriuretic peptides and B-type natriuretic peptides, which decrease rapidly after restoration of sinus rhythm [32,34]. The results of these assays should be interpreted carefully in the presence of AF. High levels of ANP and BNP may lead to diuresis and hypotension [33].

Clinical presentation

Patients who have AF have variable clinical presentations. Many patients are asymptomatic or complain of palpitations, shortness of breath, or fatigue. Some patients experience chest pain, especially when ventricular rate is not controlled well, regardless of whether they have underlying CAD. Sustained AF with rapid ventricular response may lead to tachycardia-mediated cardiomyopathy, especially in patients unaware of their condition [35]. Syncope is rare in patients without other cardiovascular conditions, but may be more common in patients who have sinus node dysfunction, an accessory pathway, hypertrophic cardiomyopathy, or aortic stenosis. Thromboembolism may be the sole presenting symptom resulting in cerebrovascular accident or ischemic extremity.

In the ICU setting, onset of AF may be associated with hemodynamic compromise and hypoxemia. Patients who have subclinical heart failure are likely to experience an exacerbation. Anticoagulation issues related to AF may complicate management of critically ill patients with trauma, malignancy, intracranial or gastrointestinal hemorrhage, platelet disorders, or history of heparin-induced thrombocytopenia.

Management

Treatment of AF is directed at three major objectives: control of ventricular rate, restoring normal sinus rhythm, and prevention of thromboembolic complications. Acute management largely depends on the clinical status of the patient. Patients who have ongoing cardiac chest pain, pulmonary edema, or who are hemodynamically unstable, should be considered for an emergent cardioversion. Management of patients who can tolerate AF initially focuses on adequate control of the ventricular rate appropriate for the hemodynamic status and underlying cardiac substrate of the ICU patient.

Acute rate control of atrial fibrillation

Agents such as beta receptor blockers, some calcium channel antagonists, and digoxin can be used acutely to control ventricular rate. Dihydropyridine calcium channel blockers such as nifedipine or amlodipine besylate have no effect on the atrioventricular node, and they are not recommended to control ventricular response. Beta-blockers are likely to be effective in postoperative patients who may have high adrenergic tone. Metoprolol is given in doses of 2.5 to 5 mg intravenously over 2 to 5 minutes. The onset of action occurs within a few minutes, and the drug can be repeated up to three times every 5 to 10 minutes as long as patient does not develop hypotension or other adverse effects. Once adequate rate control has been achieved, patients may be transitioned to oral doses of metoprolol. Esmolol, an intravenous, short-acting beta-blocker, may be very helpful in patients who are at risk for hemodynamic instability, as the drug is eliminated quickly when discontinued. Beta blockers may result in bronchospasm in patients who have chronic obstructive pulmonary disease (COPD), asthma, or reactive airway disease. In patients who do not tolerate beta-blockers, or in whom beta-blockers are insufficient to control ventricular rate, diltiazem may be administered at 0.25 mg/kg intravenously over 2 minutes followed by 5 to 10 mg/h continuous infusion, or verapamil 0.075 to 0.15 mg/kg intravenously over 2 minutes (Table 1).

Digoxin may be useful in patients with heart failure and those who have marginal blood pressures, as it increases myocardial contractility and does not result in hypotension. Digoxin can be loaded intravenously at 0.25 mg intravenously every 2 hours, up to 1.5 mg, or given orally. Caution should be exercised in patients who have kidney disease. In patients who have renal insufficiency, digitoxin, another cardiac glycoside, may be used. Unlike digoxin (which is eliminated from the body through the kidneys), digitoxin is eliminated by the liver [36].

Amiodarone causes slowing of rapid ventricular rate, most of which occurs in the first hour after administration of the drug, although other antiarrhythmic properties of this drug may not manifest until several days later [37]. This may be because of predominant beta-adrenergic and calcium channel blockade observed early after intravenous amiodarone injection.

Beta-blockers and nondihydropyridine calcium channel blockers should be avoided in patients presenting with pulmonary edema or severe LV dysfunction. Intravenous beta- blockers, nondihydropyridine calcium channel blockers, and digitalis should be used with caution in patients who have a history of pre-excitation and Wolf-Parkinson-White syndrome, because these agents can facilitate antegrade conduction over the accessory pathway and may result in acceleration of tachycardia and degeneration to ventricular fibrillation [38,39]. Patients who have ventricular pre-excitation and AF may be treated with intravenous procainamide or amiodarone. ECG during AF in a patient who has an accessory pathway may show an irregular wide complex tachycardia caused by ventricular pre-excitation of the accessory pathway (Fig. 1). In select patients who have Wolf-Parkinson-White syndrome, oral beta-blockers and calcium channel blockers may be used for rate control as chronic therapy with careful monitoring [5].

Pharmacologic cardioversion

Various agents are available for cardioversion of AF. The overall acute success rate is lower with pharmacologic cardioversion than with electrical cardioversion and ranges from 40% to 70% [40,41]. Class I antiarrhythmic agents work primarily by blocking sodium channel (Na^+) and class III agents primarily by blocking potassium slow rectifier channel (I_{kr}). Not all pharmacological agents can be employed in the intensive care setting because of their pharmacodynamics and the many comorbidities that may be contraindications for their use. Class IA (quinidine, disopyramide, procainamide) and IC agents (flecainide and propafenone) are contraindicated in patients who have structural heart disease. The Cardiac Arrhythmia Suppression Trial provided evidence against use of flecainide and encainide in patients with CAD [42]. Other agents may be available in oral preparations only, which limits their usefulness in the intensive care environment. Amiodarone and procainamide are two antiarrhythmic agents most frequently used in the ICU.

The conversion rate from AF to sinus rhythm during amiodarone load is about 30% [43]. Amiodarone often is used to maintain sinus rhythm after cardioversion in patients who have AF. Amiodarone also is used for managing ventricular arrhythmias. Its advantages include low acute adverse effect profile and a neutral effect on mortality in patients following MI and in the presence of structural heart disease. Its long-term extracardiac toxicity potential, however, is significant. Amiodarone can be administered intravenously as a bolus of 150 mg over 10 minutes, followed by a continuous drip at 1 mg/min for 6 hours, then at 0.5 mg/min for 18 hours or until the patient can take amiodarone orally. Hypotension may occur with intravenous amiodarone, especially in patients who have overt heart failure and severe LV dysfunction [37]. The maintenance dose of amiodarone for AF is usually 200 mg orally per day.

Upon initiation of therapy with amiodarone, thyroid and liver panels, and chest radiograph should be obtained. Patients who are maintained on amiodarone should undergo monitoring every 6 months and have periodic pulmonary function tests with diffusing capacity of lungs for carbon monoxide [44]. Four types of lung injury from amiodarone have been reported: chronic interstitial pneumonitis, bronchiolitis obliterans, acute respiratory distress syndrome, and a solitary lung mass. Amiodarone pulmonary toxicity correlates most closely with cumulative dose received, and it is rare in patients receiving 200 mg daily [45,46]. Acute lung injury with smaller doses of amiodarone, however, have been reported, especially following thoracotomy [47–51].

According to a recent meta-analysis, amiodarone facilitates conversion of recent-onset AF to sinus rhythm, with a 44% superiority in efficacy compared

Table 1
List of commonly used agents for rate control, their loading doses, onset of action, maintenance doses, and common adverse effects

Drug	Loading dose	Onset	Maintenance dose	Major adverse effects
Acute setting				
Esmolol	500 µg/kg intravenously over 1 min	5 min	60 to 200 µg/kg/min intravenously	↓BP, HB, ↓HR, asthma, HF
Metoprolol	2.5 to 5 mg intravenous bolus over 2 minutes, up to three doses	5 min	N/A	↓BP, HB, ↓HR, asthma, HF
Propranolol	0.15 mg/kg intravenously	5 min	N/A	↓BP, HB, ↓HR, asthma, HF
Diltiazem	0.25 mg/kg intravenously over 2 min	2 to 7 min	5 to 15 mg/h IV	↓BP, HB, HF
Verapamil	0.075 to 0.15 mg/kg intravenously over 2 min	3 to 5 min	N/A	↓BP, HB, HF
Amiodarone	150 mg over 10 min	Days	0.5 to 1 mg/min IV	↓BP, HB, pulmonary toxicity, skin discoloration, hypothyroidism, hyperthyroidism, corneal deposits, optic neuropathy, warfarin interaction, sinus bradycardia
Digoxin	0.25 mg intravenously each 2 h, up to 1.5 mg	60 min or more	0.125 to 0.375 mg intravenously daily or orally	Digitalis toxicity, HB, ↓HR
Nonacute setting and chronic maintenance therapy				
Metoprolol	Same as maintenance dose	4 to 6 h	25 to 100 mg twice a day orally	↓BP, HB, ↓HR, asthma, HF
Propranolol	Same as maintenance dose	60 to 90 min	80 to 240 mg daily in divided doses, orally	↓BP, HB, ↓HR, asthma, HF
Diltiazem	Same as maintenance dose	2 to 4 h	120 to 360 mg daily in divided doses, slow-release available, orally	↓BP, HB, HF

(*continued on next page*)

Table 1 (*continued*)

Drug	Loading dose	Onset	Maintenance dose	Major adverse effects
Verapamil	Same as maintenance dose	1 to 2 h	120 to 360 mg daily in divided doses, slow-release available, orally	↓BP, HB, HF, digoxin interaction
Amiodarone	800 mg daily for 1 wk, orally 600 mg daily for 1 wk, orally 400 mg daily for 4 to 6 wk, orally (if outpatient, should not receive more than 400 mg a day because of the need for monitoring)	1 to 3 wk	200 mg daily, orally	↓BP, HB, pulmonary toxicity, skin discoloration, hypothyroidism, hyperthyroidism, corneal deposits, optic neuropathy, warfarin interaction, sinus bradycardia
Digoxin	0.5 mg by mouth daily	2 days	0.125 to 0.375 mg daily, orally	Digitalis toxicity, HB, ↓HR

↓BP indicates hypotension; ↓HR, bradycardia.

Abbreviations: HB, heart block; HF, heart failure.

Data from Fuster V, Rydén LE, Cannom DS, et al. ACC/AHA/ESC 2006 guidelines for the management of patients with atrial fibrillation—executive summary: a report of the American College of Cardiology/American Heart Association Task Force and the European Society of Cardiology Committee for Practice Guidelines (Writing Committee to Revise the 2001 Guidelines for the Management of Patients With Atrial Fibrillation). J Am Coll Cardiol 2006;48:854–906.

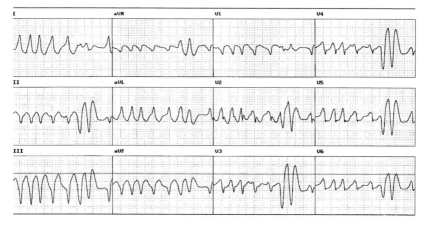

Fig. 1. Atrial fibrillation in a patient with pre-excitation may result in rapid conduction over the accessory pathway, resulting in polymorphic ventricular tachycardia (shown) and eventually ventricular fibrillation and cardiac arrest.

with placebo [52]. Its antiarrhythmic effect on AF is not apparent until 8 to 24 hours after administration. This efficacy is comparable to that of class IC agents at 24 hours after drug administration, although IC drugs showed a more rapid onset of action, with some effect already apparent at 1 to 2 hours after administration. The only significant predictors of cardioversion are the duration of AF and LA size [53].

Amiodarone potentiates the effects of warfarin (it raises international normalized ratio [INR] level); accordingly, the dose of warfarin should be reduced upon initiating amiodarone. Amiodarone also increases digoxin and cyclosporine levels. Adverse effects of amiodarone include bradycardia, hypotension, visual disturbances, nausea, or constipation after oral administration and phlebitis after peripheral intravenous administration. Amiodarone can be used in patients with poor LV function, and it has a very low risk of polymorphic ventricular tachycardia (torsades de pointes) despite QT interval prolongation. In one meta-analysis of four trials involving 738 patients who had MI and LV dysfunction treated for at least a year, low-dose amiodarone caused no cases of torsades de pointes [54]. Amiodarone is more effective than either sotalol or propafenone in maintaining sinus rhythm in patients who have paroxysmal or persistent AF [55]. Amiodarone prevented recurrence of AF in 69% of patients, while only 39% of those on sotalol or propafenone remained in sinus rhythm. Amiodarone has some beta-blocking and calcium-blocking activity, so doses of these agents also should be adjusted appropriately.

Procainamide is another intravenous agent that has been used to pharmacologically cardiovert AF. It is a class IA antiarrhythmic drug. It can be given at a rate of 30 mg/min to a maximum dose of 20 mg/kg or in 100 mg boluses every 10 minutes up to a dose of about 2 g. If hypotension or QRS complex prolongation by greater than 50% occurs, infusion of procainamide should be terminated. Procainamide also can prolong QT interval and lead to proarrhythmia. Unfortunately, its negative inotropic effects and vasodilation have limited its use in the intensive care setting. Its metabolite NAPA (N-acetylprocainamide) is cleared through the kidneys, and monitoring of NAPA levels is recommended in patients who have renal dysfunction. Procainamide also may cause bone marrow suppression, Coomb's-positive hemolytic anemia, cholestatic jaundice, and lupus-like symptoms. Procainamide is the drug of choice in patients with Wolf-Parkinson-White syndrome who present with AF.

Ibutilide is another class III antiarrhythmic drug. Ibutilide is given intravenously and may be used alone or in conjunction with direct current cardioversion. Ibutilide 1 mg is given as an infusion over 10 minutes, which can be repeated 10 to 20 minutes later if AF persists. Torsades de pointes occurs in up to 4% of patients who are given this medication, but it appears to be limited to patients who have LV dysfunction or baseline prolongation of QT interval, particularly in the presence of hypokalemia or hypomagnesaemia. Therefore ibuitilide should not be administered in patients who have a left ventricular ejection fraction less than 35% or corrected (QTc) >460 milliseconds.

Dofetilide is a newer class III oral antiarrhythmic agent that is a highly selective blocker of the rapid component of the delayed rectifier current causing action potential prolongation. It may take days to weeks before cardioversion occurs while this drug achieves therapeutic levels. This limits its use in the acute setting. Dofetilide has renal clearance. Only the oral form of the drug is available in the United States, and it is approved for both AF and atrial flutter. Inpatient initiation of therapy by certified physicians is mandated by the US Food and Drug Administration. Table 2 provides a side-by-side comparison of various antiarrhythmic agents with proven efficacy for pharmacologic cardioversion.

Electrical cardioversion of atrial fibrillation

Direct current (DC) cardioversion is the preferred initial method for termination of AF in critically ill patients because of its high acute efficacy of 67% to 94% [56–58]. Cardioversion results in immediate improvement of LV ejection fraction and stroke volume [59].

The probability of long-term maintenance of sinus rhythm is inversely related to both duration of AF before cardioversion and LA size [60,61]. If cardioversion fails, patients may be premedicated with antiarrhythmic medications before repeat cardioversion. Pretreatment with ibutilide, a class III antiarrhythmic drug, improves the success rate of DC cardioversion and is associated with a reduction in defibrillation energy requirements [62]. Other agents that can be used to enhance the success of DC cardioversion and maintenance of sinus rhythm are amiodarone, flecainide, propafenone, ibutilide, and sotalol [5].

Biphasic waveform defibrillators are more effective in cardioverting AF than are monophasic waveform defibrillators [63,64]. The energy requirement for cardioversion is usually 100 to 200 J for AF and 25 to 50 J for atrial flutter. Higher energy levels are required in patients whose BMI is high, who have had AF for a longer period of time, and whose left atrium is enlarged. Studies have failed to substantiate significant effect of high-energy defibrillation of up to 1370 J on troponin release from cardiac myocytes [65,66]. Pulmonary edema is a rare complication following cardioversion (1.2 %), and may be related to myocardial stunning, but seems not to be related to the amount of energy used [67].

DC cardioversion may be complicated by ventricular fibrillation, bradycardia or tachycardia, ST segment elevation, ventricular dysfunction, transient hypotension, pulmonary edema, and embolism. Cardioversions should be performed in the synchronized mode, in which the shock is delivered during ventricular depolarization. Shock applied during repolarization, shock on T, may result in ventricular fibrillation. Electrolyte status should be normalized when possible before cardioversion to limit proarrythmic complications. DC cardioversion should be avoided in the presence of digoxin intoxication. Ventricular fibrillation may occur following synchronous application of shock

Table 2

Recommended doses of drugs proven effective for pharmacological cardioversion of atrial fibrillation

Drug	Route of administration	Dosage		Major adverse effects
Amiodarone	Oral	Inpatient: 1.2 to 1.8 g per day in divided dose until 10 g total, then 200 to 400 mg per day maintenance or 30 mg/kg as single dose		Hypotension, bradycardia, QT interval prolongation, torsades de pointes (rare), gastroinstinal upset, constipation, phlebitis (intravenous)
		Outpatient: 600 to 800 mg per day divided dose until 10 g total, then 200 to 400 mg per day maintenance		
	Intravenous or oral	5 to 7 mg/kg over 30 to 60 min, then 1.2 to 1.8 g per day continuous intravenous dose or in divided oral doses until 10 g total, then 200 to 400 mg per day maintenance		
Dofetilide	Oral	Creatinine Clearance (mL/min)	Dose (μg twice daily)	Contraindicated if QT prolongation, torsades de pointes; adjust dose for renal function, body size, and age
		More than 60	500	
		40 to 60	250	
		20 to 40	125	
		Less than 20	Contraindicated	
Flecainide	Oral	200 to 300 mg		Hypotension, atrial flutter with high ventricular rate
	Intravenous	1.5 to 3.0 mg/kg over 10 to 20 min		
Ibutilide	Intravenous	1 mg over 10 min; repeat 1 mg when necessary		QT prolongation, torsades de pointes
Propafenone	Oral	600 mg		Hypotension, atrial flutter with high ventricular rate
	Intravenous	1.5 to 2.0 mg/kg over 10 to 20 min		
Quinidine	Oral	0.75 to 1.5 g in divided doses over 6 to 12 h, usually with a rate-slowing drug		QT prolongation, torsades de pointes, gastrointestinal upset, hypotension

Data from Fuster V, Rydén LE, Cannom DS, et al. ACC/AHA/ESC 2006 guidelines for the management of patients with atrial fibrillation—executive summary: a report of the American College of Cardiology/American Heart Association Task Force and the European Society of Cardiology Committee for Practice Guidelines (Writing Committee to Revise the 2001 Guidelines for the Management of Patients With Atrial Fibrillation). J Am Coll Cardiol 2006;48:854–906.

in patients who have digitalis toxicity, especially in the setting of hypokalemia. If cardioversion must be performed, prophylactic lidocaine should be given and low levels of energy applied. Sinus bradycardia or tachycardia occurs in up to 25% of cardioversions [68]. Patients on antiarrhythmic agents are more susceptible to bradycardia or asystole after the shock, and pacing capability should be available immediately after cardioversion [69]. In patients who have permanent pacemakers, the lowest energy necessary should be used, and the electrodes should be placed in the anteroposterior position at least 12 cm from the pacemaker generator. Most reports on damage to pacemaker circuitry refer to older devices; however, a prudent approach would be to interrogate the device to assure proper function of the pacemaker following a cardioversion.

Anticoagulation of patients with atrial fibrillation in the ICU

Management of patients with AF at risk in the ICU presents a set of challenges. Although these patients are at risk of thromboembolism, many may have relative or absolute contraindications for anticoagulation. Comorbidities that may place patients at risk for complications include postoperative state, stroke, hemorrhage, platelet disorders, renal or liver failure, acute respiratory distress syndrome (ARDS), or trauma. The clinician must make a careful assessment of the risks and benefits of anticoagulation in the individual patient. The decision about whether and when to anticoagulate patient with AF is made best in consultation of all the physicians involved in the patient's care.

If AF is of greater than 48 hours duration, or its duration is unknown, and the patient has not been anticoagulated for at least 3 weeks, cardioversion can be performed after ruling out left atrial appendage thrombus by transesophageal echocardiography (TEE) with a low risk of stroke [70]. An example of a large thrombus in the LA appendage is shown in Fig. 2. Of course, if AF is associated with hemodynamic instability in the form of angina pectoris, MI, shock, or pulmonary edema, immediate cardioversion should be done without a TEE, but intravenous unfractionated heparin or subcutaneous injection of a low molecular-weight heparin should be initiated at the time of emergency cardioversion.

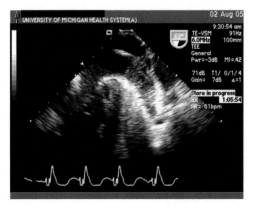

Fig. 2. A large thrombus wedged in the left atrial appendage is seen on this transesophageal echogram.

In case–control series, patients undergoing cardioversion of AF or atrial flutter have a 1% to 5% risk of thromboembolism [71,72]. According to data pooled from 32 studies, more than 80% of thromboembolic events occur during the first 3 days, and 98% occur within 10 days of cardioversion [73]. Following successful cardioversion, atrial contractile function is impaired for hours to weeks depending on the duration of AF before cardioversion. Following cardioversion, however, all patients should be anticoagulated unless there is a significant contraindication. Anticoagulation should be continued for at least 4 weeks after a successful cardioversion, and perhaps longer in patients who have a high risk profile for thromboembolic complications. Although LA thrombus and systemic embolism have been documented in patients who have AF of shorter duration, the need for anticoagulation is less clear if AF has been present for less than 48 hours.

Prevention of atrial fibrillation in ICU patients

As previously stated, atrial arrhythmias, including AF, complicate 20% to 50% of open heart surgeries. Most postoperative AF occurs in the first 5 days, especially on postoperative day 2. Risks for postoperative AF include advanced age, a history of AF, COPD, valvular heart disease, withdrawal of beta-blockers or ace inhibitors, and pericarditis. Patients who have postoperative AF have a higher inpatient mortality (4.7% versus 2.1%) and longer length of hospital stay than patients without this arrhythmia [74]. Studies on perioperative use of amiodarone, beta blockers, sotalol, and pacing showed varying degrees of benefit. A systematic Cochrane database review analyzing 8565 patients found beta-blockers to be the most efficacious [75]. Perioperative use of amiodarone starting at least 7 days before cardiac surgery has been shown to reduce the incidence of AF by about 50% compared with placebo [76,77]. Sotalol (80 or 120 mg by mouth twice daily) when given in addition to beta-blocker was more effective than beta-blockers alone in some studies [78], but was of no benefit in others. A meta analysis of 10 randomized trials of postcoronary artery bypass graft (CABG) AF suggest that atrial overdrive pacing may reduce occurrence of AF by as much as 54% [79]. Although there are some data suggesting that inhibitors of the RAAS (ACE inhibitors and angiotensin receptor blockers) and statins may reduce the incidence of AF in the general medical population, there are no data on the possible role these agents may play in preventing postoperative AF. One study suggested that withdrawal of ACE inhibitor in the perioperative period may be associated with increased incidence of AF [80].

Long term outcome of patients who develop atrial fibrillation in the ICU

AF is associated with increased risk of stroke, heart failure, and all-cause mortality, especially in women [81]. Long-term mortality rate of patients who have AF in the community is about double that of patients who have normal sinus rhythm. Data on long-term outcomes of patients who develop AF during critical illness is largely lacking, except when associated with specific disease states, such as MI and postoperative state. AF complicating acute MI doubles the in-hospital mortality [2]. In postoperative AF, on the other hand, long-term consequences of AF are more benign, and nearly 90 % of patients revert to sinus rhythm after 2 months after surgery. Patients who develop AF in the setting of thyrotoxicosis usually revert spontaneously to sinus rhythm when they become euthyroid. Antiarrhythmic drugs and DC cardioversion are generally unsuccessful until euthyroid state is restored.

Summary

AF is associated with significant morbidity and increased mortality, especially in critically ill patients or in patients who have MI and heart failure. AF is a common arrhythmia in the ICU, and its management can be challenging. Specific therapy should be individualized based on age, clinical and hemodynamic status, underlying cardiac substrate, and comorbidities. Rate control is a reasonable strategy in older patients with asymptomatic or minimally symptomatic AF. In general, rhythm control strategy may be preferred to rate control strategy in ICU patients given their usually tenuous hemodynamic status and overall condition. Anticoagulation is an important aspect of management of AF. Specific measures may be taken to prevent AF in some ICU patients.

References

[1] Reinelt P, et al. Incidence and type of cardiac arrhythmias in critically ill patients: a single-center experience in a medical–cardiological ICU. Intensive Care Med 2001;27(9):1466–73.

[2] Rathore SS, et al. Acute myocardial infarction complicated by atrial fibrillation in the elderly: prevalence and outcomes. Circulation 2000;101(9):969–74.

[3] Kannel WB, et al. Coronary heart disease and atrial fibrillation: the Framingham Study. Am Heart J 1983;106(2):389–96.

[4] Krahn AD, et al. The natural history of atrial fibrillation: incidence, risk factors, and prognosis in the Manitoba follow-up study. Am J Med 1995;98(5):476–84.

[5] Fuster V, et al. ACC/AHA/ESC 2006 guidelines for the management of patients with atrial fibrillation—executive summary: a report of the American College of Cardiology/American Heart Association Task Force on Practice Guidelines and the European Society of Cardiology Committee for Practice Guidelines (writing committee to revise the 2001 guidelines for the management of patients with atrial fibrillation). J Am Coll Cardiol 2006;48(4):854–906.

[6] Goldberg RJ, et al. Recent trends in the incidence rates of and death rates from atrial fibrillation complicating initial acute myocardial infarction: a community-wide perspective. Am Heart J 2002;143(3):519–27.

[7] Tsang TS, et al. Left ventricular diastolic dysfunction as a predictor of the first diagnosed nonvalvular atrial fibrillation in 840 elderly men and women. J Am Coll Cardiol 2002; 40(9):1636–44.

[8] Frost L, Hune LJ, Vestergaard P. Overweight and obesity as risk factors for atrial fibrillation or flutter: the Danish diet, cancer, and health study. Am J Med 2005;118(5):489–95.

[9] Wang TJ, et al. Obesity and the risk of new-onset atrial fibrillation. JAMA 2004;292(20): 2471–7.

[10] Gami AS, et al. Association of atrial fibrillation and obstructive sleep apnea. Circulation 2004;110(4):364–7.

[11] Levy S, et al. Characterization of different subsets of atrial fibrillation in general practice in France: the ALFA study. The College of French Cardiologists. Circulation 1999;99(23): 3028–35.

[12] Fioranelli M, et al. Analysis of heart rate variability five minutes before the onset of paroxysmal atrial fibrillation. Pacing Clin Electrophysiol 1999;22(5):743–9.

[13] Herweg B, et al. Power spectral analysis of heart period variability of preceding sinus rhythm before initiation of paroxysmal atrial fibrillation. Am J Cardiol 1998;82(7):869–74.

[14] Levy S, et al. International consensus on nomenclature and classification of atrial fibrillation: a collaborative project of the working group on arrhythmias and the working group of cardiac pacing of the European Society of Cardiology and the North American Society of Pacing and Electrophysiology. J Cardiovasc Electrophysiol 2003;14(4):443–5.

[15] Allessie MA, et al. Pathophysiology and prevention of atrial fibrillation. Circulation 2001; 103(5):769–77.

[16] Moe GK, Mendez C. Simulation of impulse propagation in cardiac tissue. Ann N Y Acad Sci 1966;128(3):766–71.

[17] Jalife J, Berenfeld O, Mansour M. Mother rotors and fibrillatory conduction: a mechanism of atrial fibrillation. Cardiovasc Res 2002;54(2):204–16.

[18] Scherlag BJ, Po S. The intrinsic cardiac nervous system and atrial fibrillation. Curr Opin Cardiol 2006;21(1):51–4.

[19] Haissaguerre M, et al. Spontaneous initiation of atrial fibrillation by ectopic beats originating in the pulmonary veins. N Engl J Med 1998;339(10):659–66.

[20] Oral H, et al. Mechanistic significance of intermittent pulmonary vein tachycardia in patients with atrial fibrillation. J Cardiovasc Electrophysiol 2002;13(7):645–50.

[21] Polontchouk L, et al. Effects of chronic atrial fibrillation on gap junction distribution in human and rat atria. J Am Coll Cardiol 2001;38(3):883–91.

[22] Boldt A, et al. Expression of angiotensin II receptors in human left and right atrial tissue in atrial fibrillation with and without underlying mitral valve disease. J Am Coll Cardiol 2003; 42(10):1785–92.

[23] Aviles RJ, et al. Inflammation as a risk factor for atrial fibrillation. Circulation 2003;108(24): 3006–10.

[24] Chung MK, et al. C-reactive protein elevation in patients with atrial arrhythmias: inflammatory mechanisms and persistence of atrial fibrillation. Circulation 2001;104(24):2886–91.

[25] Dudley SC Jr, et al. Atrial fibrillation increases production of superoxide by the left atrium and left atrial appendage: role of the NADPH and xanthine oxidases. Circulation 2005; 112(9):1266–73.

[26] Lamm G, et al. Postoperative white blood cell count predicts atrial fibrillation after cardiac surgery. J Cardiothorac Vasc Anesth 2006;20(1):51–6.

[27] Shiroshita-Takeshita A, et al. Effect of simvastatin and antioxidant vitamins on atrial fibrillation promotion by atrial–tachycardia remodeling in dogs. Circulation 2004;110(16): 2313–9.

[28] Marin F, et al. Statins and postoperative risk of atrial fibrillation following coronary artery bypass grafting. Am J Cardiol 2006;97(1):55–60.

[29] Pozzoli M, et al. Predictors of primary atrial fibrillation and concomitant clinical and hemodynamic changes in patients with chronic heart failure: a prospective study in 344 patients with baseline sinus rhythm. J Am Coll Cardiol 1998;32(1):197–204.

[30] Rahimtoola SH, et al. Left atrial transport function in myocardial infarction. Importance of its booster pump function. Am J Med 1975;59(5):686–94.

[31] Daoud EG, et al. Effect of an irregular ventricular rhythm on cardiac output. Am J Cardiol 1996;78(12):1433–6.

[32] Rossi A, et al. Natriuretic peptide levels in atrial fibrillation: a prospective hormonal and Doppler–echocardiographic study. J Am Coll Cardiol 2000;35(5):1256–62.

[33] Roy D, et al. Atrial natriuretic factor during atrial fibrillation and supraventricular tachycardia. J Am Coll Cardiol 1987;9(3):509–14.

[34] Mattioli AV, et al. Left atrial size and function after spontaneous cardioversion of atrial fibrillation and their relation to N-terminal atrial natriuretic peptide. Am J Cardiol 2003; 91(12):1478–81, A8.

[35] Khasnis A, et al. Tachycardia-induced cardiomyopathy: a review of literature. Pacing Clin Electrophysiol 2005;28(7):710–21.

[36] Belz GG, Breithaupt-Grogler K, Osowski U. Treatment of congestive heart failure—current status of use of digitoxin. Eur J Clin Invest 2001;31(Suppl 2):10–7.

[37] Schwartz A, et al. Hemodynamic effects of intravenous amiodarone in patients with depressed left ventricular function and recurrent ventricular tachycardia. Am Heart J 1983;106(4 Pt 2):848–56.

[38] Chen PS, Prystowsky EN. Role of concealed and supernormal conductions during atrial fibrillation in the pre-excitation syndrome. Am J Cardiol 1991;68(13):1329–34.

[39] Prystowsky EN, et al. Management of patients with atrial fibrillation. A statement for healthcare professionals. From the Subcommittee on Electrocardiography and Electrophysiology, American Heart Association. Circulation 1996;93(6):1262–77.

[40] Nichol G, et al. Meta-analysis of randomised controlled trials of the effectiveness of antiarrhythmic agents at promoting sinus rhythm in patients with atrial fibrillation. Heart 2002; 87(6):535–43.

[41] McNamara RL, et al. Management of atrial fibrillation: review of the evidence for the role of pharmacologic therapy, electrical cardioversion, and echocardiography. Ann Intern Med 2003;139(12):1018–33.

[42] Echt DS, et al. Mortality and morbidity in patients receiving encainide, flecainide, or placebo. The cardiac arrhythmia suppression trial. N Engl J Med 1991;324(12):781–8.

[43] Zimetbaum P. Amiodarone for atrial fibrillation. N Engl J Med 2007;356(9):935–41.

[44] Goldschlager N, et al. Practical guidelines for clinicians who treat patients with amiodarone. Practice Guidelines Subcommittee, North American Society of Pacing and Electrophysiology. Arch Intern Med 2000;160(12):1741–8.

[45] Effect of prophylactic amiodarone on mortality after acute myocardial infarction and in congestive heart failure: meta-analysis of individual data from 6500 patients in randomised trials. Amiodarone Trials Meta-Analysis Investigators. Lancet 1997;350(9089):1417–24.

[46] Ott MC, et al. Pulmonary toxicity in patients receiving low-dose amiodarone. Chest 2003; 123(2):646–51.

[47] Skroubis G, et al. Amiodarone-induced acute lung toxicity in an ICU setting. Acta Anaesthesiol Scand 2005;49(4):569–71.

[48] Kaushik S, et al. Acute pulmonary toxicity after low-dose amiodarone therapy. Ann Thorac Surg 2001;72(5):1760–1.

[49] Ashrafian H, Davey P. Is amiodarone an under-recognized cause of acute respiratory failure in the ICU? Chest 2001;120(1):275–82.

[50] Donaldson L, et al. Acute amiodarone-induced lung toxicity. Intensive Care Med 1998; 24(6):626–30.

[51] Hughes M, Binning A. Intravenous amiodarone in intensive care. Time for a reappraisal? Intensive Care Med 2000;26(12):1730–9.

[52] Chevalier P, et al. Amiodarone versus placebo and classic drugs for cardioversion of recent-onset atrial fibrillation: a meta-analysis. J Am Coll Cardiol 2003;41(2):255–62.

[53] Vardas PE, et al. Amiodarone as a first-choice drug for restoring sinus rhythm in patients with atrial fibrillation: a randomized, controlled study. Chest 2000;117(6):1538–45.

[54] Vorperian VR, et al. Adverse effects of low-dose amiodarone: a meta-analysis. J Am Coll Cardiol 1997;30(3):791–8.

[55] Roy D, et al. Amiodarone to prevent recurrence of atrial fibrillation. Canadian trial of atrial fibrillation investigators. N Engl J Med 2000;342(13):913–20.

[56] Lown B. Electrical reversion of cardiac arrhythmias. Br Heart J 1967;29(4):469–89.

[57] Resnekov L, McDonald L. Electroversion of lone atrial fibrillation and flutter including haemodynamic studies at rest and on exercise. Br Heart J 1971;33(3):339–50.

[58] Levy S, et al. A randomized comparison of external and internal cardioversion of chronic atrial fibrillation. Circulation 1992;86(5):1415–20.

[59] Raymond RJ, et al. Cardiac performance early after cardioversion from atrial fibrillation. Am Heart J 1998;136(3):435–42.

[60] Brodsky MA, et al. Factors determining maintenance of sinus rhythm after chronic atrial fibrillation with left atrial dilatation. Am J Cardiol 1989;63(15):1065–8.

[61] Dittrich HC, et al. Echocardiographic and clinical predictors for outcome of elective cardioversion of atrial fibrillation. Am J Cardiol 1989;63(3):193–7.

[62] Oral H, et al. Facilitating transthoracic cardioversion of atrial fibrillation with ibutilide pretreatment. N Engl J Med 1999;340(24):1849–54.

[63] Mittal S, et al. Transthoracic cardioversion of atrial fibrillation: comparison of rectilinear biphasic versus damped sine wave monophasic shocks. Circulation 2000;101(11): 1282–7.

[64] Page RL, et al. Biphasic versus monophasic shock waveform for conversion of atrial fibrillation: the results of an international randomized, double-blind multicenter trial. J Am Coll Cardiol 2002;39(12):1956–63.

[65] Neumayr G, et al. Effect of electrical cardioversion on myocardial cells in patients in intensive care. BMJ 1998;316(7139):1207–10.

[66] Saliba W, et al. Higher energy synchronized external direct current cardioversion for refractory atrial fibrillation. J Am Coll Cardiol 1999;34(7):2031–4.

[67] Lindsay J Jr. Pulmonary edema following cardioversion. Am Heart J 1967;74(3):434–5.

[68] Lemberg L, et al. Arrhythmias related to cardioversion. Circulation 1964;30:163–70.

[69] Waldecker B, et al. Dysrhythmias after direct-current cardioversion. Am J Cardiol 1986; 57(1):120–3.

[70] Klein AL, et al. Use of transesophageal echocardiography to guide cardioversion in patients with atrial fibrillation. N Engl J Med 2001;344(19):1411–20.

[71] Arnold AZ, et al. Role of prophylactic anticoagulation for direct current cardioversion in patients with atrial fibrillation or atrial flutter. J Am Coll Cardiol 1992;19(4):851–5.

[72] Naccarelli GV, et al. Cost-effective management of acute atrial fibrillation: role of rate control, spontaneous conversion, medical and direct current cardioversion, transesophageal echocardiography, and antiembolic therapy. Am J Cardiol 2000;85(10A):36D–45D.

[73] Berger M, Schweitzer P. Timing of thromboembolic events after electrical cardioversion of atrial fibrillation or flutter: a retrospective analysis. Am J Cardiol 1998;82(12):1545–7, A8.

[74] Mathew JP, et al. A multicenter risk index for atrial fibrillation after cardiac surgery. JAMA 2004;291(14):1720–9.

[75] Crystal E, et al. Interventions for preventing post-operative atrial fibrillation in patients undergoing heart surgery. Cochrane Database Syst Rev 2004;4:CD003611.

[76] Daoud EG, et al. Preoperative amiodarone as prophylaxis against atrial fibrillation after heart surgery. N Engl J Med 1997;337(25):1785–91.

[77] Mitchell LB, et al. Prophylactic oral amiodarone for the prevention of arrhythmias that begin early after revascularization, valve replacement, or repair: PAPABEAR: a randomized controlled trial. JAMA 2005;294(24):3093–100.

[78] Aranki SF, et al. Predictors of atrial fibrillation after coronary artery surgery. Current trends and impact on hospital resources. Circulation 1996;94(3):390–7.

[79] Archbold RA, Schilling RJ. Atrial pacing for the prevention of atrial fibrillation after coronary artery bypass graft surgery: a review of the literature. Heart 2004;90(2):129–33.

[80] Zaman AG, et al. The role of signal averaged P wave duration and serum magnesium as a combined predictor of atrial fibrillation after elective coronary artery bypass surgery. Heart 1997;77(6):527–31.

[81] Stewart S, et al. A population-based study of the long-term risks associated with atrial fibrillation: 20-year follow-up of the Renfrew/Paisley study. Am J Med 2002;113(5):359–64.

ELSEVIER
SAUNDERS

Crit Care Clin 23 (2007) 873–880

CRITICAL
CARE
CLINICS

Cardiopulmonary Resuscitation and Acute Cardiovascular Life Support—A Protocol Review of the Updated Guidelines

Larry M. Diamond, RPh, PharmD

*Department of Pharmacy Services, Oakwood Hospital and Medical Center,
18101 Oakwood Boulevard, Dearborn, MI 48124, USA*

For the first time in 5 years, new guidelines for cardiopulmonary resuscitation (CPR) of adults and children were introduced at the end of November 2005. The new CPR guidelines evolved from emerging evidence-based resuscitation studies and the evaluation process included the input of 281 international resuscitation experts who evaluated hypotheses, topics, and research over a 36-month period. The process included evidence evaluation, review of the literature, and focused analysis [1].

It is very difficult to perform clinical trials in CPR science because of the low survival rate of out-of and in-hospital cardiac arrest, ethical issues, and the logistics of obtaining informed consent. The greatest challenge is to complete trials with sufficient power to be able to demonstrate impact on long- or short-term outcomes. In the past, end point criteria were for the patient to survive to hospitalization and be neurologically intact by hospital discharge. These trials were small, underpowered, not randomized, and had interventions that made it hard to demonstrate a benefit. Informed consent regulations in Europe [2] and North America [3] made it also challenging.

The Emergency Cardiovascular Care (ECC) experts used the American Heart Association–American College of Cardiology (ACC/AHA) classification system for reviewing the resuscitation studies with large prospective randomized controlled trials serving as foundation of their (Class I) recommendations. Very few of the resuscitation trials had sufficient power to show an effect on mortality during hospitalization. Recommendations are based

---

E-mail address: larry.diamond@oakwood.org

therefore on human trials that are nonrandomized observational studies or inferred from animal studies and outcomes that are intermediate. The AHA/ ACC Class IIa recommendation is when the benefit is greater than the risk for a procedure/treatment or diagnostic test/assessment. Class IIb recommendations are divided into two categories: (1) optional and (2) recommended by experts despite lack of highly powered supporting evidence. Optional interventions in cardiopulmonary resuscitation are identified by terms "can be considered" or "may be useful." Interventions that the experts believe should be performed are identified as "we recommend." Class IIb recommendations were given when evidence showed only short-term benefit (eg, amiodarone for pulseless ventricular fibrillation arrest).

There are four major changes to the previous guidelines concerning CPR and sudden cardiac arrest. The most significant changes in the CPR guidelines were to increase the number of compressions delivered per minute and reduce the interruptions of the CPR cycles.

The first major recommendation relates to first exposure to an unresponsive, pulseless, and nonbreathing victim. Two rescue breaths are given over 1 second, each assuring the chest rises. The two rescue breaths are followed by 30 chest compressions. The recommendation is a 30:2 ratio for single rescuers of victims of all ages (except newborn infants). The old recommendation was for a ratio of 15:2. The 30:2 ratio is based on circulatory studies showing that over time blood flow increases with a greater amount of chest compressions [4]. If interrupted, as in the old 15:2 with two rescue breaths, blood flow decreases causing less perfusion of tissues. The 30:2 ratio of compressions to ventilation is based on a consensus opinion rather than derived from evidence. This increased ratio of chest compressions to breaths is thought to reduce hyperventilation of the patient, minimize interruptions of compressions, and simplify teaching to health care professionals and laypeople. The 30:2 ratio is based on the speed of the compressions and not the actual number of compressions per minute. There is insufficient evidence from human studies for an optimal compression rate. Animal [4] and human [5,6] studies support a chest compression rate of greater than 80 compressions per minute to achieve optimal forward blood flow during CPR. The guidelines recommend a compression rate of about 100 compressions per minute (Class IIa).

The second major recommendation is the amount of shocks given in the face of ventricular fibrillation (VF)/pulseless ventricular tachycardia (VT). The latest recommendation is for only one shock of 200 J, using a biphasic defibrillator, or 360 J if using a monophasic defibrillator. This takes the place of the three stacked shocks at 200, 300, and 360 J, as were previously recommended in the Advanced Cardiac Life Support (ACLS) guidelines. The one shock is followed by 2 minutes of CPR. The committee felt that a delay of 37 seconds or more while waiting for the defibrillator to charge, deliver a shock, and check for a pulse was delaying the administration of life-saving compressions [4]. In cases of witnessed arrest with a defibrillator on site, after two rescue breaths the health care provider should check for a pulse. If no pulse is felt in 10 seconds, the provider should turn on the defibrillator. If the patient is still in VF/pulseless VT, one shock should be delivered. If a biphasic defibrillator is available, providers should use a dose of 120 J to 200 J. If a monophasic defibrillator is supplied, one shock of 360 J is administered to the patient. Five cycles of CPR at the 30:2 ratio is resumed after the first shock. The first vasopressors that are recommended in VF/VT are intravenous (IV) or intraosseous (IO) epinephrine (1 mg), or intravenous vasopressin (40 International Units [IU]). Vasopressin can be administered as an alternate vasopressor for the first or second dose of epinephrine. Five cycles of CPR at the 30:2 ratio is reestablished. A second shock can then be administered at 360 J.

Providers should give one shock rather than three shocks, as recommended in previous ACLS guidelines [7], because of the high success rate for biphasic defibrillators [8] and fewer interruptions of CPR. There are no randomized controlled trials comparing the one-shock versus three-shock strategy. The evidence concerning the interruption of chest compressions reducing coronary perfusion pressure was strong enough for the International Committee to make the one-shock strategy a recommendation during cardiac arrest.

In pulseless VT/VF the first medication to be administered is epinephrine 1 mg every 3 to 5 minutes. There is a slight variation between the United States and Europe as to when to start the administration of epinephrine. The US guidelines recommend epinephrine to be administered before the second shock of 360 J (monophasic defibrillator). In Europe, epinephrine is administered before the third shock of 360 J.

Whether to administer epinephrine 1 mg IV every 3 to 5 minutes or one dose of vasopressin 40 IU IV during pulseless VT/VF, is disputed. One dose of vasopressin may be substituted for the first or second dose of epinephrine. A meta-analysis of five randomized control trials showed no significant difference between epinephrine and vasopressin for return of spontaneous circulation, survival for 24 hours, or survival to hospital discharge [9]. In a large in-hospital study of cardiac arrest, 200 patients were randomly assigned to epinephrine 1 mg (initial rhythm: 16% VF, 3% VT, 54% pulseless electrical activity [PEA], 27% asystole) or vasopressin 40 IU (initial rhythm: 20% VF, 3% VT, 41% PEA, 34% asystole). There was no difference in survival to 1 hour (epinephrine: 35%, vasopressin: 39%) or to hospital discharge (epinephrine: 14%, vasopressin: 12%) between groups [10]. The pharmacokinetic half-life of epinephrine is about 2 minutes as compared with vasopressin, which is 20 minutes. One dose of vasopressin 40 IU IV/IO can replace the first or second dose of epinephrine in pulseless arrest (Class Indeterminate).

The third major change in the CPR guidelines is to not interrupt chest compressions during cardiac arrest out of hospital. Delaying the start of CPR for 10 to 20 seconds can reduce the chance of successful defibrillation by automated external defibrillator (AED) in the field. The previous recommendation was for each rescue breath to be given over 2 seconds for adults, children, and infants. The advice of the committee is to give mouth-to-mouth resuscitation with two rescue breaths at 1 second per breath in adults, children, and infants. This breathing change ends up being about 8 to 10 breaths per minute.

The fourth major recommendation focuses on paramedics' response to cardiac arrest in the field. Until now the major impetus in response to pulseless VF/VT is to defibrillate the patient as soon as possible. The new guidelines recommend approximately 2 minutes of CPR before administering a shock to the patient.

There are four major rhythms encountered during cardiac arrest: (1) ventricular fibrillation (VF), (2) ventricular tachycardia (VT), (3) pulseless electrical activity (PEA, previously known as Electrical Mechanical Dissociation), and (4) asystole. For ACLS to make a difference in the above cardiac arrest rhythms, proper Basic Life Support (BLS) and attempted prompt defibrillation for VF/VT will increase the patient's chance for survival to hospital discharge. This is especially true for witnessed VF arrest.

Much time is spent intubating patients and administering medications after CPR and rescue breaths have been started. To administer the medications recommended in the algorithms of VF/VT an IV line must be inserted. A large peripheral venous catheter is recommended for IV access. Inserting a large peripheral catheter can be accomplished during CPR. This accomplishes two goals: CPR is not stopped while the IV line is being inserted and an IV access is available for administering medications during the cardiac arrest [11,12]. Medication plasma levels are lower and the onset of action is longer if a peripheral line is used. It takes 1 or 2 minutes for IV medications to get to the central plasma circulation. If spontaneous circulation has not occurred with defibrillation and the use of a peripheral IV access or IO access, a central IV line should be considered.

The proper way to administer cardiac arrest medications is to give the medication, followed by a 20-mL bolus of a large volume IV solution. This facilitates medication delivery to the central circulation. Another recommendation is to elevate the extremity where the peripheral IV is placed for 20 seconds to help deliver the medication to the central circulation [13].

The endotracheal tube is the third choice for administering medications during cardiac arrest. The first choice, as stated above, is the large peripheral venous line. The second choice is the IO cannulation that supplies access to the noncollapsible venous plexus, which is comparable to medication delivery via the central venous access. Two prospective trials, in children [14] and adults [15], and six other studies documented that IO access is safe and effective for fluid resuscitation, drug delivery, and blood sampling for laboratory evaluation.

If IV and IO cannot be achieved in the patient, an endotracheal tube must be inserted. Multiple studies show that naloxone, atropine, lidocaine, epinephrine, and vasopressin can be administered through the endotracheal tube (ET) and absorbed in the trachea. A "remembering tool" for which medications can be administered via the ET tube is "NAVEL." However, the medication levels are lower when absorbed in the trachea than if administered by the IV route. The doses of the medications administered by the ET tube are doubled. Erratic absorption occurs when epinephrine is administered by ET tube. Transient beta-adrenergic stimulation is seen with hypotension, low coronary perfusion and flow, and reduced chance for spontaneous circulation.

For VF/Pulseless VT that is witnessed in the hospital, the most important intervention is the administration of two rescue breaths while checking for a pulse. If the pulse is not felt in 10 seconds, the defibrillator should be turned on. If a manual biphasic device is available, a 120- to 200-J shock should be delivered to the patient. The most common defibrillator available in hospitals is the biphasic defibrillator. If a monophasic defibrillator is available, a 360-J shock is delivered to the patient. CPR is resumed immediately and five cycles of CPR is given. The rhythm is then checked and if the patient is in VT/VF, a 200-J shock is delivered (for this discussion, it will be presumed a biphasic defibrillator is available). CPR is resumed for five cycles and if an IV/IO access is available, epinephrine 1 mg is given every 3 to 5 minutes. Vasopressin 40 IU IV/IO can be given to replace the first or second dose of epinephrine 1 mg. CPR is continued for five cycles and if the patient continues to be in VT/VF, another 200-J shock is administered.

A number of antiarrhythmics can be considered for administration after the third shock of 200 J. In blinded randomized controlled clinical trials in adults with refractory VT/VF in the out-of-hospital hospital setting, paramedic administration of amiodarone (300 mg or 5 mg/kg) [16] improved survival to hospital admission rates when compared with administration of placebo or 1.5 mg/kg of lidocaine [17]. Additional studies documented consistent improvement in defibrillation response when amiodarone was give to humans or animals with VF or hemodynamically unstable VT [16,17]. The first antiarrhythmic to be administered in VT/VF is a bolus of amiodarone 300 mg IV. An additional 150-mg bolus can be given in 3 to 5 minutes if the first dose of 300 mg does not convert the patient from VT/VF to a sinus rhythm. Lidocaine 1 to 1.5 mg/kg IV/IO is an alternative antiarrhythmic that can be considered if the amiodarone has not successfully converted the patient. Another bolus of lidocaine 0.5 to 0.75 mg/kg can be given if the first dose of lidocaine is not successful. A maximum of three doses of lidocaine can be given. Lidocaine has no short-term or long-term benefit efficacy in VT/VF. Magnesium 1 to 2 g IV/IO for polymorphic VT (Torsades de Pointes) should be considered. If still unsuccessful, return to a 120-J shock, followed by five cycles of CPR, followed by epinephrine 1 mg every 3 to 5 minutes. CPR is continued, with no interruptions (except for shock) throughout the entire process.

The use of procainamide is no longer considered an antiarrythmic option if lidocaine is unsuccessful in breaking VF/VT given the time required for infusion of an effective dose of procainamide. The use of procainamide is only supported by one retrospective comparison study of 20 patients [18].

The precordial thump for VF/VT has not been studied in prospective trials. Given some reports of harm, no recommendations are made for or against the precordial thump in the ACLS guidelines (Class Indeterminate).

Bradycardia in the ACLS guidelines is defined as a heart rate less than 60 beats per minute. Timely intervention is warranted if the patient is symptomatic or compromised due to hypotension, such as altered mental status changes, congestive heart failure, seizures, syncope, or signs of shock related to bradycardia. If the patient is suffering from poor perfusion, the recommendation is to apply transcutaneous pacing. This is a Class I recommendation for symptomatic bradycardias. It is to be started immediately for patients who are unstable with Mobitz Type II second-degree block or third-degree block. The down side of transcutaneous pacing is that it may not be effective and can be very painful to the patient. While preparing for transcutaneous pacing, atropine at a dose of 0.5 mg every 3 to 5 minutes, to a maximum of 3 mg should be given (Class IIa, based on one clinical trial for atropine in adults [19] and additional lower-level studies [20,21]). Transcutaneous pacing is also indicated for bradycardia if the patient fails to respond to atropine.

Two non–first-line drugs that are used in symptomatic bradycardia, are epinephrine and dopamine. Isoproterenol has been omitted from the list of medications to be used in bradycardia. Epinephrine is used when atropine and transcutaneous pacing have failed to work (Class IIb). The infusion for epinephrine is 2 to 10 μg/min and titrated to the patient's blood pressure. Dopamine is an inotrope with alpha- and beta-adrenergic stimulation. The dopamine infusion rate is 2 to 10 μg/kg/min and can be added to the epinephrine infusion if needed. There has been one case series of glucagon [22] improving heart rate and symptoms. The dose of glucagon is a 3-mg bolus, followed by an infusion at 3 mg/h for patients with beta-blocker or calcium-blocker overdose in the above case series.

In summary, there have been four major changes to the 2005 guidelines. First, the chest compression ratio has been changed from 15:2 to 30:2 to increase the circulation blood flow. Second, when using a monophasic defibrillator, one shock is given at 360 J. One shock is given at 200 J when using a biphasic defibrillator. The "three stacked shocks," from past ACLS Guidelines for VT/VF has become "one shock." The US ACLS Committee recommends giving epinephrine 1 mg before the second shock of 360 J if the patient has not responded to CPR and one dose of epinephrine. The third major change is to not interrupt chest compressions. There should be very little if any interruptions of CPR to ensure maintenance of circulatory blood flow. Interruptions during CPR of 10 to 20 seconds can reduce the chance of successful defibrillation when VT/VF is present. Fourth, it is now recommended for the paramedics to give a few minutes of CPR before attempting defibrillation. Changes are currently being made in the training of all new and recertifying ACLS health care providers.

References

[1] Zaritsky A, Morley P. 2005 American Heart Association guidelines for Cardiopulmonary Resuscitation and emergency Cardiovascular Care. Editorial: the evidence evaluation process for the 2005 International Consensus on Cardiopulmonary Resuscitation and emergency Cardiovascular Care Science With Treatment recommendations. Circulation 2005; 112:III-128–30.

[2] Lemaire F, Bion J, Blanco J, et al. The European Union Directive on Clinical Research: present status of implementation in EU member states' legislations with regard to the imcompetent patient. Intensive Care Med 2005;31:476–9.

[3] Hsieh M, Dailey MW, Callaway CW. Surrogate consent by family members for out-of-hospital cardiac arrest research. Acad Emerg Med 2001;8:851–3.

[4] Yu T, Weil MH, Tang W, et al. Adverse outcomes of interrupted precordial compression during automated defibrillation. Circulation 2002;106:368–72.

[5] Swenson RD, Weaver WD, Niskanen RA, et al. Hemodynamics in humans during conventional and experimental methods of cardiopulmonary resuscitation. Circulation 1988;78: 630–9.

[6] Kern KBV, Sanders AB, Raife J, et al. A study of chest compression rates during cardiopulmonary resuscitation in humans: the importance of rate-directed chest compressions. Arch Intern Med 1992;152:145–9.

[7] American Heart Association in collaboration with the International Liason Resuscitation and Emergency Cardiovascular Care. International consensus on science. Circulation 2000;102:I1–384.

[8] Martens PR, Russell JK, Wolcke B, et al. Optimal Response to Cardiac Arrest study: defibrillation waveform effects. Resuscitation 2001;49:233–43.

[9] Aung K, Htay T. Vasopressin for cardiac arrest: a systematic review and meta-analysis. Arch Intern Med 2005;165:17–24.

[10] Stiell IG, Heberft PC, Wells GA, et al. Vasopressin versus epinephrine for in-hospital cardiac arrest: a randomized controlled trial. Lancet 2001;358:105–9.

[11] Barsan WG, Levy RC, Weir H. Lidocaine levels during CPR: differences after peripheral venous, central venous, and intracardiac injections. Ann Emerg Med 1981;10:73–8.

[12] Kuhn GJ, White BC, Swetnam RE, et al. Peripheral vs. central circulation times during CPR: a pilot study. Ann Emerg Med 1981;10:417–9.

[13] Emerman CL, Pinchak AC, Hancock D, et al. Effect of injection site on circulation times during cardiac arrest. Crit Care Med 1988;16:1138–41.

[14] Banerjee S, Singhi SC, Singh S, et al. The intraosseous route is a suitable alternative to intravenous route for fluid resuscitation in severely dehydrated children. Indian Pediatr 1994;31: 1511–20.

[15] Brickman KR, Krupp K, Rega P, et al. Typing and screening of blood from intraosseous access. Ann Emerg Med 1992;21:414–7.

[16] Kudenchuk PJ, Cobb LA, Copass MK, et al. Amiodarone for resuscitation after out-of-hospital cardiac arrest due to ventricular fibrillation. N Engl J Med 1981;10:462–7.

[17] Dorian P, Cass D, Schwartz B, et al. Amiodarone as compared with lidocaine for shock-resistant ventricular fibrillation. N Engl J Med 2002;346:884–90.

[18] Stiell IG, Wells GA, Hebert PC, et al. Association of drug therapy with survival in cardiac arrest: Limited role of advanced cardiac life support drugs. Acad Emerg Med 1995;2:264–73.

[19] Smith I, Monk TG, White PF. Caomparison of transesophageal atrial pacing with anticho-linergic drugs for the treatment of intraoperative bradycardia. Anesth Analg 1994;78: 245–52.

[20] Brady WJ, Swart G, DeBehnke DJ, et al. The efficacy of atropine in the treatment of hemo-dynamically unstable bradycardia and atrioventricular block: prehospital and emergency department considerations. Resuscitation 1999;41:47–55.

[21] Chadda KD, Lichstein E, Gupta PK, et al. Effects of atropine in patients with bradyarrhyth-mia complicating myocardial infarction: usefulness of an optimum dose for overdrive. Am J Med 1977;63:503–10.

[22] Love JN, Sachdeva DK, Bessman ES, et al. A potential role for glucagons in the treatment of drug-induced symptomatic bradycardia. Chest 1998;114:323–6.

ELSEVIER
SAUNDERS

Crit Care Clin 23 (2007) 881–900

CRITICAL
CARE
CLINICS

Delirium, Depression, and Other Psychosocial and Neurobehavioral Issues in Cardiovascular Disease

Oliver G. Cameron, MD, PhD

*Department of Psychiatry, University of Michigan Medical Center,
c/o 1215 Southwood Court, Ann Arbor, MI 48103-9735, USA*

A merry heart makes a cheerful countenance, but by sorrow of the heart the spirit is broken.

Proverbs 15:13

The belief that there is a connection between the heart and the emotions is illustrated well in the epigraph from the Old Testament of the Bible. This belief has been around for a very long time. The Book of Proverbs was written no later than the third century B.C.E., and at least some of it possibly as early as the tenth century B.C.E. Despite this longstanding and widespread belief, supported by a substantial amount of correlative research results, the fact of a linkage between psychosocial factors and physical disease, so-called psychosomatic medicine, is not accepted fully in all quarters. This doubt seems to remain, because the putative mechanisms, the how of such relationships, are just beginning to be understood.

This article addresses behavioral and psychosocial factors in heart disease, focusing on practical clinical information, and especially discussing delirium and depression. Some mechanistic information is provided along the way. At the end of the article, additional relevant topics are reviewed briefly.

Delirium

Delirium (sometimes referred to as an organic brain syndrome) is a common and problematic syndrome frequently associated with various medical disorders, including cardiovascular conditions such as acute myocardial infarction, congestive heart failure, acute coronary syndrome, and stroke.

E-mail address: ocameron@umich.edu

Although postoperatively, any major surgical procedure is a risk factor for developing delirium, some have considered that individuals who have had open-heart procedures are particularly prone [1]. Psychiatrically, delirium is defined as one of the cognitive disorders [2], the others being dementia and other amnestic disorders. Delirium is a medical condition that can occur as the result of virtually any diffuse and substantial impairment of cerebral function. Thus, systemic metabolic changes or intracerebral changes (eg, increased intracranial pressure caused by an intracerebral bleed or a tumor) can produce delirium, as can various psychoactive drugs (Box 1). It is important to recall that over-the-counter medications and prescription drugs, especially if not being taken correctly, as well as drugs of abuse, can produce, or be a contributing factor to delirium. Individuals with pre-existing impairments of cerebral function (eg, age-related impairment, Alzheimer's disease, or cerebrovascular disease) are at increased risk. Further, delirium can be caused by the accretion of several small insults, such that no one abnormality need be severe enough to produce delirium if several are present; thus, in these situations, no one easily identifiable cause can be isolated.

The *Diagnostic and Statistical Manual of Mental Disorders, Fourth Edition (DSM-IV)* [2] definition of delirium includes four criteria:

1. Disturbance of level of consciousness and attention
2. Cognitive and/or perceptual changes, including memory or language disturbance, disorientation, and/or illusions or hallucinations
3. Relatively rapid development (hours to days) with fluctuating severity
4. Evidence that the disturbance is caused by the physiological consequences of a medical condition or a substance (effect of the drug or its withdrawal)

Dementia is also a cognitive disorder, and differentiating dementia from delirium is often difficult but very important, because delirium is typically treatable. (Although some dementias are treatable, most are not.) Helpful differentiating features are:

- Delirium develops much more rapidly than dementia
- Delirium more strongly affects attention, while dementia more strongly disrupts short-term memory
- In delirium, cognitive defects can be more focal, while in dementia they tend to be more global [3].

Because of the characteristic fluctuating severity of delirium, which is less common in dementia, it is essential to assess a person suspected of being delirious more than once, at least hours apart, to determine severity, and especially to avoid incorrectly concluding that the person is not delirious, based on one assessment, because the person was assessed when symptoms were less prominent.

There are numerous changes commonly associated with delirium that are not part of the definition. Psychomotor activity often is perturbed, either with increases such as motor agitation or hyperarousal and seemingly purposeless behavior, or decreased. The sleep–wake cycle can be disrupted, sometimes to the extent of complete reversal of the day–night pattern. (So-called sundowning might reflect an aspect of a circadian rhythm abnormality, and/or be caused by the typical evening and night decrease in orienting sensory input needed to diminish confusion.) Emotional disturbances are common, often manifesting as anxiety or fearfulness, but other changes also can occur. Although delirium is a diagnosis based on clinical features, laboratory testing to identify underlying medical causes is essential. There is no precise list of required tests to assess the delirious patient. One common finding is an abnormal electroencephalogram (EEG). A careful and thorough neurological examination and mental status testing are always necessary, as is a complete physical examination, especially focusing on systems thought to be dysfunctional (eg, detection of hypotension or signs of congestive heart failure in cardiac patients). Routine laboratory tests (eg, blood chemistries, blood count, ECG) are almost always necessary [1]. Need for an EEG or a brain scan, for example, should be based on the clinical presentation. History and concomitant symptoms often will lead to the diagnosis of the specific underlying disorder. Frequently, delirious individuals cannot give reliable histories, so information must be obtained from family or staff who are familiar with the person's condition, especially about behavior at night when symptoms of delirium are often most prominent.

The major risk factor for the development of delirium is the severity, and possibly acuteness, of the underlying medical condition(s). Risk of developing delirium in the presence of medical impairment is increased by any preexisting disruption of higher cerebral functions. The actual prevalence of delirium in medically hospitalized individuals might be as high as 25% [4], including patients who have cardiac disease [5], and episodes of delirium occur outside of hospitals also, although at a lower rate. For especially prone individuals such as severely acutely ill elderly persons, the rate might be even substantially higher. Delirium lengthens hospitalization and increases mortality in hospitalized elderly individuals [6]. The differential psychiatric diagnosis of delirium includes, in addition to dementia and other amnestic disorders, psychotic disorders, depression, and, quite rarely, malingering or factitious disorder. Typically, delirious states last only days to weeks, in part because there is usually a relatively prompt (positive or negative) resolution to clinical conditions severe enough to produce delirium. Occasionally, however, especially in delirium-prone individuals, a state of quiet hypoactive delirium can persist for longer periods, overlooked, and possibly be less responsive to drug treatment.

It is essential to distinguish between the treatment of delirium and its management. The treatment of delirium is the treatment of the underlying medical condition. Of course, risk factors such as old age cannot be changed, and coexisting dementia usually cannot be treated, but the acute cause of the delirium itself usually can. Whether done by internists,

Box 1. Causes of delirium

Disorders
Acute central nervous system (CNS) vascular changes
  Thrombosis
  Bleed
  Transient ischemic attack (TIA)
  Vasculitis
Acute metabolic abnormalities Hypoglycemia
  Renal failure
  Liver failure
Cardiac
  Congestive heart failure
  Shock
  Acute coronary syndrome
  Recent myocardial infarction
  Cardiac rhythm disturbance
CNS space-occupying lesions
  Tumor
  Hematoma
Electrolyte changes
  Acidosis
  Hyperkalemia
  Hyponatremia (water intoxication)
Endocrinopathies
  Adrenal cortex
  Thyroid
  Parathyroid
Hypotension or hypertension
Hypoxia
Infectious
Nutritional deficiencies
  Thiamine
Seizure and postictal state
Trauma
  Closed head injury
  Postconcussive state

Drugs
CNS stimulant intoxication
Antihypertensives
Anticholinergics
Drug withdrawal
  Benzodiazepines

Alcohol
Heavy metal intoxication
Lithium intoxication
Narcotics
  Sedative hypnotics
    benzodiazepine
  Alcohol

The box lists medical disorders and drugs that are associated with delirium. The lists are illustrative, not inclusive. Any systemic condition or any drug (or drug withdrawal) that produces significant diffuse disturbance of cerebral function potentially can produce delirium.

surgeons, psychiatrists, or other physicians, the treatment of delirium is always medical, and should be done in a medically appropriate setting.

Some delirious individuals require management of the syndrome while awaiting resolution of the causative medical condition. Usually, this is necessitated by behavioral problems, but many of the nonpharmacological techniques would be part of optimal care for any delirious person. Although there are certain factors in management particularly relevant to cardiac disease (eg, cardiovascular side effects of some of the drugs used), most of the principles of both nonpharmacological and pharmacological management apply to delirium generally.

Nonpharmacological techniques to manage delirium are focused mainly on avoiding conditions that increase the likelihood of confusion or agitation. Primarily, that entails providing an optimum level of sensory input. As much as possible, a quiet and calm environment is best, avoiding excessive stimulation. Familiar persons and surrounding should be provided. Orienting stimuli (eg, large readable clocks and calendars) are often helpful. Music at a low level and low illumination are sometimes useful, but complete darkness (or light that promotes shadows) should be avoided. because lack of any sensory input promotes confusion and fear. The individual should receive reassurance, and all procedures or other changes in the environment should be explained simply. Of course, do not neglect general measures of supportive care, for example, adequate hydration and nourishment.

When agitation or other behavioral problems occur, physical or chemical restraints often are needed. Physical restraint should be applied by experienced personnel and monitored frequently. (In addition to the obvious clinical reasons for providing optimal care, there are in many venues now close scrutiny of the appropriateness and expertise of physical restraint from a medical–legal perspective.) Psychiatric hospitalization, along with other benefits, provides staff knowledgeable in behavioral management. That option, however, usually should be considered only when the underlying medical condition causing the delirium has been diagnosed, and treatment has been initiated and been shown to be effective. The delirious person sometimes is cognitively incapacitated to the extent that it becomes doubtful if he or she can give informed consent. Psychiatric assessment usually is indicated when: initial treatment is not successful; treatment with standard medication is contraindicated, and/or evaluation for competence is needed.

In addition to physical restraint, pharmacological methods are also available. Before deciding that more drugs are needed, however, all unnecessary medications should be discontinued, because medications that the person already is receiving could be contributing to the delirium (see Box 1).

It might appear that sedation would be an appropriate means of behavioral control in delirious individuals, although some consider the target as calming rather than actual sedation [7]. Although there is a place for sedation in the management program of some of these individuals, sedation can make the situation worse [8]. Because delirium is in large part a disorder of impairment of cognition and the ability to process incoming sensory stimuli, mild to moderate levels of sedation (ie, undertreatment) sometimes will increase that impairment. If sedation is to be used, a dose must be determined that is medically safe for that person (eg, does not suppress respiration significantly), while also providing an adequate sedative benefit without significantly contributing to confusion. As a corollary of this principle, drugs of all kinds with sedative properties that are not explicitly part of the behavioral management program should be stopped, or at least the dose lowered, if that can be done safely.

The mainstay of pharmacological management of delirium (and other similar behavioral dysfunctions) is the family of antipsychotic drugs. There are numerous groups of antipsychotic drugs now called typical antipsychotics that differ in chemical structure, but have the common property of high-affinity binding to brain dopamine receptors. These drugs differ in potency (ie, dose needed to obtain maximal effect) but not in efficacy. Potency differences do relate to different side effect profiles.

In the past two decades, numerous antipsychotic drugs now referred to as atypical have become available. These drugs are called atypical because the receptor-binding pattern in brain relevant to effect involves not only the dopamine receptors but also serotonin receptors. The prototype drug in this class is clozapine (Clozaril). Clozapine itself has a minimal place in the management of delirium, but other drugs in this class can play a major role.

Before the availability of the atypical antipsychotic agents, the drug most used for management of delirium was haloperidol (Haldol). It is still probably the most commonly agent used in the intensive care setting. It is a high potency typical antipsychotic with low levels of sedative, hypotensive, anticholinergic, and respiratory depressive effects. It is considered to be safe in patients who have cardiovascular disorders, although rare cases of sudden death have been reported, thought to be associated in part with a prolonged QT interval (Box 2) [9]. Lower-potency antipsychotics generally are avoided, because they have more hypotensive and anticholinergic properties.

Box 2. Psychotropic drugs that prolong the QT interval and raise risk for torsades de Pointes

Antidepressants [11]
   Tricyclic antidepressants (all)
   Serotonin reuptake inhibitors (SSRIs), perhaps especially:
      citalopram (Celexa, Lexapro)
   Other antidepressants less clear
Stimulant agents
Appetite suppressants
Antipsychotics

Antipsychotics
   Typical antipsychotics, especially:
      Chlorpromazine (Thorazine)
      Thioridazine (Mellaril)
      Haloperidol (Haldol) generally safe but sudden death has
      been reported
   Atypical antipsychotics
      Olanzapine (Zyprexa, aripiprazole (Abilify), and clozapine
      (Clozaril)
      Might be safer than the others

   There are many nonpsychotropic drugs that can prolong the QT interval, or raise the risk of torsades de pointes, as well. A summary of those is beyond the scope of this article. In situations in which there is a risk of one of these adverse events occurring, both psychotropic and nonpsychotropic agents must be considered, including additive or synergistic risk and drug–drug interactions.

Haloperidol also became the drug of choice in part because it is available by oral, intramuscular, and intravenous route of administration [10].

   Like all drugs, dosage should be appropriate to the individual. Because many delirious persons are elderly, lower doses are sometimes, but not always, indicated. In less acutely ill elderly patients, haloperidol doses as low as 0.5 mg orally might be sufficient. On the other hand, in younger severely ill individuals, doses as high 5 mg/h intravenously can be necessary in rare situations to control symptoms. In all cases, titration should be done to determine the lowest effective dose. All patients receiving this drug should be monitored closely for the emergence of extrapyramidal adverse effects, including muscle rigidity, acute dystonias, akathisia, and the rare occurrence of neuroleptic malignant syndrome. The restlessness of akathisia can be mistaken easily for worsening delirium, leading to increasing dosing when decreasing or discontinuing is called for, sometimes with substitution with an atypical antipsychotic drug. Finally, as with all drugs, drug–drug interactions need consideration, especially when large numbers of drugs are being used. Review of the drug–interaction literature is beyond the scope of this article.

As of the writing of this article, in addition to clozapine, five other atypical antipsychotic drugs are available in the United States: risperidone (Risperdal), olanzapine (Zyprexa), quetiapine (Seroquel), ziprasidone (Geodon), and aripiprazole (Abilify). These drugs have fewer adverse effects and different adverse effect profiles than the typical antipsychotics. For example, the risk of extrapyramidal effects is considerably lower with these drugs, although they can occur. One problem is the lack of liquid oral or injectable formulations, but a few are available (eg, oral liquid for risperidone, injectable forms for olanzapine and ziprasidone), and likely more will be available over time. From an efficacy perspective, it is likely that these drugs (at appropriate doses) should work as well as haloperidol.

From an adverse effect perspective, in the acute setting, the most important adverse effects are sedative, and especially cardiovascular. Quetiapine is perhaps the most sedating, possibly without as much risk from sedation-related cognitive change as the benzodiazepines. All of these drugs can produce postural hypotension, generally less with the higher potency drugs. It is usually mild.

A major concern with this group of drugs is prolongation of the QT interval and increased risk of torsades de pointes, obviously especially important in patients who have pre-existing cardiac disease [11–14]. Ziprasidone and risperidone are more likely to do this, while olazapine and aripiprazole appear less likely to. (The US Food and Drug Administration has identified an increased risk of death, including from cardiovascular causes, in elderly demented patients treated with atypical antipsychotics. Whether such an increased risk would be found with treatment of delirium—or with any brief treatment regimen—is not clear.) The QT increase is usually less than 5 milliseconds. Judgment as to the significance of this potential adverse effect should be made on a case-by-case basis.

Sometimes, use of sedation is necessary for adequate behavioral control. Benzodiazepines are the usual drugs of choice, although some clinicians are using opioids successfully. Again, when used, the basic principle is to determine the dose that provides adequate sedation without problematic increases in confusion or other adverse effects (ie, avoid both under-sedation and over-sedation). Because of their sedative properties, some clinicians are choosing especially quetiapine or other atypical antipsychotics instead of benzodiazepines. In very rare instances, only with expert consultation, general anesthetic drugs (or ECT [electroconvulsive therapy]) have been used for severely ill individuals with refractory delirious states.

There are a few situations in which a specific kind of pharmacological agent is indicated explicitly. The most common is alcohol withdrawal, including delirium tremens. Sedative–hypnotic drugs, specifically intermediate to long-acting benzodiazepines, are the treatment of choice. Usually, a dosage taper of 4 to 7 days is effective. The initial dose should be sufficient to counteract signs of withdrawal such as tremor, hyperactive reflexes, or elevated heart rate or blood pressure. Alcohol withdrawal and delirium tremens can increase blood pressure [15] and affect numerous cardio–respiratory functions (cardiac index and cardiac work and oxygen delivery and consumption) [16]. Monitoring of these parameters during the taper is indicated to assure that the rate of dosage decrease is not too rapid. Typically, lower doses are needed to prevent rather than reverse withdrawal. Lorazepam (Ativan) is a common and appropriate choice, starting at 1 to 2 mg three to four times per day. It has the advantages of being safe in people who have liver disease and having a parenteral dosage form.

There are also situations in which use of drugs with specific pharmacological effects should be minimized or avoided. Probably the most common are drugs with anticholinergic effects, because such effects can make delirium worse. Finally, pharmacological control of associated disorders should provide benefit. For example, because dementia is a risk factor for the development of delirium, use of cognition enhancers might reduce the likelihood of delirium in mildly to moderately demented individuals. It is not likely that these drugs would have a role in the acute management of delirium. They might be useful, however, as prophylaxis in susceptible individuals. Because new drugs and new routes of administration frequently are being developed, and because new effects and adverse effects of these drugs are being identified as greater experience is gained, it is necessary for every clinician to review this field for these new developments periodically.

The pathophysiology of delirium is complex and not understood in detail. The abnormal slowing often observed in the EEG and disruption in cerebral metabolism demonstrate the involvement of the cerebral cortex [17]. Abnormalities of several neurotransmitter systems and synapses, especially cholinergic, are implicated, as are dysfunctions of the blood–brain barrier [18]. It has been hypothesized that inflammatory processes might play a role, as might changes in activity of the hypothalamic-pituitary-adrenocortical (HPA) axis [19]. Although it generally is considered that delirium results from diffuse brain dysfunction involving both hemispheres, there is some evidence for specific dysfunction of the right hemisphere [20]. Specific anatomical regions implicated include prefrontal, fusiform, posterior parietal, and temporal cortices, thalamus, and basal ganglia [21]. Dysfunction in these structures and systems often take hours to days to recover after removal of the offending process, and infrequently take longer or, rarely, might not be fully reversible at all.

Depression

The capacities to experience sadness (depression) and apprehension and fear (anxiety) are normal [22–24]. There is a threshold for severity and dysfunction, however, beyond which sadness or depression is considered a disorder [2]. The epigraph at the start of this article relates not just broadly to emotion, but more specifically to the very longstanding belief in the relationship between mood and the heart to sorrow (depression). This observation is supported by recent research. For example, two symptoms of major depression, sad mood and hopelessness, were associated with ischemic heart disease [25]. In another study [26] 20% of individuals who had congestive heart failure reached criteria for major depression, and 50% had some depressive symptoms. Conversely, in one study, approximately one third of individuals admitted for chest pain had a diagnosable psychiatric disorder [27]. This section addresses the relationship between depression and diseases of the heart, including an attempt to answer the question, "Why in the setting of acute and chronic heart diseases such as myocardial infarction, should the nonpsychiatric physician be concerned with the patient's mood?"

There are five defined psychiatric mood disorders primarily associated with depression—major depressive disorder, dysthymic disorder, depressive disorder NOS (not otherwise specified), mood disorder caused by a general medical condition, and substance-induced mood disorder. Research in the 25 years has used these diagnostic definitions, and major depression has been the focus of the most study. Two points about diagnosis are of particular importance to this article. First, the sine-qua-non criteria for diagnosing major depression include the presence of either sad mood or anhedonia (markedly diminished interest or pleasure in most or all activities). In other words, major depression can be present even if sadness is not. Second, all seven of the remaining diagnostic symptoms—weight change, sleep disturbance, psychomotor disruption, fatigue or loss of energy, decreased ability to think or concentrate, and even feelings of worthlessness, or recurrent thoughts of death—can be caused by a co-occurring medical disorder. Thus, in the setting of a coexisting medical illness, it is essential to attempt to determine the source of those symptoms that are present.

Prior research has identified an extensive list of medical conditions and drugs that are associated with depressive symptoms, including cardiovascular disorders (eg, myocardial infarction, stroke) and numerous drugs used in the setting of cardiovascular disease. It is beyond the scope of this article to review this literature. In using the results of those studies, it is important to recognize that most such results are correlative and not based on controlled studies.

In a widely cited study reported somewhat more than a decade ago [28], more than 200 individuals were studied soon after myocardial infarction. Depression was found to be an independent risk factor for mortality in the first 6 months. Subsequent follow-up demonstrated that depression remained a risk out to 18 months [29]. Mortality at 1 year did not differ between men and women [30]. Of note, there was a suggested association among depression, mortality, and the occurrence of frequent premature ventricular contractions. Anxiety symptoms in these subjects also played a role in predicting subsequent cardiac events [31]. A later study by a different group [32] did not find anxiety associated with 3-year changes in carotid intima–media thickness in an elderly community sample. Depression also is associated with poorer outcomes in heart failure more generally [33].

Documentation of the importance of depression to the occurrence and prognosis of patients who have myocardial infarction and other cardiovascular disorders has led to substantial interest in determining if treatment of depression in these individuals could change the cardiovascular prognosis. Among the studies that have been reported, two are probably of most interest: the Sertraline Anti-Depressant Heart Attack Trial (known as SADHAT or SADHEART), and the ENhanced Recovery In Coronary Heart Disease (referred to as ENRICHD).

The primary goal of the SADHEART trial [34], a randomized double-blind placebo-controlled clinical trial, was to demonstrate the efficacy and safety of sertraline (Zoloft), a selective serotonin reuptake inhibitor (SSRI) antidepressant, for 24 weeks in 369 people with major depression hospitalized acutely for unstable angina (25%) or a myocardial infarction (75%). The primary cardiac outcome measure was left ventricular ejection fraction. Sertraline was found to be safe and effective for depression. Roughly 50% of the episodes of depression started before the index cardiac event, and these were more responsive to drug treatment [35]. The study did not have sufficient power to determine if depression treatment also improved the cardiac prognosis, but there was a trend in that direction. It is important to note that, if successful depression treatment were correlated with improved cardiac prognosis, that association would not necessarily demonstrate that this improved prognosis was a result of the successful depression treatment. They could occur by different mechanisms.

The ENRICHD study [36], also a clinical trial, involved almost 2500 individuals who had myocardial infarction and major or minor depression. The experimental group received nonpharmacological cognitive–behavioral therapy (CBT) plus usual care, while the other subjects received usual care only. (Severely depressed subjects also received an SSRI antidepressant.) Although patients in the experimental group showed improvement of depression, at follow-up out to 29 months, no difference in cardiac prognosis was observed. Subjects in the subgroup of white males did show benefit [37]. The presence of medical comorbidity in these individuals raised the likelihood of having depression [38]. Patients whose treatment for depression was not effective had a poorer cardiac prognosis [39]. Interestingly, consistent with the effect suggested in the SADHEART study, those individuals who received sertraline in this study did show benefit in cardiac prognosis [40]. Of note, sertraline has effects on platelet function, which might mediate its beneficial effects in these studies [41].

Before the late 1980s, first-line pharmacological treatment for major depression was the class of drugs called the tricyclic antidepressants, so named because of communality in their chemical structure. Since the introduction of fluoxetine (Prozac), followed by several other SSRI drugs, so-named because of the communality of pharmacological mechanism, these antidepressants have become the accepted first-line medications in most situations for depression treatment. There are, of course, effective nonpharmacological methods of depression treatment, such as CBT, but these are beyond the scope of this article.

Concerns with the safety of the tricyclic drugs in people who have cardiac disorders [42] has motivated investigators to assess the safety of the class of SSRI drugs in such individuals. Numerous studies, including SADHEART, have documented the safety and efficacy of these medications administered to patients with subacute and more chronic cardiovascular disease. Of note, several of the SSRI medications, because of their effects on the P450 metabolic system, are implicated in increasing the risk of drug–drug interactions, an essential issue in the setting of cardiovascular and other medical comorbidity. The least risk appears to occur with citalopram and its isomer (Celexa and Lexapro). Sertraline also has a lower risk than the remaining SSRIs.

Results of the SADHEART and ENRICHD studies begin to address the question of why clinicians caring for patients who have cardiovascular disease should be concerned with the presence of depression. Although the primary purpose of the SADHEART trial was not to address this issue, the results suggested that medication treatment of depression might improve the cardiovascular prognosis. The results of the ENRICHD study from the subgroup that received sertraline were consistent with this very preliminary conclusion. The main results of the ENRICHD study indicated that effective nonpharmacological treatment of depression did not change the cardiovascular prognosis (although CBT nonresponders had poorer cardiovascular status at follow up). Thus, although these results are too tentative to justify firm conclusions, they raise the possibility that the change in cardiac prognosis from the drug treatment (if substantiated) might be caused by mechanisms different than those producing the improvement in depression (ie, that resolution of depression per se was not sufficient). In other words, the answer to the question posed is:

1. Evaluation and treatment of the depression is called for, if present, because of the seriousness of the depressive disorder itself. The clinician providing care for the cardiovascular disease should either provide treatment for the depression or refer the patient for such intervention.
2. Relevant to the cardiovascular treatment, SSRI drug treatment of the depression *might* improve cardiovascular prognosis, even if by mechanisms independent of the depression improvement. A recent review concluded that the evidence is strong that depression is related etiologically to coronary heart disease, while the prognostic relationship is likely, but negative studies have been reported [43].

The association between depression and cardiovascular disease could be caused by

- Cardiovascular disease, increasing the likelihood of depression (perhaps, a so-called reactive depression)
- Depression, raising the likelihood of cardiovascular disease, including affecting the prognosis of individuals who have cardiovascular disorders
- The association caused by a third factor that affects the likelihood of both, including the possibilities that successful treatment of either depression or cardiovascular disorder does not affect this third factor and therefore does not affect the risk for the other disorder. It is also possible that treatment could affect the prognosis of both, but by different (and possibly completely unrelated) mechanisms.

There are numerous potential mechanisms by which depression and cardiovascular disorder could be associated. Several of them are behavioral, such as continued poor health habits (eg, smoking, lack of exercise) or lack of adherence with medical care. There are also a number that a more specifically physiological. Although the behavioral mechanisms are important issues, much research has shown that the behavioral mechanisms do not account for the association fully.

The possible physiological mechanisms potentially abnormal in both depression and cardiovascular disease include:

- Autonomic (possibly either sympathetic and/or parasympathetic) dysfunctions [44], including cardiac rhythm disturbances such as frequent premature ventricular contractions [29] and diminished heart rate variability [45]
- Inflammatory changes [46] and endothelial dysfunction [47]
- HPA hyperactivity [48]
- Platelet dysfunction [48,49]
- Changes in serotonin and its gene control [50,51]
- Sleep and circadian rhythm dysfunctions [52–54]
- Common genetic variability [55]

Review of the details of these possibilities is beyond the purview of this article. Each of these is very tentative, especially because the etiology and pathophysiology of depression itself are poorly understood. Drug treatment of depression might affect any of these that turn out to be relevant by pharmacological mechanisms independent of mechanism of depression relief, but producing an apparent association nonetheless. There is now a great deal of interest in these questions, and the research literature is likely to increase rapidly.

Because depression is a disease of the brain, linkages between the brain and the cardiovascular system should be highly relevant to an understanding of the relationship between cardiovascular disorders and depression. Neuroimaging and associated studies are beginning to understand brain regions and circuits related to depression [56,57]. Prefrontal cortex, striatal systems, and limbic structures are implicated primarily, including cingulate cortex, thalamus, amygdala, and hippocampus. Studies are appearing that relate brain structures to cardiac function, although there do not yet seem to be any yet that did so specifically in depressed individuals.

Heart beat EEG-evoked potentials correlated with frontal cortical brain activity [58]. Behavioral tasks that increased heart rate and blood pressure activated prefrontal cortex, thalamus, and insular cortex [59]. Coronary vasodilation produced with dipyridamole activated prefrontal cortex and thalamus [60]. Central plus peripheral sympathetic activation with yohimbine activated medial frontal cortex, thalamus, insular cortex, and cerebellum [61], while sympathetic activation only in the periphery activated cingulate cortex, somatosensory cortex, and insula [62]. Breathlessness (dyspnea) activated only the insula [63]. Finally, Rosen and colleagues found that dobutamine-induced angina activated prefrontal cortex and cingulate, along with hypothalamus and peri-aqueductal gray [64]. This same investigative group found that painful ischemia differed from painless ischemia by activation of frontal cortex, cingulate, and temporal cortex in the painful group only [65]. Thus, there is substantial overlap between regions activated in these studies and several implicated in the pathophysiology of depression, although these regions also are involved in various functions not necessarily directly related to either cardiovascular function or depression, so it cannot be stated that this overlap has specificity. Of note, the insula, a region of brain highly implicated in visceral sensation (interoception) was activated in a number of these studies [66].

Other factors and issues

Numerous other behavioral/psychosocial factors and psychiatric disorders have been implicated in cardiovascular dysfunction. The literature on many of these issues is extensive. They will be described here, but only briefly.

Stress (eg, specific recent stressful life events and the organismic responses to those events), inadequate social support, and low socioeconomic status appear to raise the risk of cardiovascular disorders (eg, acute coronary heart disease episodes) [67–70]. The observation that so-called type A behavior might increase cardiac risk goes back 50 years [71]. There is a long history of research into this issue, including efforts to identify more precisely which aspects of the type A constellation are most relevant. Anger and hostility have been recognized as the possible relevant factors [68,72–75]. Finally, a relatively new personality construct, called type D behavior, has been described, involving inhibition of negative emotion and a tendency toward social isolation, and possibly associated with increased risk [76].

Recent studies and reviews have come to different conclusions about the status of these variables:

- The Interheart study [77] reported that hostility, depression, and anxiety all raised cardiovascular risk.
- A review of systematic reviews [69] concluded that depression and social support were independent risks but that life events, type A behavior, hostility, and anxiety were not.
- A third review [78] concluded that anxiety was a relevant risk, although data for anger were less conclusive.

Clearly, there are data supporting numerous psychosocial factors in the occurrence and prognosis of cardiovascular disease, but the details are far from being clarified fully.

The literature on psychophysiological factors of potential relevance to cardiovascular disease is far too extensive to review, and beyond the purview of this article. A few issues will be mentioned briefly to give a sense of the breadth of this field of research.

Studies in animals of the effects of social group competition on emotional arousal and resulting dysfunction of the cardiovascular system [79,80], including sustained high blood pressure and sudden death, go back at least 25 years [81]. As noted previously, reductions in heart rate variability are likely to be involved, as are inflammatory mechanisms [82]. Animal models have studied ventricular dysrhythmias and T-wave alternans as potentially relevant [83]. Consideration of the involvement of vasospasm mediated by behavioral factors also has a long-standing history [84]. Endocrine changes (HPA axis and sympatho–adrenal) are implicated [85]. Blockade of fronto-cortical brainstem connections, or intracerebral inhibition of beta-adrenergic receptors (and the other heart-brain linkages discussed previously) can influence this effect [86]. Overall, perhaps the most extensive and consistent findings implicate abnormalities in the heart–brain connections mediated through the autonomic nervous system, and other physiological processes that directly or indirectly affect the functions of those connections.

Summary

It has been observed for many years, indeed many centuries, and verified by many correlative data, that cardiovascular disease is associated with many psychosocial factors and behavioral disorders, including delirium and depression.

Delirium is a behavioral condition produced by diffuse cerebral dysfunction from either systemic metabolic changes and/or intracerebral pathology; it often is associated with cardiovascular disorders.

Major risk factors for delirium development include overall medical illness severity, presence of multiple disorders, pre-existing cognitive impairment, and use of drugs that predispose (especially sedative and anticholinergic drugs; drug-drug interactions). Specific cardiovascular factors include acute coronary syndrome, recent myocardial infarction, cardiac rhythm distur-bance, significant high or low blood pressure, congestive heart failure, stroke, and/or respiratory abnormalities.

Treatment of delirium requires treatment of the underlying medical disorder, but often also requires behavioral management involving both nonpharmacological measures and pharmacological intervention with anti-psychotic, and sometimes sedative, medications.

Depression is associated with, and changes the prognosis for, cardiovas-cular disorders, especially myocardial infarction.

Clinical trials have demonstrated that treatment of depression with sertraline (and probably other SSRI antidepressants) is safe and effective in individuals who have cardiovascular disorders. Nonpharmacological treatment of depression with CBT does not improve cardiac prognosis after myocardial infarction (except possibly in the subgroup of white males). Sertraline (or other SSRI) treatment might improve cardiac prognosis.

Several other psychosocial factors also are associated with cardiovascular diseases, including anxiety, stress, social support, anger/hostility, and other personality factors.

References

[1] Glick RL, Riba M. Common psychiatric emergencies in the office setting. In: Knesper DJ, Riba MB, Schwenk TL, editors. Primary care psychiatry. Philadelphia: WB Saunders; 1997. p. 45–60.

[2] American Psychiatric Association. Diagnositic and statistical manual of mental disorders. 4th edition. Washington, DC: American Psychiatric Association; 1994. p. 317–91.

[3] Beers MH, Berkow R. The Merck manual of diagnosis of therapy. 17th edition. Washington Station (NJ): Merck Research Laboratories; 1999. p. 1390–3.

[4] Caine ED, Grossman H, Lyness JM. Delirium, dementia, and amnestic and other cognitive disorders and mental disorders due to a general medical condition. In: Kaplan HI, Sadock BJ, editors. Comprehensive textbook of psychiatry, vol. 1. 6th editionBaltimore (MD): Williams and Wilkins; 1995. p. 705–54.

[5] Rolfson DB, McElhaney JE, Rockwood K, et al. Incidence and risk factors for delirium and other adverse outcomes in older adults after coronary artery bypass graft surgery. Can J Cardiol 1999;15(7):771–6.

[6] Edlund A, Lundstrom M, Karlsson S, et al. Delirium in older patients admitted to general internal medicine. J Geriatr Psychiatry Neurol 2006;19(2):83–90.

[7] Allen MH, Currier GW, Carpenter D, et al. Treatment of behavioral emergencies, 2005. J Psychiatr Pract 2005;11(Suppl 1):5–108.

[8] Pandharipande P, Shintani A, Peterson J, et al. Lorazepam is an independent risk factor for transitioning to delirium in intensive care unit patients. Anesthesiology 2006;104(1):21–6.

[9] Hassaballa HA, Balk RA. Torsades de pointes associated with the administration of intra-venous haloperidol: a review of the literature and practical guidelines for use. Expert Opin Drug Saf 2003;2(6):543–7.

[10] Shapiro BA, Warren J, Egol AB, et al. Practical parameters for intravenous analgesia and sedation for adult patients in the intensive care unit: an executive summary. Crit Care Med 1995;23(9):1596–600.

[11] Sala M, Coppa F, Cappucciati C, et al. Antidepressants: their effects on cardiac channels, QT prolongation, and Torsades de Pointes. Curr Opin Investig Drugs 2006;7(3):256–63.

[12] Stollberger C, Huber JO, Finsterer J. Antipsychotic drugs and QT prolongation. Int Clin Psychopharmacol 2005;20(5):243–51.

[13] H.J., Hancox JC, Nutt DJ. Psychotropic drugs, cardiac arrhythmia, and sudden death. J Clin Psychopharmacol 2003;23(1):58–77.

[14] Pigott TA, Carson WH, Saha AR, et al. Aripiprazole for the prevention of relapse in stabilized patients with chronic schizophrenia: a placebo-controlled 26-week study. J Clin Psychiatry 2003;64(9):1048–56.

[15] Saunders JB, Beevers DG, Paton A. Alcohol-induced hypertension. Lancet 1981;2(8248):653–6.

[16] Abraham E, Shoemaker WC, McCartney SF. Cardiorespiratory patterns in severe delirium tremens. Arch Intern Med 1985;145(6):1057–9.

[17] Blass JP, Nolan KA, Black RS, et al. Delirium: phenomenology and diagnosis—a neurobiologic view. Int Psychogeriatr 1991;3(2):121–34.

[18] van der Mast RC. Pathophysiology of delirium. J Geriatr Psychiatry Neurol 1998;11(3):138–45.

[19] Flacker JM, Lipsitz LA. Neural mechanisms of delirium: current hypotheses and evolving concepts. J Gerontol Series A Biol Sci Med Sci 1999;54(6):B239–46.

[20] Trzepacz PT. Update on the neuropathogenesis of delirium. Dementia Geriatr Cogn Disord 1999;10(5):330–4.

[21] Trzepacz PT. Is there a final common neural pathway in delirium? Focus on acetylcholine and dopamine. Semin Clin Neuropsychiatry 2000;5(2):132–48.

[22] Wiessman MM, Prusoff B, Pincus C. Symptom patterns in depressed patients and depressed normals. J Nerv Ment Dis 1975;160(1):15–23.

[23] Hodiamont P. How normal are anxiety and fear? Int J Soc Psychiatry 1991;37(1):43–50.

[24] Finley-Jones R, Brown GW. Types of stressful life events and the onset of anxiety and depressive disorders. Psychol Med 1981;11(4):803–15.

[25] Anda R, Williamson D, Jones D, et al. Depressed affect, hopelessness, and the risk of ischemic heart disease in a cohort of US adults. Epidemiology 1993;4(4):285–94.

[26] Freedland KE, Rich MW, Skala JA, et al. Prevalence of depression in hospitalized patients with congestive heart failure. Psychosom Med 2003;65(1):119–28.

[27] Kisely SR. The relationship between admission to hospital with chest pain and psychiatric disorder. Aust NZ J Psychiatry 1998;32(2):172–9.

[28] Frasure-Smith N, Lesperance F, Talajic M. Depression following myocardial infarction. Impact on 6-month survival. JAMA 1993;270(15):1819–25.

[29] Frasure-Smith N, Lesperance F, Talajic M. Depression and 18-month prognosis after myocardial infarction. Circulation 1995;91(4):999–1005.

[30] Frasure-Smith N, Lesperance F, Juneau M, et al. Gender, depression, and one-year prognosis after myocardial infarction. Psychosom Med 1999;61(1):26–37.

[31] Frasure-Smith N, Lesperance F, Talajic M. The impact of negative emotions on prognosis following myocardial infarction: is it more than depression? Health Psychol 1995;14(5):388–98.

[32] Stewart JC, Janicki DL, Muldoon MF, et al. Negative emotions and 3-year progression of subclinical atherosclerosis. Arch Gen Psychiatry 2007;64(2):225–33.

[33] Rutledge T, Reis VA, Linke SE, et al. Depression in heart failure: a meta-analytic review of prevalence, intervention effects, and association with clinical outcomes. J Am Coll Cardiol 2006;48(8):1527–37.

[34] Glassman AH, O'Connor CM, Califf RM, et al. Sertraline treatment of major depression in patients with acute MI or unstable angina. JAMA 2002;288(6):701–9.

[35] Glassman AH, Bigger JT, Gaffney M, et al. Onset of major depression associated with acute coronary syndrome: relationship to onset, major depressive disorder history, and episode severity to sertraline treatment. Arch Gen Psychiatry 2006;63(3):283–8, A.

[36] Berkman LF, Bumenthal J, Burg M, et al. Effects of treating depression and low perceived social support on clinical events after myocardial infarction: the enhanced recovery in coronary heart disease patients (ENRICHD) randomized trial. JAMA 2003;289(23):3106–16, A.

[37] Schneiderman N, Saab PG, Catellier DJ, et al. Psychosocial treatment within gender by ethnicity subgroups in the Enhancing Recovery in Coronary Heart Disease (ENRICHD) clinical trial. Psychosom Med 2004;66:475–83, A.

[38] Watkins LL, Schneiderman N, Blumenthal JA, et al. Cognitive and somatic symptoms of depression are associated with medical comorbidity in patients after acute myocardial infarction. Am Heart J 2003;146(1):48–54, A.

[39] Carney RM, Blumenthal JA, Freedland KE, et al. Depression and late mortality after myocardial infarction in the Enhancing Recovery in Coronary Heart Disease (ENRICHD) study. Psychosom Med 2004;66(4):466–74, A.

[40] Taylor CB, Youngblood ME, Catellier D, et al. Effects of antidepressant medication on morbidity and mortality in depressed patients after myocardial infarction. Arch Gen Psychiatry 2005;62:792–8, A.

[41] Markovitz JH, Shuster JL, Chitwood WS, et al. Platelet activation in depression and effects of sertraline treatment: an open-label study. Am J Psychiatry 2000;157:1006–8, B.

[42] Glassman AH. Cardiovascular effects of antidepressant drugs: updated. J Clin Psychiatry 1998;59(Suppl):13–8.

[43] Frasure-Smith N, Lesperance F. Recent evidence linking coronary heart disease and depression. Can J Psychiatry 2006;51(12):730–7.

[44] Cameron OG. Depression increases post-MI mortality: how? Psychosom Med 1996;58(2):111–2.

[45] Carney RM, Blumenthal JA, Freedland KE, et al. Low heart rate variability and the effect of depression on postmyocardial infarction mortality. Arch Intern Med 2005;165(13):1486–91, A.

[46] Lesperance F, Frasure-Smith N, Theroux P, et al. The association between major depression and levels of soluble intracellular adhesion molecule 1, interleukin-6, and C-reactive protein in patients with recent acute coronary syndromes. Am J Psychiatry 2004;161:271–7, A.

[47] Zellweger MJ, Osterwalder RH, Langewitz W, et al. Coronary artery disease and depression. Eur Heart J 2004;25(1):3–9.

[48] Malhotra S, Tesar GE, Franco K. The relationship between depression and cardiovascular disorders. Curr Psychiatry Rep 2000;2(3):241–6.

[49] Serebruany VL, Glassman AH, Malinin AI, et al. Enhanced platelet/endothelial activation in depressed patients with acute coronary syndrome: evidence from recent clinical trials. Blood Coagul Fibrinolysis 2003;14(6):563–7, A.

[50] Caspi A, Sugden K, Moffitt TE, et al. Influence of life stress on depression: moderation by a polymorphism in the 5-HTT gene. Science 2003;301:386–9.

[51] Grabe HJ, Lange M, Volzke H, et al. Mental and physical distress is modulated by a polymorphism in the 5-HT transporter gene interacting with social stressors and chronic disease burden. Mol Psychiatry 2005;10:220–4.

[52] Koskenvuo M. Cardiovascular stress and sleep. Ann Clin Res 1987;19(2):110–3.

[53] Deedwania PC. Hemodynamic changes as triggers of cardiovascular events. Cardiol Clin 1996;14(2):229–38.

[54] Muller JE. Circadian variation and triggering of acute coronary events. Am Heart J 1999;137:(4 Pt 2):S1–8.

[55] McCaffery JM, Frasure-Smith N, Dube MP, et al. Common genetic vulnerability to depressive symptoms and coronary artery disease: a review and development of candidate genes related to inflammation and serotonin. Psychosom Med 2006;68(2):187–200.

[56] Drevets WC. Neuroimaging and neuropathological studies of depression: implications for the cognitive–emotional features of mood disorders. Curr Opin Neurobiol 2001;11:240–9.

[57] Seminowicz DA, Mayberg HS, McIntosh AR, et al. Limbic–frontal circuitry in major depression: a path modeling meta-analysis. Neuroimage 2004;22(1):409–18.

[58] Schandry R, Montoya P. Event-related brain potentials and the processing of cardiac activity. Biol Psychol 1996;42(1–2):75–85.

[59] King AB, Menon RS, Hachinski V, et al. Human forebrain activation by visceral stimuli. J Comp Neurol 1999;413(4):572–82.

[60] Ito H, Yokoyama I, Tamura Y, et al. Regional changes in human cerebral blood flow during dipyridamole stress: neural activation in the thalamus and prefrontal cortex. Neuroimage 2002;16(3 Pt 1):788–93.

[61] Cameron OG, Minoshima S. Regional brain activation due to pharmacologically induced adrenergic interoceptive stimulation in humans. Psychosom Med 2002;64(6):851–61.

[62] Cameron OG, Zubieta JK, Grunhaus L, et al. Effects of yohimbine on cerebral blood flow, symptoms, and physiological functions in humans. Psychosom Med 2000;62(4):549–59.

[63] Banzett RB, Mulnier HE, Murphy K, et al. Breathlessness in humans activates insular cortex. Neuroreport 2000;11(10):2117–20.

[64] Rosen SD, Paulesu E, Frith CD, et al. Central nervous pathways mediating angina pectoris. Lancet 1994;344(8916):147–50.

[65] Rosen SD, Paulesu E, Nihoyannopoulos P, et al. Silent ischemia as a central problem: regional brain activation compared in silent and painful myocardial ischemia. Ann Int Med 1996;124(11):939–49.

[66] Cameron OG. Visceral sensory neuroscience: interoception. New York: Oxford University Press; 2002.

[67] Tennant C. Life stress, social support, and coronary heart disease. Aust NZ J Psychiatry 1999;33(5):636–41.

[68] Krantz DS, McCeney MK. Effects of psychological and social factors on organic disease: a critical assessment of research on coronary heart disease. Annu Rev Psychol 2002;53: 341–69.

[69] Bunker SJ, Colquhoun DM, Esler MD, et al. Stress and coronary heart disease: psychosocial risk factors. Med J Aust 2003;178(6):272–6.

[70] Ramachandruni S, Handberg E, Sheps DS. Acute and chronic psychological stress in coronary disease. Curr Opin Cardiol 2004;19(5):494–9.

[71] Friedman M, Rosenman RH. Comparison of fat intake of American men and women: possible relationship to incidence of clinical coronary artery disease. Circulation 1957;16: 339–47.

[72] Verrier RL, Mittleman MA. Life-threatening cardiovascular consequences of anger in patients with coronary heart disease. Cardiol Clin 1996;14(2):289–307.

[73] Inbarren C, Sidney S, Gild DE, et al. Association of hostility with coronary artery calcification in young adults. JAMA 2000;283:2546–51.

[74] Scherwitz LW, Perkins LL, Chesney MA, et al. Hostility and health behaviors in young adults: the CARDIA study: Coronary Artery Risk Development in Young Adults study. Am J Epidemiol 1992;15:136–45, A.

[75] Siegler IC, Peterson BL, Barefoot JC, et al. Hostility during late adolescence predicts coronary risk factors at midlife. Am J Epidemiol 1992;136:146–54.

[76] Sher L. Type D personality: the heart, stress, and cortisol. QJM 2005;98(5):323–9.

[77] Das S, O'Keefe JH. Behavioral cardiology: recognizing and addressing the profound impact of psychosocial stress on cardiovascular health. Curr Atheroscler Rep 2006;8(2):111–8.

[78] Kubzansky LD, Kawachi I. Going to the heart of the matter: do negative emotions cause coronary heart disease? J Psychosom Res 2000;48(4–5):323–37.

[79] Kaplan JR, Manuck SB, Clarkson TB, et al. Social status, environment, and atherosclerosis in cynomolgus monkeys. Arteriosclerosis 1982;2:359–68.

[80] McCabe PM, Gonzales JA, Zaias J, et al. Social environment influences the progression of atherosclerosis in the Watanabe heritable hyperlipidemic rabbit. Circulation 2000;105: 354–9.

[81] Henry JP. The induction of acute and chronic cardiovascular disease in animals by psychosocial stimulation. Int J Psychiatry Med 1975;6(1–2):147–58.

[82] Parissis JT, Fountaoulaki K, Paraskevaidis I, et al. Depression in chronic heart failure: novel pathophysiological mechanisms and therapeutic approaches. Curr Opin Invest Drugs 2005; 14(5):567–77.

[83] Krantz DS, Quigley JF, O'Callahan M. Mental stress as a trigger of acute cardiac events: the role of laboratory studies. Ital Heart J 2001;2(12):895–9.

[84] Hellstrom HR. Coronary artery vasospasm: the likely immediate cause of acute myocardial infarction. Br Heart J 1979;41(4):426–32.

[85] Eliot RS, Buell JC. Role of emotions and stress in the genesis of sudden death. J Am Coll Cardiol 1985;5(6 Suppl):95B–8B.

[86] Skinner JE. Regulation of cardiac vulnerability by the cerebral defense system. J Am Coll Cardiol 1985;5(6 Suppl):88B–94B.

ELSEVIER
SAUNDERS

CRITICAL
CARE
CLINICS

Crit Care Clin 23 (2007) 901–909

Index

Note: Page numbers of article titles are in **boldface** type.

A

AAD. See *Acute aortic dissection (AAD)*.

ACC/AHA. See *American Heart Association/American College of Cardiology (ACC/AHA)*.

ACE inhibitors. See *Angiotensin-converting enzyme (ACE) inhibitors*.

ACLS. See *Acute Cardiac Life Support (ACLS)*.

Acute aortic dissection (AAD), **779–800**
 aortography in, 787
 biomarkers in, 785–786
 classification of, 780–781
 clinical manifestations of, 782–786
 CT in, 788–789
 differential diagnosis of, 785
 echocardiography in, 787–788
 imaging of, 786–790
 incidence of, 780
 intradural hematomas, 782
 MRI in, 789–790
 pathophysiology of, 779
 physical findings in, 784–785
 predisposing factors for, 780
 symptoms of, 782–784
 TEE in, 788
 treatment of
  long-term, 796
  medical, 790–794
  surgical, 794–796

Acute Cardiac Life Support (ACLS), review
 of updated guidelines for, **873–880**
 bradycardia, 878
 medication administration, 876–877
 rescue breaths, 877

Acute decompensated heart failure
 (ADHF), **737–758**
 ancillary evaluation of, 742–746
 clinical evaluation of, 740–742
 clinical presentation of, 740
 defined, 737–739
 hemodyamic monitoring in, 746
 hospitalizations due to, 737

 precipitating factors in, 738
 treatment of, 746–753
  ACE inhibitors in, 752
  Bi PAP in, 747
  ß-blockers in, 752
  CPAP in, 747
  device therapy in, 751
  digoxin in, 753
  diuretics in, 747–748
  dobutamine in, 750
  in-hospital, 746–748
  inotropes in, 749–751
  long-term, 752–753
  milrinone in, 750–751
  morphine sulfate in, 747
  nesiritide in, 749
  nitroglycerin in, 748–749
  nitroprusside in, 749
  oxygen in, 747
  postdischarge management
   in, 753
  spironolactone in, 753
  ultrafiltration in, 751
  vasodilators in, 748–749

Acute pulmonary embolism, 836–841
 described, 836
 diagnosis of, CTPA in, 837–841
 in critical care setting, diagnosis of,
  836–841
 treatment of, 817–818

Acute thoracic cardiovascular emergencies,
 CT and MRI of, **835–853**

ADHERE study, 748

ADHF. See *Acute decompensated heart
 failure (ADHF)*.

Alcohol withdrawal, sedative-hypnotics
 for, 888–889

American College of Cardiology/American
 Heart Association, ST elevation
 myocardial infarction guidelines, 767

American Heart Association/American
 College of Cardiology (ACC/AHA),
 873–874

Amiodarone
  for atrial fibrillation, 860–864, 866
  for cardiac arrest, 877
  for cardiogenic shock, 765

Aneurysm(s), left ventricular, STEMI
    and, 701

Angiography
  coronary, in UA/NSTEMI evaluation,
      715–716
  pulmonary, in pulmonary
      thromboembolic disease
      evaluation, 814

Angiotensin-converting enzyme (ACE)
    inhibitors
  for acute STEMI, 698–699
  for ADHF, 752

Antiarrhythmic agents, for cardiac arrest,
    876–877

Anticoagulant(s), for UA/NSTEMI,
    724–727

Anti-ischemic agents, for UA/NSTEMI,
    718–727

Antiplatelet agents, for UA/NSTEMI,
    720–724

Antiplatelet therapy, for acute STEMI,
    696–697

Antithrombin agents, for UA/NSTEMI,
    724–727

Antithrombotic agents, for acute STEMI,
    697–698

Aortic dissection, 841–845
  clinical presentation of, 841–842
  described, 841
  diagnosis of, 842–845

Aortography, in AAD, 787

Aripiprazole, in delirium management, 888

Arrhythmia(s)
  cardiac, atrial fibrillation, in critically
      ill patients, 855–872. See also
      Atrial fibrillation, in critically ill
      patients.
  STEMI and, 702
  treatment of, 823

Aspirin, for UA/NSTEMI, 720–721

Atrial fibrillation
  causes of, 855–857
  clinical presentation of, 859
  conditions associated with,
      855–857
  defined, 855, 856
    hemodynamic consequences of,
        858–859
    in critically ill patients, **855–872**
    management of
      acute rate control
          in, 860–861
      anticoagulation in ICU,
          867–868
      biphasic waveform
          defibrillators in, 865
      ß-blockers in, 860
      calcium channel blockers in,
          860
      digoxin in, 860–861
      electrical cardioversion
          in, 865–866
      pharmacologic
          cardioversion in,
          861–865
    in ICU, long-term outcome of,
        868–869
    management of, 859–868
    pathophysiology of, 856, 858
    prevalence of, 855
    prevention of, 868
    STEMI and, 702

Atrial flutter, STEMI and, 702

B

Benzodiazepine(s), in alcohol withdrawal,
    888–889

Bi PAP. See Biphasic positive airway
    pressure (Bi PAP).

Biochemical markers, in UA/NSTEMI
    evaluation, 713–714

Biomarker(s)
  cardiac, in acute STEMI evaluation,
      688
  in AAD, 785–786

Biphasic positive airway pressure (Bi PAP),
    for ADHF, 747

Biphasic waveform defibrillators, for atrial
    fibrillation, 865

ß-blockers
  for acute STEMI, 698
  for ADHF, 752
  for atrial fibrillation, 860
  for UA/NSTEMI, 720

Bradycardia
  defined, 878
  treatment of, 878

Bumetanide, for cardiogenic shock, 765

C

Calcium channel blockers
for atrial fibrillation, 860
for UA/NSTEMI, 720

Cardiac arrest
medications for, administration
of, 876–877
rhythms encountered during, 876

Cardiac arrhythmias, atrial fibrillation,
in critically ill patients, **855–872.**
See also *Atrial fibrillation,*
in critically ill patients.

Cardiac biomarkers, in acute STEMI
evaluation, 688

Cardiac catheterization, in UA/NSTEMI
evaluation, 715–716

Cardiogenic shock
criteria for, 759–760
defined, 759
management of
conventional, 764
mechanical support devices in,
771–772
new approaches in,
772–773
pharmacologic, 765–766
myocardial infarction complications
of, **759–777**
clinical presentation of, 761–763
incidence of, 760
initial stabilization of, 763–766
management of
IABP in, 766–767
reperfusion strategies in,
767–771
pathogenesis of,
760–761
STEMI and, 701–702

Cardiopulmonary resuscitation (CPR)
review of updated guidelines for,
873–880
amount of shocks, 874–875
interruption of chest
compressions, 875–876
number of compressions, 874
paramedics' response to cardiac
arrest in field, 876

Cardiovascular disease
abnormal physiologic mechanisms
in, 893
drugs for, depression resulting
from, 890–893

Cardiovascular system, stress effects
on, 894–895

Cardioversion
electrical, for atrial fibrillation,
865–866
pharmacologic, for atrial fibrillation,
861–865

Catheterization, cardiac, in UA/NSTEMI
evaluation, 715–716

Chest radiography, in AAD, 786–787

Chronic thromboembolic pulmonary
hypertension (CTEPH), treatment
of, 818–819

Clopidogrel, for acute STEMI, 697

Clopidogrel in Unstable Angina to Prevent
Recurrent Events (CURE) trial, 721

Clozapine, in delirium management, 888

Computed tomography (CT)
in AAD, 788–789
of acute thoracic cardiovascular
emergencies, **835–853**
pulmonary embolism protocol, in
pulmonary thromboembolic
disease evaluation, 813–814

Computed tomography pulmonary
angiography (CTPA), in acute
pulmonary embolism diagnosis,
837–841

Continuous positive airway pressure
(CPAP), for ADHF, 747

Coronary angiography, in UA/NSTEMI
evaluation, 715–716

Coronary artery bypass, for acute STEMI,
696

Coronary artery disease, prevalence of, 709

Coronary disease, in critical care setting,
advanced imaging for, 845–849

Coronary revascularization,
for UA/NSTEMI, 727–729

CPAP. See *Continuous positive airway*
pressure (CPAP).

CPR. See *Cardiopulmonary resuscitation*
(CPR).

CT. See *Computed tomography (CT).*

CTEPH. See *Chronic thromboembolic*
pulmonary hypertension (CTEPH).

CTPA. See *Computed tomography*
pulmonary angiography (CTPA).

CURE trial. See *Clopidogrel in Unstable*
Angina to Prevent Recurrent Events
(CURE) trial.

D

Defibrillator(s), biphasic waveform,
for atrial fibrillation, 865

Delirium, **881–889**
causes of, 884–885
changes associated with, 882–883
defined, 882
described, 881–882
management of, 883–885
haloperidol in, 886–888
nonpharmacologic, 885–886
pharmacologic, 886–889
side effects of, 886–889
vs. treatment, 884–885
risk factors for, 883

Delirium tremens, sedative-hypnotics
for, 888–889

Depression, **889–894**
abnormal physiologic mechanisms in,
893
cardiovascular disease and, 890–894
described, 889–890
drugs causing, 890
mood disorders associated with, 890
myocardial infarction and, 890–894

Device therapy, for ADHF, 751

Digoxin, 860–861
for ADHF, 753
for atrial fibrillation, 862, 863

Diltiazem, for atrial fibrillation, 862

Diuretic(s), for ADHF, 747–748

Dobutamine
for ADHF, 750
for cardiogenic shock, 765–766

Dofetilide, for atrial fibrillation, 864–866

Dopamine
for bradycardia, 878
for cardiogenic shock, 765, 766

Drug(s)
for cardiogenic shock, 765–766
in delirium management, 886–889

E

ECC. See *Emergency Cardiovascular Care
(ECC)*.

ECG. See *Electrocardiogram (ECG)*.

Echocardiography
in AAD, 787–788
in pulmonary hypertension diagnosis,
812–813

ECLS. See *Extracorporeal life support
(ECLS)*.

Efficacy and Safety of Subcutaneous
Enoxaparin in Non-Q-wave Coronary
Events (ESSENCE) trial, 725

Electrical cardioversion, for atrial
fibrillation, 865–866

Electrocardiography (ECG)
in acute STEMI evaluation, 687
in pulmonary hypertension diagnosis,
809–811
in UA/NSTEMI evaluation, 713

Embolism(i), pulmonary, acute, 836–841.
See also *Acute pulmonary embolism*.

Emergency Cardiovascular Care (ECC), 873

Endothelin antagonists, for pulmonary
hypertension, 826

ENhanced Recovery In Coronary Heart
Disease (ENRICHD), 891–892

ENRICHD. See *ENhanced Recovery In
Coronary Heart Disease (ENRICHD)*.

Epinephrine
for bradycardia, 878
for cardiogenic shock, 766

Esmolol, for atrial fibrillation, 862

ESSENCE trial. See *Efficacy and Safety
of Subcutaneous Enoxaparin in
Non-Q-wave Coronary Events
(ESSENCE) trial*.

European Society of Cardiology, 856

Extracorporeal life support (ECLS), in
cardiogenic shock management, 772

F

Factor X inhibitors, for UA/NSTEMI,
726–727

Fast Revascularization During Instability in
Coronary Artery Disease (FRISC)
trial, 726

Fibrillation(s), ventricular, STEMI and,
702–703

Fibrinolysis, for acute STEMI,
contraindications to, 695

Fibrinolytic therapy
for acute STEMI, 691–694
in cardiogenic shock management,
767–768

Flecainide, for atrial fibrillation, 866

Fondaparinux, for UA/NSTEMI, 726–727

Food and Drug Administration, 725

Free wall rupture, left ventricular, STEMI and, 700–701

FRISC trial. See *Fast Revascularization During Instability in Coronary Artery Disease (FRISC) trial.*

Furosemide, for cardiogenic shock, 765

G

Gas exchange, in pulmonary hypertension diagnosis, 811–812

Glycoprotein IIb/IIIa inhibitors
 for acute STEMI, 698
 for UA/NSTEMI, 721–724

H

Haloperidol, in delirium management, 886–888

Hematoma(s), intradural, 782

Hemodynamic parameters, normal, 809

Heparin
 low-molecular-weight,
  for UA/NSTEMI, 725–726
 unfractionated, for UA/NSTEMI, 724–725

Hirudin, for UA/NSTEMI, 726

Hypertension
 pulmonary, in critical care setting, **801–834.** See also *Pulmonary hypertension, in critical care setting.*
 pulmonary arterial, treatment of, 820–823

Hypotension, treatment of, 820–823

Hypoxemia, treatment of, 823

Hyupertension, pulmonary arterial, adjunctive therapy for, 823–825

I

IABP. See *Intra-aortic balloon pump (IABP).*

Ibutilide, for atrial fibrillation, 864, 866

ICTUS study. See *Invasive versus Conservative Treatment in Unstable Coronary Syndrome (ICTUS) study.*

Inotrope(s), for ADHF, 749–751

Intra-aortic balloon pump (IABP)
 for acute STEMI, 699
 in cardiogenic shock management, 766–767

Intradural hematomas, 782

Invasive versus Conservative Treatment in Unstable Coronary Syndrome (ICTUS) study, 728

K

Kussmaul's sign, 763

L

Left ventricular aneurysm, STEMI and, 701

Left ventricular failure, STEMI and, 701–702

Left ventricular free wall rupture, STEMI and, 700–701

Low-molecular-weight heparin,
 for UA/NSTEMI, 725–726

M

Magnetic resonance imaging (MRI)
 in AAD, 789–790
 of acute thoracic cardiovascular emergencies, **835–853**

Metoprolol, for atrial fibrillation, 862

Milrinone
 for ADHF, 750–751
 for cardiogenic shock, 765, 766

Mitral regurgitation, STEMI and, 699–700

Mood disorders, depression and, 890

Morphine sulfate, for ADHF, 747

MRI. See *Magnetic resonance imaging (MRI).*

Myocardial infarction
 acute, causes of, nonatherosclerotic, 686
 cardiogenic shock complicating, **759–777.** See also *Cardiogenic shock, myocardial infarction complications of.*
 drugs for, depression resulting from, 893

N

National Heart Attack Alert Program, 689–690

Nesiritide, for ADHF, 749

Nitrate(s), for UA/NSTEMI, 718–720

Nitroglycerin
    for ADHF, 748–749
    for cardiogenic shock, 765

Nitroprusside
    for ADHF, 749
    for cardiogenic shock, 765

Nitrous oxide (NO), inhaled, for pulmonary
    hypertension, 831

NO. See Nitrous oxide (NO).

Norepinephrine, for cardiogenic shock, 765,
    766

North American Society of Pacing and
    Electrophysiology, 856

O

OASIS-5 trial. See Organization to Assess
    Strategies for Ischemic Syndromes
    (OASIS)-5 trial.

Olanzapine, in delirium management, 888

Organization to Assess Strategies for
    Ischemic Syndromes (OASIS)-5 trial,
    727

Oxygen, for ADHF, 747

P

Percutaneous cardiopulmonary bypass, in
    cardiogenic shock management, 772

Percutaneous coronary intervention, in
    cardiogenic shock management,
    768–771

Pericarditis, STEMI and, 703–704

Pharmacologic cardioversion, for atrial
    fibrillation, 861–865

Phenylephrine, for cardiogenic shock, 765

Phosphodiesterase-5 inhibitor, for
    pulmonary hypertension, 826–827

Physical restraint, in delirium management,
    885–886

Pravastatin or Atorvastatin Evaluation and
    Infection Therapy (PROVE IT)–TIMI
    22 study, 728

Primary PCI, for acute STEMI, 694–696

Procainamide
    for atrial fibrillation, 864
    for cardiac arrest, 878

Propafenone, for atrial fibrillation, 866

Propranolol, for atrial fibrillation, 862

Prostacyclin analogues, for pulmonary
    hypertension, 827–831

PROVE IT–TIMI 22 study, 728

Psychotropic drugs, torsades de Pointes due
    to, 886–887

Pulmonary angiography, in pulmonary
    thromboembolic disease evaluation,
    814

Pulmonary arterial hypertension
    adjunctive therapy for, 823–825
    treatment of, 820–823

Pulmonary embolism, acute, 836–841. See
    also Acute pulmonary embolism.

Pulmonary embolism protocol CT, in
    pulmonary thromboembolic disease
    evaluation, 813–814

Pulmonary function testing, in pulmonary
    hypertension diagnosis, 811–812

Pulmonary hypertension
    chronic thromboembolic, treatment of,
        818–819
    in critical care setting, **801–834**
        biomarkers in, 815
        classification of, 801–804
        clinical assessment of,
            805–813
        clinical characteristics of,
            805–813
        defined, 801–804
        diagnosis of, 805–813
            ECG in, 809–811
            echocardiography in,
                812–813
            gas exchange in, 811–812
            pulmonary function testing
                in, 811–812
        hemodynamics in, 816–817
        hypoxemia in, acute worsening
            of, causes of, 810
        pathogenesis of, 804–805
        physiology of, 801–804
        pulmonary arterial hypertension
            adjunctive therapy for,
                823–825
            treatment of, 820–823
        pulmonary thromboembolic
            disease, evaluation for,
                813–815
        rapid deterioration in, causes of,
            810
        thromboembolic disease,
            treatment of, 817–819

treatment of
endothelin antagonists
in, 826
inhaled NO in, 831
phosphodiesterase-5
inhibitor in, 826–827
prostacyclin analogues in,
827–831
surgical, 831–832
WHO classification of, 803–804, 808

Pulmonary thromboembolic disease,
evaluation for, 813–815

Q

Quetiapine, in delirium management, 888

Quinidine, for atrial fibrillation, 866

R

Radiography, chest, in AAD, 786–787

Regurgitation, mitral STEMI and, 699–700

Reperfusion strategies
for acute STEMI, 691
in cardiogenic shock management,
767–771
fibrinolytic therapy, 767–768
percutaneous coronary
intervention, 768–771
surgical revascularization, 771

Restraint(s), physical, in delirium
management, 885–886

Revascularization
coronary, for UA/NSTEMI, 727–729
surgical, in cardiogenic shock
management, 771

Right ventricular infarction, STEMI
and, 701

Risperidone, in delirium management, 888

Rupture, ventricular septal, STEMI
and, 700

S

SADHAT. See Sertraline Anti-Depressant
Heart Attack Trial (SADHAT).

SADHEART. See Sertraline
Anti-Depressant Heart Attack Trial
(SADHAT).

Sedative-hypnotics, in alcohol withdrawal,
888–889

Sertraline Anti-Depressant Heart Attack
Trial (SADHAT), 891–892

Shock, cardiogenic. See Cardiogenic shock.

SHOCK trial, 768, 769, 772–773

SMASH trial. See Swiss Multicenter of
Angioplasty Shock (SMASH) trial.

Spironolactone, for ADHF, 753

Statin(s), for UA/NSTEMI, 728–729

STEMI. See ST-segment myocardial
infarction (STEMI).

Stress, cardiovascular system effects of,
894–895

ST-segment myocardial infarction (STEMI)
acute
arrhythmias in patients with, 702
atrial fibrillation/flutter due to,
702
cardiac biomarkers in, 688
cardiogenic shock due to,
701–702
clinical presentation of,
686–687
complications of, 699–704
critical care perspective on,
685–707
differential diagnosis of, 688, 689
ECG in, 687
evaluation of, 686–687
imaging in, 688
left ventricular aneurysm due to,
701
left ventricular failure due to,
701–702
left ventricular free wall rupture
due to, 700–701
mitral regurgitation due to,
699–700
pericarditis due to, 703–704
physical examination in, 687
prognosis of, 704
recurrent ischemic events due to,
703
right ventricular infarction due
to, 701
symptoms of, 686–687
tachycardia due to, 702–703
treatment of, 688–699
ACE inhibitors in, 698–699
adjunctive therapy in, 696
antiplatelet therapy in,
696–697
antithrombotic agents in,
697–698
ß-blockers in, 698
coronary artery bypass in,
696
discharge care in, 704–705

ST-segment myocardial (*continued*)
    fibrinolysis in,
        contraindications to, 695
        fibrinolytic therapy in, 691–694
        glycoprotein IIb/IIIa inhibitors in, 698
        IABP in, 699
        in-hospital, 704–705
        primary PCI in, 694–696
        reperfusion strategy in, 691
        ventricular fibrillation due to, 702–703
        ventricular septal rupture due to, 700
    causes of, 685–686
    prevalence of, 685
    prognosis of, 685

Superior Yield of the New Strategy of Enoxaparin, Revascularization and Glycoprotein IIb/IIIa Inhibitors (SYNERGY) trial, 725

Swiss Multicenter of Angioplasty Shock (SMASH) trial, 768

SYNERGY trial. See *Superior Yield of the New Strategy of Enoxaparin, Revascularization and Glycoprotein IIb/IIIa Inhibitors (SYNERGY) trial.*

T

Tachycardia, STEMI and, 702–703

TACTICS trial. See *Thrombolysis and Counterpulsation to Improve Cardiogenic Shock Survival (TACTICS) trial.*

TEE. See *Transesophageal echocardiography (TEE).*

Thienopyridine(s), for UA/NSTEMI, 721

Third World Symposium of Pulmonary Hypertension, 803–804

Thrombin inhibitors, for UA/NSTEMI, 726–727

Thromboembolic disease, treatment of, 817–819

Thrombolysis and Counterpulsation to Improve Cardiogenic Shock Survival (TACTICS) trial, 766

Tilarginine Acetate Injection in a Randomized International Study in Unstable MI Patients with

Cardiogenic Shock (TRIUMPH) trial, 773

Torsades de Pointes, psychotropic drugs and, 886–887

Transesophageal echocardiography (TEE), in AAD, 788

Transthoracic echocardiography (TTE), in AAD, 787

TRIUMPH trial. See *Tilarginine Acetate Injection in a Randomized International Study in Unstable MI Patients with Cardiogenic Shock (TRIUMPH) trial.*

TTE. See *Transthoracic echocardiography (TTE).*

U

UA/NSTEMI. See *Unstable angina/non–ST elevation myocardial infarction.*

Ultrafiltration, for ADHF, 751

Unfractionated heparin, for UA/NSTEMI, 724–725

Unstable angina/non–ST elevation myocardial infarction (UA/NSTEMI), **709–735**
    complications of, 716
    described, 709
    diagnostic evaluation of, 713–716
        cardiac catheterization in, 715–716
        coronary angiography in, 715–716
        ECG in, 713
        noninvasive testing in, 714–715
    pathogenesis of, 710–711
    signs and symptoms of, 711–713
    treatment of, 716–730
        anticoagulants in, 724–727
        anti-ischemic agents in, 718–727
        antiplatelet agents in, 720–724
        antithrombin agents in, 724–727
        aspirin in, 720–721
        ß-blockers in, 720
        calcium channel blockers in, 720
        coronary revascularization in, 727–729
        factor X inhibitors in, 726–727
        follow-up care, 729–730
        fondaparinux in, 726–727
        general measures in, 717–718
        glycoprotein IIb/IIIa inhibitors in, 721–724
        hirudin in, 726
        long-term, 729–730
        low-molecular-weight heparin in, 725–726

nitrates in, 718–720
statins in, 728–729
thienopyridines in, 721
thrombin inhibitors in, 726–727
unfractionated heparin in,
724–725

V

VADs. See *Ventricular assist devices
(VADs)*.

Value of First Day Angiography/
Angioplasty in Evolving Non–ST
Segment Elevation Myocardial
Infarction: An Open Multicenter
Randomized Trial (VINO), 728

Vasodilator(s), for ADHF, 748–749

Ventilation/perfusion scanning, in
pulmonary thromboembolic disease
evaluation, 814

Ventricular assist devices (VADs), in
cardiogenic shock management, 772

Ventricular fibrillation, STEMI and,
702–703

Ventricular septal rupture, STEMI and, 700

Verapamil, for atrial fibrillation, 862, 863

VINO. See *Value of First Day Angiography/
Angioplasty in Evolving Non–ST
Segment Elevation Myocardial
Infarction: An Open Multicenter
Randomized Trial (VINO)*.

W

WHO. See *World Health Organization
(WHO)*.

World Health Organization (WHO),
classification of pulmonary
hypertension, 803–804, 808

Z

Ziprasidone, in delirium management, 888